MW01056475

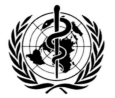

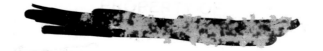

World Health Organization Classification of Tumours

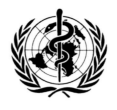

WHO   OMS

International Agency for Research on Cancer (IARC)

Pathology and Genetics of Skin Tumours

Edited by

Philip E. LeBoit

Günter Burg

David Weedon

Alain Sarasin

IARC*Press*

Lyon, 2006

World Health Organization Classification of Tumours

Series Editors   Paul Kleihues, M.D.
Leslie H. Sobin, M.D.

Pathology and Genetics of Skin Tumours

Editors   Philip E. LeBoit, M.D.
Günter Burg, M.D.
David Weedon, M.D.
Alain Sarasin, Ph.D.

Coordinating Editors   Wojciech Biernat, M.D.
Hiroko Ohgaki, Ph.D.

Editorial assistants   Asiedua Asante
Agnès Meneghel

Layout   Marlen Grassinger
Stephan Rappo
Sibylle Söring

Illustrations   Nobert Wey
Thomas Odin

Printed by   Team Rush
69603 Villeurbanne, France

Publisher   IARC*Press*
International Agency for
Research on Cancer (IARC)
69008 Lyon, France

This volume was produced in collaboration with the

International Academy of Pathology (IAP)

European Organization for Research and Treatment of Cancer (EORTC)

and the

Department of Pathology, University Hospital, Zurich, Switzerland

The WHO Classification of Skin Tumours
presented in this book reflects the views of a Working Group that convened for an
Editorial and Consensus Conference in Lyon, France,
September 22-25, 2003.

Members of the Working Group are indicated
in the List of Contributors on page 295.

Published by IARC Press, International Agency for Research on Cancer,
150 cours Albert Thomas, F-69008 Lyon, France

Format for bibliographic citations:
LeBoit P.E., Burg G., Weedon D, Sarasain A. (Eds.): World Health Organization
Classification of Tumours. Pathology and Genetics of Skin Tumours. IARC Press:
Lyon 2006

IARC Library Cataloguing in Publication Data

Pathology and genetics of skin tumours/ edited by Philip E. LeBoit... [et. al.].

(World Health Organization classification of tumours ; 10)

1. Skin Neoplasms – genetics
2. Skin Neoplasms – pathology

 I. LeBoit, P.E.
II. Series

ISBN   92 832 2414 0   (NLM Classification: WR 500)

Contents

CHAPTER 1

Keratinocytic Tumours

Keratinocytic tumours are derived from epidermal and adnexal keratinocytes and comprise a large spectrum of lesions ranging from benign proliferations (acanthomas) to malignant squamous cell carcinomas which occasionally show aggressive growth and even metastatic potential. Keratinocytic tumours are very frequent and, despite their low mortality rate, pose a significant public health problem. The main etiologic factor is solar radiation which causes DNA alterations, including pyrimidine dimers which during DNA replication may lead to CC:TT mutations in the *TP53* tumour suppressor gene. Other genes involved in the multistep formation of skin cancer include *PTCH* and the *RAS* oncogene.

Verrucas, epidermal proliferations produced by infection with human papilloma viruses (HPV), are also included in this section.

WHO histological classification of keratinocytic skin tumours

Keratinocytic tumours	
Basal cell carcinoma	8090/3
Superficial basal cell carcinoma	8091/3
Nodular (solid) basal cell carcinoma	8097/3
Micronodular basal cell carcinoma	8090/3
Infiltrating basal cell carcinoma	8092/3
Fibroepithelial basal cell carcinoma	8093/3
Basal cell carcinoma with adnexal differentiation	8098/3
Basosquamous carcinoma	8094/3
Keratotic basal cell carcinoma	8090/3
Squamous cell carcinoma	8070/3
Acantholytic squamous cell carcinoma	8075/3
Spindle-cell squamous cell carcinoma	8074/3
Verrucous squamous cell carcinoma	8051/3
Pseudovascular squamous cell carcinoma	8075/3
Adenosquamous carcinoma	8560/3
Bowen disease	8081/2
Bowenoid papulosis	

Actinic keratosis	
Arsenical keratosis	
PUVA keratosis	
Verrucas	
Verruca vulgaris	
Verruca plantaris	
Verruca plana	
Acanthomas	
Epidermolytic acanthoma	
Warty dyskeratoma	
Acantholytic acanthoma	
Solar lentigo	
Seborrhoeic keratosis	
Melanoacanthoma	
Clear cell acanthoma	
Large cell acanthoma	
Keratoacanthoma	8071/1
Lichen planus-like keratosis	

[1] Morphology code of the International Classification of Diseases for Oncology (ICD-O) {786} and the Systematized Nomenclature of Medicine (http://snomed.org). Behaviour is coded /0 for benign tumours, /3 for malignant tumours, /2 for in situ carcinoma and /1 for borderline or uncertain behaviour.

TNM classification of skin carcinomas

TNM classification [1,2]

T – Primary tumour

TX	Primary tumour cannot be assessed
T0	No evidence of primary tumour
Tis	Carcinoma in situ
T1	Tumour 2 cm or less in greatest dimension
T2	Tumour more than 2 cm but no more than 5 cm in greatest dimension
T3	Tumour more than 5 cm in greatest dimension
T4	Tumour invades deep extradermal structures, i.e., cartilage, skeletal muscle, or bone

Note: In the case of multiple simultaneous tumours, the tumour with the highest T category is classified and the number of separate tumours is indicated in parentheses, e.g., T2(5).

N – Regional lymph nodes

NX	Regional lymph nodes cannot be assessed
N0	No regional lymph node metastasis
N1	Regional lymph node metastasis

M – Distant metastasis

MX	Distant metastasis cannot be assessed
M0	No distant metastasis
M1	Distant metastasis

Stage grouping

Stage 0	Tis	N0	M0
Stage I	T1	N0	M0
Stage II	T2, T3	N0	M0
Stage III	T4	N0	M0
	Any T	N1	M0
Stage IV	Any T	Any N	M1

[1] {894,2219}.
[2] A help desk for specific questions about the TNM classification is available at www.uicc.org/index.php?id=508 .

Keratinocytic tumours: Introduction

D. Weedon
R. Marks
G. F. Kao
C.A. Harwood

The keratinocytic tumours are a clinically and histopathologically diverse group of lesions derived from the proliferation of epidermal and adnexal keratinocytes. At one end of the spectrum the proliferations are benign (acanthomas) and usually of cosmetic importance only, while at the other there are malignant tumours, which uncommonly may be aggressive with metastatic potential, as seen with some squamous cell carcinomas. Included in the spectrum are the epidermal dysplasias (actinic keratosis, arsenical keratosis and PUVA keratosis) and intraepidermal carcinomas (Bowen disease and bowenoid papulosis). Ackerman and others have proposed that solar keratoses should be regarded as squamous cell carcinoma de novo and not as pre-malignancies or pre-cancers that evolve into squamous cell carcinoma {994,1443,1701}.

Epidemiology

Keratinocytic tumours are an important public health problem, despite their comparatively low mortality rate {2484}. The lifetime risk for the development of skin cancer in the USA is now 1 in 5 {1937}. It is much higher in subtropical Australia. There is an increasing incidence of squamous cell carcinoma of the skin in some countries {2462}. Keratinocytic tumours account for approximately 90% or more of all skin malignancies, of which approximately 70% are basal cell carcinomas. The latter exceed squamous cell carcinomas in frequency by a factor of approximately 5:1 although in lower latitudes the incidence of squamous cell carcinoma increases and this ratio becomes 3:1. If solar keratoses are regarded as squamous cell carcinomas (see above), then squamous cell carcinoma becomes the more common tumour {300}.

Precursor lesions

There are no known precursor lesions to basal cell carcinoma. On the other hand, there are a number of intra-epidermal proliferative disorders (dysplasias) that may be precursors of squamous cell carcinoma. These include actinic keratosis and Bowen disease (intraepidermal carcinoma/squamous cell carcinoma in-situ).

Actinic keratoses are erythematous, scaling lesions occurring on heavily sunlight exposed areas that increase in prevalence with increasing age in fair skinned people. Histologically, they demonstrate confluent keratinocytic atypia involving predominantly the keratinocytes in the basal layer of the epidermis {2475}.

It is difficult to determine the incidence of actinic keratoses as they come and go over time {788}. Longitudinal studies suggest that they are likely to be a precursor of squamous cell carcinoma, although the malignant transformation rate is small, certainly less than one in a hundred per year {1517}. Data suggest, also, that remission of these lesions will occur if sunlight exposure can be reduced. Thus the majority of lesions do not progress to squamous cell carcinoma {1516,2349}.

Bowen disease demonstrates keratinocyte atypia involving the full thickness of the epidermis. There is also involvement of the hair follicle and rarely the sweat duct. Although Bowen disease has been classified as a full thickness in-situ squamous cell carcinoma, there are no longitudinal studies published on the frequency of malignant transformation. Even if invasive squamous cell carcinoma does occur within one of these lesions, it is believed that the in-situ phase may be very prolonged, lasting many years {1203}.

Etiology

Findings regarding the genetic basis of non-melanoma skin cancer (NMSC) have confirmed that UV radiation, especially UVB (290-320 nm in the solar spectrum), contributes to the formation of squamous {1336} and basal cell carcinomas {602}. Squamous cell carcinomas (SCCs) of the skin develop through a multistep process that involves activation of proto-onco-genes and/or inactivation of tumour suppressor genes in the human skin keratinocytes. NMSCs are caused by genetic abnormalities, most often induced by UVB exposure. Actinic keratoses, which lead to SCCs, have gene mutations in K-ras {2235}. H-rasV12 and cyclin dependent kinase 4 (CDK4) produce human epidermal neoplasia. Therefore, a combination of these genetic abnormalities might be crucial to the carcinogenesis at least in a subset of SCCs {1336}.

High doses of ultraviolet light can also lead to skin cancers by inducing reactive oxygen species (ROS) that play an important role in tissue injury. Increased production of ROS and/or decreased efficiency of antioxidant defence system contribute to a number of degenerative processes including cancer {1161}. UV induces pyrimidine dimers and loss of heterozygosity (LOH). TP53 and PTCH, two tumour suppressor genes, have LOH which lead to basal cell carcinoma (BCC) {1265}. LOH in TP53 is related to elevated microsatellite instability at selected tetranucleotide repeats {587}. LOH at 9q22 loci in PTCH genes causes non-melanoma skin cancer tumours {1265}. The type of mutations for TP53 and PTCH are predominantly UV-signature transitions, C->T and CC->TT at dipyrimidine sites {1265}. SCCs have mutations of H-Ras gene and the INK4a locus whereas BCC has missense mutations leading to rasGTPase activating protein {168}. Further, mutations have been found in both TP53 tumour suppressor gene and ras in patients with xeroderma pigmentosum (XP), a disease of DNA repair deficiencies {1717}.

Common exogenous carcinogenic agents in addition to UV radiation include 1) tobacco use {2457}, 2) human papilloma viruses {1703}, 3) arsenic {2184}, 4) industrial chemicals such as vinyl chloride {1362}, polycyclic aromatic hydrocarbons {1086}, 5) MNNG (N-methyl-N'-nitro-N-nitrosoguanidine), an alkylating agent {335}, and 6) exposure to gasoline or gasoline vapours {1567}.

Clinical features

Keratinocytic tumours vary in their clinical appearance depending on the type of lesion and stage of development.

Histopathology

The histopathologic changes noted in keratinocytic proliferative lesions involve disturbance of normal surface maturation. The degree and extent of keratinocytic atypia vary in these lesions. The atypical keratinocytes show enlarged nuclei with hyperchromasia, dyskeratosis and mitoses in any layer of the epidermis. In lesions of epidermal dysplasias (AK, arsenical, and PUVA keratoses), surface keratinocytic maturation is present, i.e. a granular cell layer is usually noted.

In intraepidermal carcinomas (Bowen disease, bowenoid papulosis), there is full-thickness involvement of the epidermis by the atypical keratinocytes.

Molecular markers

A number of potentially useful molecular markers or tests have been proposed. These include the demonstration of a different pattern of basic fibroblast growth factor expression in neoplastic keratinocytes by in situ hybridization and the persistence of integrated HPV sequences in the host cell genome of HPV associated keratinocytic lesions detected by ligation mediated PCR assay. The lower level of TIG-3 mRNA expression in SCC is visualized by immunohistochemistry or by in situ mRNA hybridization. Upregulation of S100 protein subtypes in specific keratinocyte disorders is confirmed by immunohistochemistry.

Prognosis and predictive factors

Most patients with primary cutaneous non-melanoma skin cancer (NMSC) have an excellent prognosis. The overall mortality rates are generally low, on average approximately 0.1% of the incidence rates, but significantly higher for SCCs than BCCs {2483}. Invasive SCC has the potential to recur and metastasize with an overall 5-year rate of recurrence for primary tumours of 8%. With the exception of lip tumours, sqamous cell carcinomas arising in actinic keratoses have a frequency of metastatic spread of 0.5-3% {1459,1630}. For those with metastatic disease the long-term prognosis is poor; 10-year survival rates are <20% for patients with regional lymph node involvement and <10% for patients with distant metastases {50}. More than 70% of SCC recurrences and metastases develop within 2 years of treatment of the primary tumour {635}, and 95% within 5 years {1985}. The 3-year cumulative risk of non-melanoma skin cancer developing in an individual diagnosed with SCC is 35-60% and the risk of melanoma is also increased {1507}. Five-year cure rates for BCC of up to 99% are obtainable with surgical techniques {1617, 1984}, and metastasis is extremely rare, occurring in approximately 0.05% of cases {1440}. As with SCC, patients with BCC are at high risk of further primary BCCs; in patients with one lesion the 5-year risk is 27%, and in those with 10 lesions the risk is 90% {1208}, and the risk of SCC and malignant melanoma is also increased {1208,1430}.

Basal cell carcinoma

S. Kossard
E.H. Epstein, Jr.
R. Cerio
L.L. Yu
D. Weedon

Definition
A group of malignant cutaneous tumours characterized by the presence of lobules, columns, bands or cords of basaloid cells ("germinative cells").

ICD-O code
8090/3

Synonyms
Basal cell epithelioma, trichoblastic carcinoma.

Epidemiology
Basal cell carcinomas (BCC) develop predominantly in sun-damaged skin in individuals who are fair skinned and prone to sunburn {330,888,889}. Migration of such individuals particularly as children, to countries with high UV radiance is associated with increased rates of skin cancer. Although basal cell carcinomas typically occur in adults, the tumours also develop in children {1873}. Arsenic exposure {924} and ionizing radiation may also induce basal cell carcinomas.

Nodular basal cell carcinomas occur at a later age than superficial basal cell carcinomas and are more frequently on the head whereas the trunk is the most frequent site for superficial tumours {1550, 2121}.

Basal cell carcinomas are very frequent tumours particularly in light-skinned individuals living in countries at low latitudes. Incidences of 2000 per 100,000 population have been recorded in Queensland, Australia. The rate of basal cell carcinomas has increased in the older age groups. Older men have a higher incidence of basal cell carcinoma than women, but women have been found to outnumber men in younger age groups. The latter may be due to increased sun exposure in younger women in association with tanning bed use as well as smoking {293}.

Clinical features
Basal cell carcinomas typically have a pearly appearance with telangiectasia that may appear as a papule or nodule that can be eroded or ulcerated. These features may be more subtle in the superficial forms that appear as erythematous patches resembling an area of dermatitis. Pale scar-like lesions may also be a presentation of basal cell carcinoma and these slowly grow over years. Pigmented basal cell carcinomas may masquerade as melanomas but usually can be distinguished by the presence of a pearly component. Dermatoscopy is also helpful in analysing pigmented basal cell carcinoma and distinguishing these from melanocytic tumours {1587}. Erosive lesions on the lower limbs may be mistaken for slowly healing traumatic wounds. Delays in clinical diagnosis may occur for basal cell carcinomas that are localized within non-sun exposed sites {225} such as the perianal area {1312} or between the toes, young age of onset, tumours with very slow growth, or superficial erythematous patches that appear as a dermatitis or tumours complicating vaccination scars, rhinophyma or a venous ulcer. The clinical capacity to differentiate some basal cell carcinomas from squamous cell carcinoma or even melanoma may be impossible without skin biopsy. In countries with a high incidence of basal cell carcinomas it is not unusual to have individuals with multiple basal cell carcinomas, and regular review is required to deal with new skin tumours. Incomplete removal of basal cell carcinoma may result in delayed recurrences that may not be recognized for years, particularly if the tumour recurrence is deep or masked by skin grafts.

Genetics
Genetic analysis of sporadic basal cell carcinoma {2024} has been propelled by the identification of mutations in PTCH1 (chromosome 9q22.3) as the cause of the basal cell naevus syndrome (BCNS), a rare autosomal dominant disorder {110, 1146,2395}. These patients develop multiple basal cell carcinomas which may appear in childhood (see Chapter 2). PTCH1 encodes a protein that functions as an inhibitor of the hedgehog signaling pathway, and BCCs, whether sporadic or occurring in BCNS patients, all have abnormalities of this signaling pathway {110,1146,2272,2395}. In most sporadic BCCs this is due to somatically-acquired mutations in PTCH1 {802}, and in many

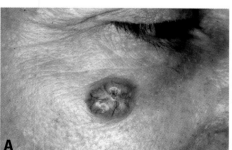 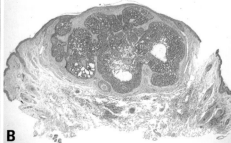 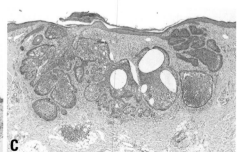

Fig. 1.1 Basal cell carcinoma, nodular type. **A** and **B** The epidermis is raised with flattening of the rete ridges overlying solid and cystic groups of atypical basaloid cells with peripheral palisading showing invasion of the deep dermis in a nodular pattern. **C** High power view of nodular basal cell carcinoma showing focal cystic change, peripheral palisading and cleft between tumour nests and stroma.

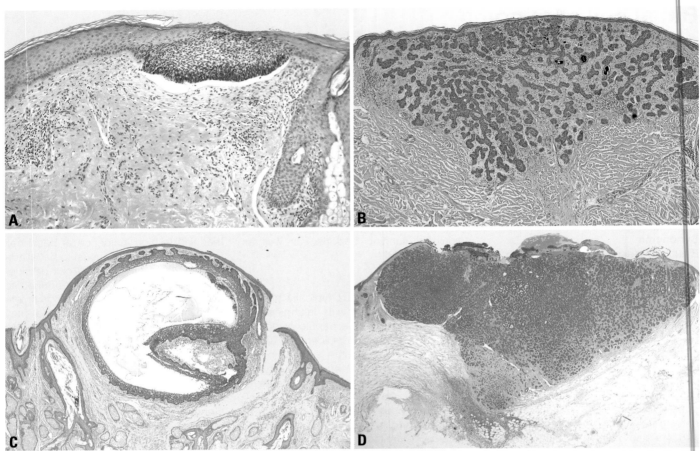

Fig. 1.2 A Basal cell carcinoma, superficial type. A solid group of atypical basaloid cells is present at the dermo-epidermal junction showing peripheral palisading and cleft formation between tumour nest and dermis. The dermis shows fibrosis and a patchy lymphocytic infiltrate which frequently accompany basal cell carcinoma of the superficial type. **B** Basal cell carcinoma, nodular type, pigmented. The appearances are those of typical nodular basal cell carcinoma with the additional feature of melanin pigmentation of the tumour nests. **C** Basal cell carcinoma, cystic type. There is extensive cystic change in an otherwise nodular basal cell carcinoma. The cystic space contains connective tissue type mucin. In the purely cystic variant, tumour cells may be compressed to only 1 to 2 cell layers thick. **D** Basal cell carcinoma, micronodular type. The tumour cell nests are tightly packed, with a diameter of 3 to 10 cells across with deep dermal invasion. In this example, there is also tumour-associated amyloid in the stroma.

tumours the type of PTCH1 mutations are those expected from UV-mutagenesis {108,1265}. Approximately 10% of sporadic BCCs have mutations in SMOOTHENED which encodes the protein whose function is inhibited by the PATCHED1 protein {2553}. Thus it appears that the relevant dysfunction driving BCCs is abnormal hedgehog signaling, irrespective of which gene controlling that signaling is mutated. The identification of hedgehog signaling abnormalities as crucial to BCC formation has stimulated the development of genetically-engineered mice with hedgehog signaling abnormalities {109,708, 1716,2163}. Unlike previously studied mouse carcinogenesis models, which uniformly produce tumours of the squamous cell lineage, these mice develop BCCs and either spontaneously or in response to environmental mutagens (i.e. UV or ionizing radiation) develop BCCs and adnexal basaloid tumours.

Histopathology

The multiple variants of basal cell carcinoma are connected by the common histological feature of lobules, columns, bands and cords of basaloid cells ("germinative cells") associated with scant cytoplasm and a characteristic outer palisade of cells associated with a surrounding loose fibromucinous stroma {2147, 2282}. Artefactual retraction spaces between the tumour and stroma are often present. The tumour-stromal interaction is weakened by the characteristic lack of the hemidesmosomes that anchor the normal epidermis to the dermis {475}.

Apoptosis is usually apparent. The release of keratin into the stroma as a result of apoptosis may lead to the formation of amyloid deposits {2067}. Mucinous cystic degeneration, focal vacuolation with lipid or ductular differentiation, and in rare cases, sebocytes or follicular differentiation with squamous eddies, trichohyaline granules and blue-grey corneocytes may be seen. Melanocytes may proliferate within some tumours and produce pigmentation by melanin production that can be stored in tumour cells or in surrounding melanophages {1365}.

Problematic lesions include tumours that merge with squamous cell carcinoma (basaloid squamous cell carcinoma) or those that share adnexal differentiation demonstrating trichilemmal or sebaceous areas. Some examples of morphoeic or sclerotic basal cell carcinoma may resemble desmoplastic trichoepithelioma or microcystic adnexal carcinoma particularly when a small sample is obtained for analysis. The growth pattern of the basal cell carcinoma should be included in the pathology report as well as the presence of perineural involvement and excision margins particularly if less than 1 mm. Although the majority of basal cell carcinomas can be classified into the nodular, micronodular, superficial, sclerosing/morphoeic or infiltrative subtypes, it is not unusual to have a mixed pattern.

Immunoprofile

Occasionally in curette specimens, differentiation from small cell melanoma may require the use of a combination of light-weight keratin markers and S-100 acidic protein to differentiate the tumours. BerEP4, a keratin marker, has been used to differentiate basal cell carcinoma from squamous cell carcinomas {2334}. CK20, a marker for Merkel cells, has been used to differentiate some forms of trichoblastoma, trichoepithelioma or fibroepitheliomas as these have scattered CK20 positive Merkel cells compared to basal cell carcinoma where they are rare or absent {13,2104}.

Prognosis and predictive factors

Basal cell carcinomas are locally invasive tumours and metastases occur in less than 1 in 10,000 tumours {1440, 1950,2443}. Morbidity is increased with deeply invasive tumours which may extend into the deep tissue to bone and follow fusion planes particularly on the face where they follow nerves through bony channels. Morbidity also increases with neglected tumours that may measure more than 10 cm in diameter and have been described as giant basal cell carcinomas {1502,2009}. Multiple recurrences with deep residual tumour on the head may be associated with particular morbidity as basal cell carcinomas can ultimately penetrate the cranium. Increased recurrences are associated with infiltrative, morphoeic and micronodular basal cell carcinomas as surgical margins may be underestimated {639, 1940}. The possibility of the BCNS should be considered in children who develop BCCs. Families can be screened for mutations of the PTCH1 gene. Low bcl-2 protein expression has been found to correlate with clinically aggressive basal cell carcinomas with infiltrative, sclerosing/morphoeic patterns as compared to superficial and nodular tumours {296,1883}.

BCC recurrences are more common in lesions on the nose and nasolabial fold, but this may be in part due to the difficulty in achieving adequate margins in these sites {638,651}. Tumours recurring after radiotherapy are usually aggressive and infiltrative {2209}. Lesions which metastasize are usually large, ulcerated, deeply infiltrating and recurrent {70}. The risk of further primary BCCs is increased by male gender, age over 60 years and truncal site {1208,1378}.

Rarely, extensive perineural invasion is seen in infiltrative primary BCCs of the face, presenting life-threatening complications of CNS extension {317,946}. Distance to the closest resection margin is an important predictor of BCC recurrence {639}.

Superficial basal cell carcinoma

ICD-O code   8091/3

Clinical features

This variant appears as erythematous patches that are often multiple and may vary from a few millimetres to over 10 cm in diameter. A fine pearly border or central superficial erosions with a history of contact bleeding may be present. Areas of regression may appear as pale patches or fibrosis. This variant makes up 10-30% of basal cell carcinomas and occurs most frequently on the trunk.

Histopathology

The histopathology consists of superficial lobules of basaloid cells which project from the epidermis or from the sides of follicles or eccrine ducts into the dermis and are surrounded by loose myxoid stroma. The lobules are usually confined

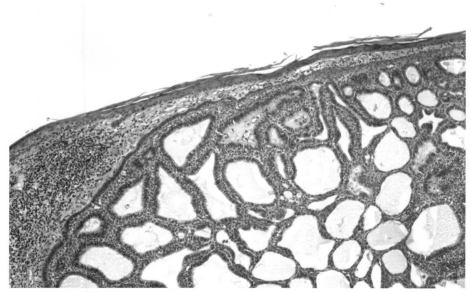

Fig. 1.3 Nodular BCC. Cribriform nodular basal cell carcinoma.

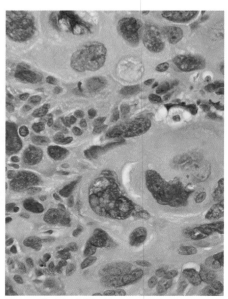

Fig. 1.4 Nodular BCC with monster giant cells.

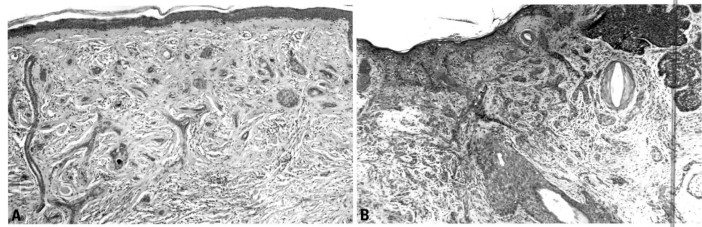

Fig. 1.5 A Infiltrative basal cell carcinoma. **B** Mixed nodular and infiltrative basal cell carcinoma.

to the papillary dermis. Some examples of superficial basal cell carcinoma appear multifocal on vertical sections but may be connected by a stroma when reconstructed by three-dimensional techniques using digital image analysis. There are, however, examples of multi-focal superficial basal cell carcinoma where the lobules are separated by large distances and represent discrete tumours that are truly multifocal and may measure only a few millimetres in diameter. Mixed patterns with a nodular, micronodular or infiltrative component may be seen in some tumours.

Nodular basal cell carcinoma

ICD-O code   8097/3
Clinical features
Nodular (solid) basal cell carcinomas often appear as elevated pearly nodules associated with telangiectasia but may become ulcerated or cystic. Endophytic nodules may present as flat indurated lesions. Haemorrhagic lesions may resemble haemangiomas or melanoma when pigmented. Nodular basal cell carcinomas make up 60-80% of tumours and occur most frequently on the head.

Histopathology
Histopathology shows large lobules of basaloid cells ("germinative cells") with peripheral palisading nuclei that project into the reticular dermis or deeper. The lobules may have associated mucinous degeneration with cysts or have an adenoid (cribriform) pattern. Some nodules may have an organoid appearance with smaller basaloid lobules that are connected by loose fibromucinous stroma. The periphery of such nodules should be scanned to ensure that an outlying micronodular pattern has not developed.

Micronodular basal cell carcinoma

ICD-O code   8090/3

Clinical features
Micronodular basal cell carcinoma presents as elevated or flat infiltrative tumours. The most common site is the back.

Histopathology
This variant has small nodules that permeate the dermis {1010}. Individual nodules may appear to be separated by normal collagen. The tumour nodules may approximate the size of follicular bulbs and form subtle extensions into deep tissue. In contrast to nodular basal cell carcinoma the surgical margins of micronodular basal cell carcinoma may be underestimated. Perineural extension may be seen.

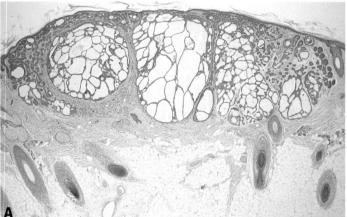
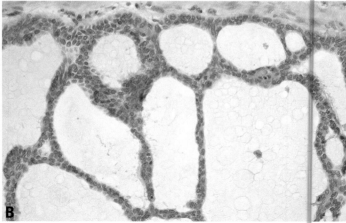

Fig. 1.6 Nodular cystic BCC **A** There are well circumscribed cystic nodules of atypical basaloid cells pushing into the deep dermis in a nodular pattern. **B** High power view of nodulocystic basal cell carcinoma showing cribriform cystic spaces filled with stromal mucin.

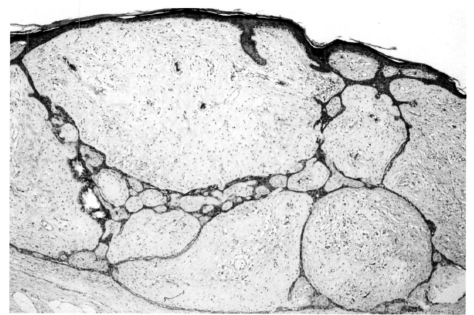

Fig. 1.7 Fibroepithelial basal cell carcinoma (fibroepithelioma of Pinkus).

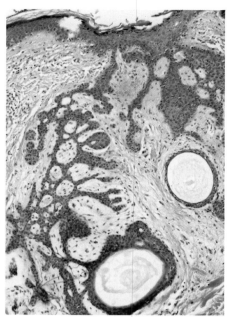

Fig. 1.8 BCC with adnexal differentiation; basaloid follicular hamartoma.

Infiltrating basal cell carcinoma

Definition
This variant of BCC is composed of thin strands, cords and columns of basaloid cells that infiltrate between the collagen bundles of the dermis and may extend into deeper tissues.

ICD-O code
8092/3

Clinical features
The infiltrative basal cell carcinoma presents as a pale, indurated poorly-defined plaque. These tumours are usually found on the upper trunk or face. Paraesthesia or loss of sensation may develop rarely as a manifestation of perineural extension, particularly in lesions on the face. This variant is important in that the margins at the time of surgery may be frequently underestimated.

Histopathology
Infiltrative patterns of basal cell carcinoma appear as strands, cords and columns of basaloid cells with scant cytoplasm. Peripheral palisading and retraction spaces are usually not seen. There is no fibrosis/sclerosis as seen in the sclerosing/morphoeic variant. The infiltrative pattern is particularly associated with perineural invasion. Low molecular-weight keratin markers are useful in highlighting subtle groups of tumour cells (that may consist of 1-2 keratinocytes on cross section), in assessing clearance of the tumour and in confirming perineural involvement.

Differential diagnosis
Due to the cord-like arrangement of this variant there is a morphological overlap with the tumour pattern seen in microcystic adnexal carcinoma (sclerosing sweat duct carcinoma), desmoplastic squamous cell carcinoma and desmoplastic trichoepithelioma.

Fibroepithelial basal cell carcinoma

Definition
This variant of BCC is characterized by a unique clinicopathological presentation and an indolent behaviour.

ICD-O code
8093/3

Synonyms
Fibroepithelioma of Pinkus, Pinkus tumour

Clinical features
These tumours usually appear as an elevated flesh coloured or erythematous nodule that may resemble a seborrhoeic keratosis or acrochordon. The lesions are most often found on the back and are rarely multiple {1834}. Prior radiotherapy may predispose to these tumours.

Histopathology
The histopathology is characterized by an arborising network of cords of basaloid cells that extend downwards from the epidermis and create a fenestrating pattern. There are strands of basaloid cells that surround fibrovascular stroma. Ductules may be present in some of the cords which may represent extension of the tumour down pre-existing eccrine ducts {2263}. The cords also are associated with small follicle-like bulbs which project into the surrounding connective tissue.

Histogenesis
Fibroepitheliomas, like BCCs, may be best classified as a form of appendageal tumour. These tumours have mutations of the PTCH1 gene. In some fibroepitheliomas transition to classical basal cell carcinomas may be seen, and this conversion may reflect a further mutation. A variant of fibroepithelioma with extramammary Paget cells has been described in the perianal area {2461}.

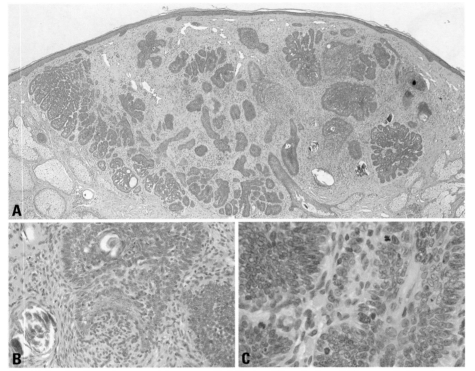

Fig. 1.9 Basal cell carcinoma, nodular type, with follicular differentiation. **A** The overall view shows a resemblance to typical nodular basal cell carcinoma, with the addition of a cellular fibrous stroma. **B** There is follicular bulbar differentiation in parts of the tumour, with formation of hair bulb accompanied by mesenchymal bodies. Focal dystrophic calcification. **C** High power view showing groups of atypical basaloid cells with peripheral palisading with trichohyaline granules and abrupt trichilemmal keratinization.

Basal cell carcinoma with adnexal differentiation

Definition
This variant is characterized histologically by adnexal differentiation in a BCC.

ICD-O code
8098/3

Clinical features
This variant has no distinguishing clinical features.

Histopathology
This variant is characterized by the presence of adnexal differentiation including basaloid buds, ductal, sebaceous and trichilemmal elements. Follicular differentiation may be prominent in more superficial BCCs. Eccrine or apocrine differentiation has also been observed in some basal cell carcinomas {997,2022}. It is important to distinguish such tumours from sweat gland carcinomas which have an increased risk for metastases. Some forms of adnexal basal cell carci-nomas show overlap and may be better classified as benign adnexal tumour such as a basaloid follicular hamartoma, trichoepithelioma, trichoblastoma or trichilemmoma.

Histogenesis
The cytokeratin profile of basal cell carcinoma is essentially identical to that of trichoblastomas (immature trichoepithelioma) and developing foetal hair follicles linking all basal cell carcinomas to the pilosebaceous pathway of differentiation {2086}. It has been proposed that basal cell carcinoma be renamed trichoblastic carcinoma {1623}.

Prognosis and predictive factors
These patterns of adnexal differentiation do not appear to have any prognostic implications.

Basosquamous carcinoma

Definition
Basosquamous carcinoma is a term used to describe basal cell carcinomas that are associated with squamous differentiation {285,2102}.

ICD-O code
8094/3

Synonyms
Metatypical carcinoma, basosquamous cell carcinoma.

Clinical features
This variant has no distinguishing clinical features.

Histopathology
The tumour cells have more abundant cytoplasm with more marked keratinization than typical basal cell carcinomas. The nuclei have vesicular chromatin with pleomorphism and palisading may be focally lost. Some examples of this variant may merge with sebaceous carcinoma as lipid vacuoles or ducts may be focally apparent. This tumour may also have central fibrosis and a radiating peripheral rim of infiltrative cells extending into the deep dermis or subcutis.

Prognosis and predictive factors
This variant has a more aggressive behaviour and has been associated with regional or widespread metastases {1525}.

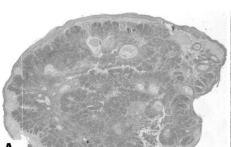
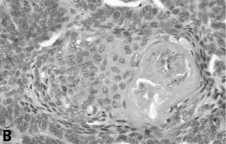

Fig. 1.10 Basal cell carcinoma, keratotic type. **A** Prominent keratin horn cysts in the center of the tumour nests. **B** Detail of trichilemmal keratinization.

Keratotic basal cell carcinoma

Definition
This variant is characterized by the presence of prominent keratin formation (horn cysts) in the centre of tumour islands.

ICD-O code   8090/3

Clinical features
This variant characteristically appears pearly and may be studded with small keratin cysts (milia).

Histopathology
These tumours share the overall architectural features of a nodular BCC. Keratinization may be laminated and infundibular in type or hyaline and trichilemmal in type or consist of keratinised shadow cells representing pilomatricomal differentiation {66}. Dystrophic calcification is frequently present. Trichilemmal keratin may be associated with accentuated apoptosis in surrounding tumour cells and the presence of pale keratinocytes.

Differential diagnosis
This variant is distinguished from basosquamous carcinoma by the presence of numerous, superficial small keratin cysts. Basosquamous carcinoma is usually larger and less well circumscribed.

Other variants

Other variants account for less than 10% of all basal cell carcinomas. Many of them do not have distinctive clinical features.

Cystic
One or more cystic spaces, of variable size, are present near the centre of the tumour nests. There is sometimes increased mucin between the cells bordering the central space {2112}.

Adenoid
There are thin strands of basaloid cells in a reticulate pattern. Stromal mucin is often present. The adenoid type may occur in association with the nodular (solid) type.

Sclerosing / morphoeiform
Strands and nests of tumour cells are

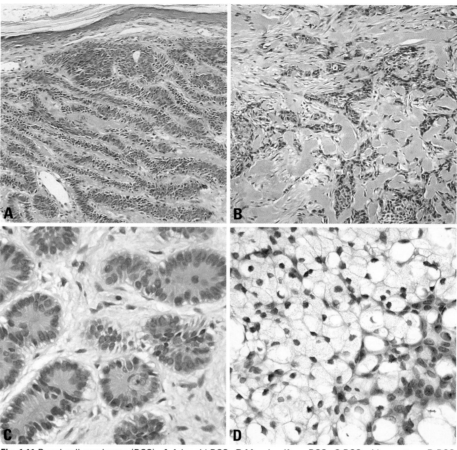

Fig. 1.11 Basal cell carcinoma (BCC). **A** Adenoid BCC. **B** Morphoeiform BCC. **C** BCC with rosettes. **D** BCC with sebaceous differentiation.

embedded in a dense fibrous stroma {1932}. Some authors use the term morphoeic for any BCC with a fibrous stroma, while others restrict it to those BCC's with keloidal collagen bundles in the stroma {1923}. Enhanced procollagen gene expression has been found in this variant {1657}. Furthermore, smooth muscle α-actin is often present in the stroma. This variant usually presents as an indurated, pale plaque with a slightly shiny surface and indistinct margins.

Infundibulocystic
Often confused with the keratotic type, this variant is composed of small infundibular-like structures with a central keratinous plug and a peripheral component of basaloid cells {1218}. The nests are arranged in an anastomosing pattern. Multiple lesions are sometimes present {1178}.

Pigmented
Pigmentation may occur in several of the

variants including the nodular, micronodular, multifocal superficial and keratotic types. Melanocytes are scattered through the tumour nests, while melanophages are present in the stroma {1495}. This variant can be misdiagnosed clinically as malignant melanoma.

Miscellaneous
Other rare variants, subject to isolated case reports, include the clear-cell {165}, "signet-ring"-cell {1269,2503}, granular-cell {1659} and giant ("monster")-cell {680} types. Adamantanoid {1403}, neuroendocrine {817} and schwannoid {2032} variants have also been described.

Squamous cell carcinoma

D. Weedon
M.B. Morgan
C. Gross
E. Nagore
L.L. Yu

Definition

Squamous cell carcinoma is a malignant neoplasm of epidermal (and mucous membrane) keratinocytes in which the component cells show variable squamous differentiation.

ICD-O code   8070/3

Epidemiology

Most cases arise on the sun-exposed skin of elderly people. They can occur on all cutaneous surfaces and mucous membranes, and in younger patients, especially those with a fair complexion who tan poorly. Its incidence in an Australian study was 166 cases per 100,000 of the population, the highest in the world {828}. It is relatively uncommon in Black people.

Etiology

Ultraviolet-B radiation is the most important etiological factor. Less important factors include radiation therapy, previous burns, arsenic, coal tar {1759}, industrial carcinogens, immunosuppresion, HPV infection, and inflammatory lesions and ulcers of long standing (see Introduction). Organ transplant recipients are particularly prone to develop these tumours. Most of the fatal cases have been reported from Australia, suggesting that sunlight, which also has a profound effect on the cutaneous immune system plays a role in the formation of these aggressive tumours {1974}. HPV infection is commonly found in these immunosuppressed patients {264}.

Localization

Most SCCs arise in areas of direct exposure to the sun, such as the forehead, face, ears, scalp, neck and dorsum of the hands. The vermilion part of the lower lip is another common site.

Clinical features

Squamous cell carcinomas present as shallow ulcers, often with a keratinous crust and elevated, indurated surrounds, or as plaques or nodules. The surrounding skin usually shows changes of actinic damage.

Histopathology

Squamous cell carcinoma consists of nests, sheets and strands of squamous epithelial cells which arise from the epidermis and extend into the dermis for a variable distance. The cells have abundant eosinophilic cytoplasm and a large, often vesicular, nucleus. There are prominent intercellular bridges. There is variable central keratinization and horn pearl formation, depending on the differentiation of the tumour.

The degree of anaplasia in the tumour nests is used to grade the tumours. A rather subjective assessment is usually made using the categories of 'well,' 'moderately' and 'poorly' differentiated. Most squamous cell carcinomas arise in solar keratoses and evidence of this lesion is usually present at the periphery of the invasive tumour.

Squamous cell carcinomas occasionally infiltrate along nerve sheaths, the adventitia of blood vessels, lymphatics, fascial planes and embryological fusion plates {218}. The presence of perineural lymphocytes is a clue to the likely presence of perineural invasion in deeper sections {2289}.

There may be a mild to moderate chronic inflammatory cell infiltrate at the periphery of the tumours. This infiltrate sometimes includes eosinophils {1455}.

Rare histological variants of SCC include clear-cell {1344}, signet-ring {1557}, pigmented {451}, basaloid {573}, inflammatory, infiltrative {1395}, desmoplastic {1546} and rhabdoid {1534} types.

The cells in SCC are positive for epithelial membrane antigen and cytokeratin. The keratins are of higher molecular weight than those found in basal cell carcinoma {1672}.

Prognosis and predictive factors

The majority of squamous cell carcinomas are only locally aggressive and are cured by several different modalites {1656}. SCC developing in patients who are immunocompromised, including those infected with the human immunodeficiency virus {1704}, are usually more aggressive. Tumours with deep invasion, poor differentiation, perineural invasion and acantholytic features are more likely to recur or metastasize. Narrow surgical margins are another risk factor for recurrence {2389}.

The clinical setting in which the SCC arises also influences the risk of metastasis. Tumours arising in sun-damaged skin have the lowest risk, in the order of 0.5% or less, while for those arising in skin not exposed to the sun, the risk is 2-3%. The risk is further increased for tumours arising in Bowen disease {1203}, on the lip, vulvar, perineal and penile skin and in a Marjolin ulcer, radiation scar or thermal burn. Tumour thickness is a prognostic variable, just as it is for melanoma. SCCs less than 2 mm in thickness rarely metastasize, while those between 2 and 5 mm thick are of intermediate risk (about 5%). Tumours greater than 5 mm in thickness have a risk of metastasis of about 20% {1254}. Tumours greater than 2 cm in diameter are more likely to recur and metastasize than smaller lesions {1985}.

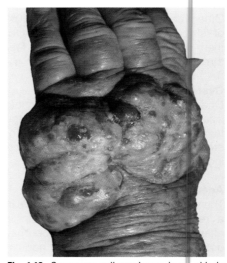

Fig. 1.12 Squamous cell carcinoma in an elderly male with delayed medical treatment. This is an unusually large neoplasm which spread to the regional lymph nodes.

Acantholytic squamous cell carcinoma

Definition
Acantholytic squamous cell carcinoma (ASCC) is a histologic variant of cutaneous squamous cell carcinoma (SCC) that is histologically defined by loosening of the intercellular bridges resulting in acantholysis. These tumours may present as intraepidermal (in-situ) or invasive SCC.

ICD-O code   8075/3

Synonyms
Adenoid squamous cell carcinoma, pseudoglandular squamous cell carcinoma.

Epidemiology
The acantholytic variant accounts for 2-4% of all cutaneous SCC {1149,1687, 1819,2549}. The age range is wide but it usually affects aged individuals with a male predominance.

Etiology
As in conventional SCC, ultraviolet light constitutes the most important etiologic risk factor.

Localization
The tumour involves predominantly the skin of the head and neck region, particularly on and around the ears {1149, 1687,1819,2549}.

Clinical features
ASCC presents similarly to conventional SCC, as a slowly growing scaly and occasionally ulcerated papule/plaque on the sun-exposed skin.

Histopathology
Invasive lesions typically show a thickened, and/or ulcerated epithelium. Scanning magnification reveals a flattened thinned, normal or hyperplastic epidermis with or without asymmetric and infiltrating dermal tumour islands. At intermediate power, prominent suprabasilar or intratumoural acantholysis is seen. Zones of acantholysis are capable of producing large intraepidermal cavities. Acantholytic areas may extend down adjacent follicular structures involving the follicular epithelium and rarely, circumscribe the follicle simulating a glandular arrangement. Acantholytic foci may also produce a pseudovascular pattern mimicking angiosarcoma (pseudovascular SCC) {139,1675,1688}. At high power typical features of squamous malignancy are identified including dyskeratosis, keratinocytic atypia, consisting of an increased nuclear-to-cytoplasmic ratio and nuclear hyperchromasia, altered maturation within the epithelium, and increased typical and atypical mitotic figures.

Immunoprofile
The lesional cells in ASCC stain for cutaneous epithelial markers that include high molecular weight keratins such as AE-2/3. Involucrin, vimentin and EMA immunostains may also be positive {1808,2011}. Low-molecular weight keratins such as AE-1, CAM 5.2 are typically negative. Various intercellular peptides have been invoked in the pathogenesis of acantholysis including the intercellular adhesion molecule syndecan, E-cadherin and the anhidrotic ectodermal dysplasia gene product {183,1635}. It has also been shown recently that decreased TP53 and PCNA expression correlated with a decrement in desmosomes seen ultrastructurally {1889}.

Differential diagnosis
The changes described above constitute an important histologic means of separating this entity from acantholytic disorders. The differential also includes true adenosquamous cell carcinoma of the skin that exhibits squamous and glandular differentiation on ultrastructural examination and histochemical staining {2482}.

Prognosis and predictive factors
The behaviour of ASCC like other SCCs is depth-dependent and may be more aggressive than conventional SCC {461, 1097,1149,1687,1819,1985}. In-situ lesions are capable of recurrence and in up to 10% of cases, may show microinvasion. The overall rate of metastases with lesions greater than 2.0 cm of invasion ranges from 5-19%.

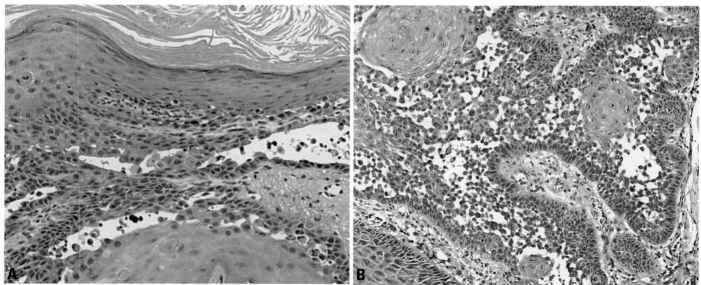

Fig. 1.13 Acantholytic squamous cell carcinoma (SCC). **A** Intermediate-power photomicrograph and **B** higher magnification depicting acantholysis extending down adjacent follicle epithelium.

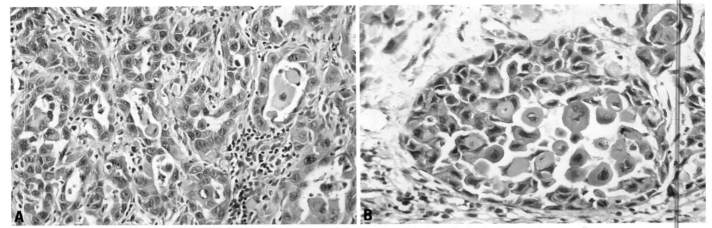

Fig. 1.14 Squamous cell carcinoma (acantholytic) **A**, **B** Note the pseudoglandular pattern and the loss of cohesion between tumour cells.

Spindle-cell squamous cell carcinoma

Definition
This is an uncommon variant of squamous cell carcinoma that exhibits a prominent spindle cell morphology.

ICD-O code   8074/3

Etiology
Lesions usually arise in sun-damaged or irradiated skin. A case has been reported in association with lichen sclerosus of the vulva {2057}. The incidence of this variant may be higher in immunosuppressed patients.

Clinical features
Spindle-cell squamous cell carcinoma presents as a plaque or nodule on the skin. It may be clinically indistinguishable from the more usual type of squamous cell carcinoma. Sometimes there is a history of rapid growth.

Histopathology
It may be composed entirely of spindle cells, or have a variable component of more conventional squamous cell carcinoma. The spindle cells have a large vesicular nucleus and scanty eosinophilic cytoplasm, often with indistinct cell borders. There is variable pleomorphism, usually with many mitoses.

Differential diagnosis
It may be difficult to separate from other cutaneous spindle cell neoplasms including spindle cell melanoma, atypical fibroxanthoma and, less often, leiomyosarcoma. Some cases can only be confirmed ultrastructurally, as all keratin markers are negative {2180}. CK5/6 is positive in two-thirds of all cases, a higher figure than obtained with AE1/3,

CAM5.2 or MNF116. Some tumours may coexpress cytokeratin and vimentin, suggesting metaplastic change to a neoplasm with mesenchymal characteristics {1116}.

Prognosis and predictive factors
Spindle-cell squamous cell carcinoma is a poorly differentiated variant of squamous cell carcinoma that may be associated with an aggressive clinical course {2180}. These tumours account for slightly over one-third of cutaneous squamous cell carcinomas which metastasize {1985}. Metastases usually occur to the regional lymph nodes in the first instance.

Verrucous squamous cell carcinoma

Definition
Verrucous squamous cell carcinoma is a rare variant of well-differentiated squamous cell carcinoma with low malignant potential.

ICD-O code   8051/3

Synonyms
Oral florid papillomatosis, Ackerman tumour {32,348}, epithelioma cuniculatum {41,2096,2108}, giant condyloma acuminatum, Buschke-Löwenstein tumour {359,1347,1947,2124,2570}, papillomatosis cutis carcinoides {218,870, 2108}.

Epidemiology
Verrucous carcinoma comprises 2-12%

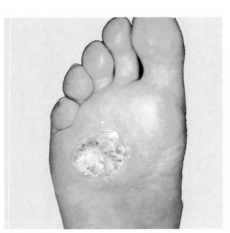

Fig. 1.15 Verrucous squamous cell carcinoma

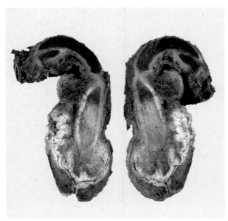

Fig. 1.16 Verrucous squamous cell carcinoma

of all oral carcinomas, and is found predominantly in men (age peak in 5th decade, range 34-85) {348}. Verrucous carcinoma of the extremities (epithelioma cuniculatum) most often affects men in the 6th decade {2108}. The incidence of the genital type (Buschke-Löwenstein tumour) varies between 5- and 24% of all penile cancers; the tumour tends to occur in men younger than 50 years (range 18-86) {218}.

Etiology
Leading theories of the pathogenesis include chronic irritation, inflammation and impaired immune response {2096, 2108}. Important factors for the development of oral verrucous carcinomas are poor oral hygiene with ill-fitting dentures or decaying teeth, chewing of tobacco or betel nuts, and use of snuff. In genital lesions poor hygiene and phimosis play a major role. Other theories include HPV infection (mostly HPV 6, 11) {898} and chemical carcinogens {2096,2108}.

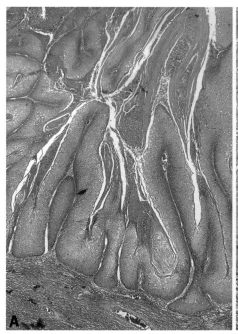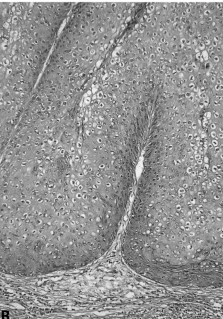

Fig. 1.17 Verrucous squamous cell carcinoma **A, B** Note the well-differentiated proliferative process and the bulbous nature of the squamous downgrowths.

Localization
Common sites include buccal and retromolar mucosa, gingiva, floor of mouth, tongue and hard palate. They also arise on the soles, rarely the palms and distal fingers, and on amputation stumps. Genital lesions occur primarily on the glans and prepuce of the penis {778, 2108,2570}. It is uncommon in the vagina and the perianal region {1347,1947, 2124}. Rare cases have been described on the scalp, face, back and extremities, sometimes associated with long-standing ulcerations or scars, especially in the pretibial area (papillomatosis cutis carcinoides) {218,870,2096,2108}.

Clinical features
These lesions show cauliflower-like appearance with exophytic and endophytic growth, and a papillomatous surface. They are pale in colour and sometimes have draining sinuses. Some are tender and painful, particularly on the sole of the foot. There is slow but relentless growth over the course of a long time {2570}.

Histopathology
In all cases a well-differentiated proliferative epithelial process is visible, the malignant nature of which may easily be overlooked, particularly if the biopsy is small and superficial. The squamous

epithelium shows an asymmetric exo- and endophytic growth pattern with pushing rather than destructive or infiltrative margins. Usually, there is deep penetration below the level of the surrounding epidermis / mucosa. Tumour cells exhibit only minimal atypia and very low mitotic activity. The presence of neutrophils is an important diagnostic clue; they may form small intraepidermal abscesses. Draining sinuses containing inflammatory cells and keratin debris may also be present. No foci of the usual squamous cell carcinoma should be found {1833}.

Differential diagnosis
The separation from benign reactive processes and SCC of the more usual type can be difficult. The presence of blunted projections of squamous epithelium in the mid and/or deep dermis is suspicious for verrucous carcinoma. The squamous downgrowths are bulbous. Small collections of neutrophils may extend into the tips. Clinicopathological correlation and adequate sampling are often helpful.

Precursor lesions
Oral lesions may develop in areas of previous leukoplakia, lichen planus, lupus erythematosus or candidiasis {218}.

Prognosis and predictive factors
If the tumour is completely excised, prognosis is excellent; after inadequate excision, the recurrence rate is high and the survival decreases. In long-standing cases or after irradiation and / or chemotherapy the biologic character of the disease may change into a metastasizing squamous cell carcinoma {1216}.

Pseudovascular squamous cell carcinoma

Definition
Pseudovascular SCC is an aggressive variant of SCC with marked acantholysis resulting in angiosarcoma-like areas {139,1688}.

ICD-O code   8075/3

Synonyms
Pseudoangiosarcomatous SCC, pseudoangiomatous SCC

Epidemiology
The tumour is exceedingly rare.

Clinical features
It usually presents as a circumscribed white-grey ulcer or a nodular tan-red/pink tumour, most often located on sun-

exposed areas of middle-aged or elderly patients.

Histopathology

It is characterized by areas of anastomosing cord-like arrays of polygonal or flattened tumour cells, with internal pseudolumina that contain detached tumour cells and amorphous basophilic material {550,1675,2558}. Erythrocytes may also be seen in pseudovascular spaces. Immunohistochemical examination is essential to differentiate it from angiosarcoma. Pseudovascular SCC is positive for one or more monoclonal antibodies to cytokeratin and consistently negative for CD31 and factor VIII-related antigen.

Differential diagnosis

In classical angiosarcoma vascular markers are positive, keratin staining is negative; in epithelioid angiosarcoma in addition to vascular markers epithelial markers are frequently expressed.

Prognosis and predictive factors

The prognosis is worse than it is for other variants of SCC, with a mortality up to 50%. Large size may confer a worse prognosis {1675}.

Adenosquamous carcinoma

Definition

Adenosquamous carcinoma is a rare variant of squamous cell carcinoma arising from pluripotential cells related to acrosyringia, characterized by the formation of mucin secreting glands.

ICD-code   8560/3

Epidemiology

Most reported cases occurred on the head and neck of elderly patients, with male predominance {120,140,572, 1933,2482}. The penis can also be involved {120}.

Clinical features

It can present as an asymptomatic smooth surfaced dermal nodule or a large ulcerated deeply invasive tumour indistinguishable from squamous cell carcinoma or basal cell carcinoma.

Histopathology

The tumour consists of invasive tongues, sheets, columns and strands of atypical dyskeratotic squamous cells, merging with glandular structures with epithelial mucin secretion, which can be demonstrated by a PAS, mucicarmine or alcian blue stain at pH 2.5. The mucin is hyaluronidase resistant and sialidase sensitive. Intracytoplasmic neolumina containing targetoid mucin secretions can also be seen. The tumour cells are positive for cytokeratin and epithelial membrane antigen, whereas those cells forming glands stain with carcinoembryonic antigen. There may be connection between tumour cells and acrosyringia, as well as perineural invasion.

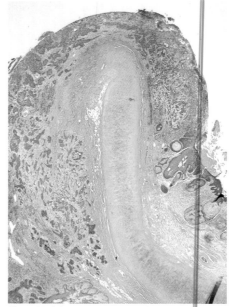

Fig. 1.18 Adenosquamous carcinoma of the ear. There are deeply invasive tongues, columns and strands of atypical dyskeratotic squamous cells abutting the cartilage.

Differential diagnosis

Adenosquamous carcinoma should be distinguished from mucoepidermoid carcinoma, which had been reported as adenosquamous carcinoma in early reports. Adenosquamous carcinoma has well formed glands with mucin secretion and no goblet cells. Mucoepidermoid carcinoma consists of polygonal squamous cells and goblet cells without glands. Signet ring squamous

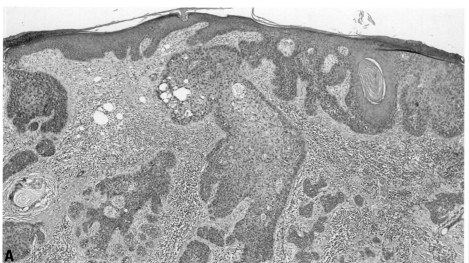
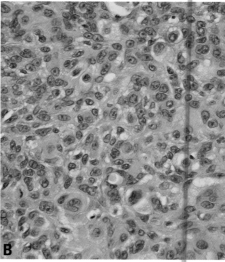

Fig. 1.19 Adenosquamous carcinoma. **A** Overt squamous differentiation in parts of the tumour. **B** Sheets of atypical dyskeratotic squamous cells from the squamous area of the tumour.

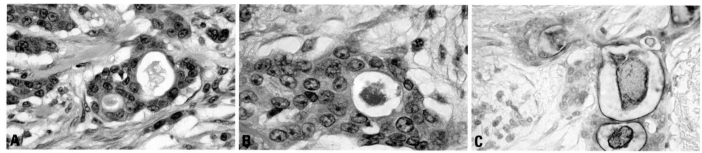

Fig. 1.20 Adenosquamous carcinoma. **A** Well formed glandular structures containing mucinous secretion in the glandular area of the tumour. **B** PAS stain. Intracytoplasmic targetoid PAS positive and diastase sensitive globules in the glandular areas of the tumour. **C** CEA immunohistochemical stain. Positive luminal staining in glandular structures.

cell carcinoma has foamy cytoplasmic mucin globules with displacement of the cell nucleus but no glands. Microcystic adnexal carcinoma (syringomatous carcinoma, sclerosing sweat duct carcinoma) shows a more ductal appearance with prominent tubular structures but no mucin secretion. Metastatic adenosquamous carcinoma from other primary sites such as the lung, salivary gland, female genital tract should also be excluded.

Prognosis and predictive factors
The tumours usually follow an aggressive course with the capacity for metastasis and local recurrence. Early superficially located tumours tend to have a better prognosis.

Bowen disease

G.F. Kao
R. Cerio
R. Salom
S. Pala

Definition
Bowen disease (BD) is a form of squamous cell carcinoma in situ. It is a distinct clinicopathologic entity of the skin and mucocutaneous junction.

ICD-O code   8081/2

Synonyms
Squamous cell carcinoma in situ (SCCIS), intraepidermal carcinoma, bowenoid dysplasia, bowenoid squamous carcinoma in situ (BSCIS), vulvar intraepithelial neoplasia (VIN III).
The terms bowenoid dysplasia and BSCIS are customarily applied to cutaneous and mucocutaneous lesions of the male and female external genitalia. BD is no longer used in gynaecological pathology. It has been replaced by the concept of vulvar intraepithelial neoplasia (VIN). The degree of epithelial atypia seen in BD corresponds to VIN, grade III (VIN III) {362,1580}.

Epidemiology
Bowen disease occurs predominantly in fair-complexioned Caucasian men, but both sexes are affected. One in five patients (20%) is a woman. The disease commonly affects patients in the 6-8th decades of life. However, the average age at onset of the disease is 48 years, and the average age at first biopsy is 55 years. Both exposed and non-exposed skin sites are equally affected. The disease uncommonly affects black skin, in which it is found more commonly on non-sun-exposed areas.

Etiology
The exact underlying cause of BD remains unclear, although multiple factors are likely to be responsible for it. Many lesions arise without an apparent cause. However, it is known that chronic sun damage disrupts normal keratinocytic maturation, causes mutation of the tumour suppressor gene protein (TP53) {375,1075}, and results in the development of keratinocytic atypia as seen in lesions of BD. The predilection for anatomic sites affected by BD on sun-exposed glabrous skin and lesions being reported more commonly in patients with a history of PUVA or UVB therapy {1410}, attest to the critical role of causal relationship between UV damage and BD. Ingestion of inorganic arsenic may play a role, as lesions of arsenical keratosis (As-K) may display identical histopathologic features to BD. A large number of cases of As-K with associated invasive carcinoma have been reported in a rural population using well water containing a high concentration of inorganic arsenic {2567,2572}. Human papillomavirus (HPV) genomes have been demonstrated by in situ hybridization in the nuclei of keratinocytes in the stratum malpighii and stratum corneum of the BD lesions. HPV types 16 and 18 have been linked to lesions of genital BD and non-condylomatous genital warts, i.e., bowenoid papulosis {1098}. HPV is less commonly associated with nongenital BD. HPV types 15 and 16 have been identified in some cases of BD of the distal extremities. Evidence of other papillomavirus types, including HPV31, 54, 58, 61, 62 and 73, have also been identified in some cases of BD. Aberrations in local and systemic immunity, trauma, chronic irritation, mutagenic factors, and tobacco exposure are other possible etiologies of BD.

Localization
Based upon a large series of 1001 biopsy-proven BD in Australia, most lesions occurred on a sun-exposed glabrous area {1315}. About one-third (33%) of the lesions occured in the head and neck areas, especially the face. Men had predominance of lesions on the scalp and ears, whereas women had a predominant involvement of the legs and cheeks. BD rarely affects the nail bed and periungual area {2070}.

Clinical features
The classic appearance of cutaneous BD is a single or multiple erythematous, rounded to irregular, lenticular, scaly, keratotic, fissured, crusty, nodular, eroded, pigmented patches or plaques. The plaques are devoid of hair, and usually appear sharply demarcated from the surrounding unaffected skin. Areas of normal-appearing skin may occur within the boundaries of larger lesions of BD. The plaques vary from 1-5 cm in overall dimensions. In intertriginous areas, BD may appear as moist patches without scale. In anogenital locations, the lesions appear polypoid or verrucoid, frequently pigmented. Erythroplasia of Queyrat (EPQ) presents as an asymptomatic,

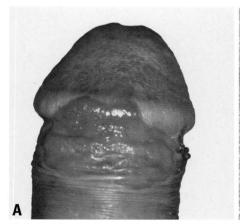
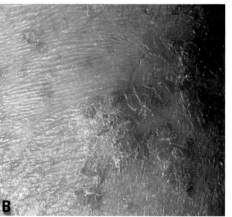

Fig. 1.21 A Bowen disease. Sharply circumscribed, bright red plaque of erythroplasia of Queyrat (EPQ).
B Bowen disease. Erythematous, scaly, fissuring plaques of BD on lower leg of a middle-aged woman.

26 Keratinocytic tumours

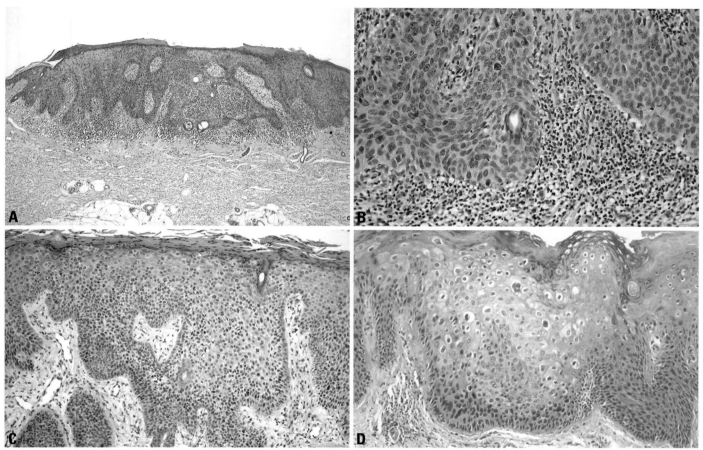

Fig. 1.22 Bowen disease (BD). **A** Low-power photomicrograph of BD. Note hyperkeratosis, full-thickness of epidermal atypia, extensive pilar epithelial involvement, and a lichenoid upper dermal mixed chronic inflammatory infiltrate. **B** Atypical keratinocytes encircle an acrosyringium. **C** Atypical squamous cells extend along acrosyringia. **D** Prominent vacuolated atypical cells, focally mimicking koilocytotic change and pagetoid appearance seen in BD.

bright red, velvety to shiny, sharply circumscribed plaque. The mucocutaneous junction of the glans penis, coronal sulcus, or undersurface of the foreskin is involved, and lesions are usually found in older, uncircumcised men.

There are two clinical variants of BD: those involving glabrous skin, and those of the anogenital area. On the glabrous skin, BD manifests as asymptomatic, slowly enlarging, scaly patches or plaques. The average duration of the lesion is 6.4 years. Plaques of BD enlarge slowly, and expand centrifugally, sometimes for decades. Anogenital BD involves the mucocutaneous junction and adjacent mucosa. If untreated, 5-8% of patients may develop invasive carcinoma. The invasive carcinomas are larger (up to 15 cm), rapidly growing tumours that occur in pre-existing scaly plaques {1203}.

The clinical entity of erythroplasia of Queyrat (EPQ) is regarded as BD of the

glans penis. Such lesions have a greater potential for developing into invasive carcinoma than does BD involving glabrous skin {875}. Although evidence for the association of BD and internal malignancies is reported in earlier studies, more recent population-based cohort studies do not confirm the link {484}.

Histopathology

The typical low-power microscopic features of BD are hyperkeratosis, parakeratosis, hypo- or hypergranulosis, plaque-like acanthosis with increased cellularity, and a chronic inflammatory infiltrate in the upper corium. The epidermis exhibits loss of normal polarity and progression of normal surface keratinocytic maturation. A "windblown" appearance of crowding of atypical keratinocytes, with hyperchromatism, pale-staining to vacuolated cells, occasional multinucleated cells, individual cell keratinization (dyskeratosis), and abnormal mitoses are noted.

These changes are confined by an intact dermoepidermal basement membrane. Lesions of BD from hair-bearing areas invariably demonstrate involvement of the pilar acrotrichium, infundibulum, and sebaceous gland. In some lesions, prominent vacuolated atypical cells focally mimic koilocytotic viral cytopathic change and exhibit a pagetoid appearance. The acrosyringium is occasionally involved. An inflammatory infiltrate of lymphocytes, macrophages, and plasma cells is seen in the upper dermis. Capillary ectasia is commonly noted. Prominent solar elastosis is also present in lesions on sun-exposed skin. An invasive carcinoma arising in BD shows variable histologic differentiation, with squamous, basosquamous, pilar, sebaceous {1120}, pilosebaceous, poorly-differentiated, and occasionally ductal features {1203,2016}. The atypical vacuolated keratinocytes are negative for cytoplasmic mucin; some, however, contain glycogen. Melanin pigment may be present in the atypical cells, and in the pigmented genital lesions, melanophages are numerous. The abnormal keratinizing cells are intensely reactive with glucose-6-phosphate dehydrogenase. Ultrastructural changes of BD include decrease in tonofilament-desmosomal attachments, aggregated tonofilaments and nuclear substance, and absence of keratohyaline granules {1204}.

Differential diagnosis

Bowenoid solar keratosis differs from BD by its clinically smaller size, exclusive location on sun-exposed skin, and presence of superficial keratinocytic maturation. Bowenoid papulosis is distinguished from BD by its clinical appearance of multiple papular to coalescing lesions on the anogenital areas, and the typical microscopic salt and pepper distribution of atypical keratinocytes and mitoses in the affected cutaneous and mucocutaneous lesions, as well as frequent HPV positive koilocytotic cells {1790}. The pagetoid variant of BD is sometimes difficult to distinguish from extramammary Paget disease. In the latter, mucicarmine, Cam 5.2 and CEA positive tumour cells are present in the epidermis, individually or in small nests, forming glandular structures at the dermoepidermal junction. These features are absent in BD. The vacuolated cells in BD contain glycogen and not mucin. In malignant melanoma in situ, the basilar keratinocytes are replaced by neoplastic melanocytes. The presence of intercellular bridges and prominent dyskeratotic keratinocytes are features favouring the diagnosis of BD. Melanoma cells do not contain cytokeratins of 54 and 66 kilodaltons (kd); the reverse applies with the cells in BD.

Histogenesis

It has been suggested that BD most likely originates from germinal cells of the pilar outer root sheath and the pluripotential epidermal cells of the acrotrichium. This concept is substantiated by the findings of various types of histologic differentiation in carcinoma arising in BD {1120,1203,2016}. Using immunohistochemical localization of keratins and involucrin, the atypical cells of BD exhibit a diversity of differentiation {1093}.

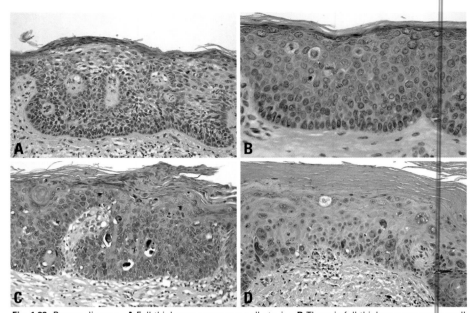

Fig. 1.23 Bowen disease. A Full thickness squamous cell atypia. B There is full thickness squamous cell atypia with apparent sparing of the basal keratinocytes and hyperpigmentation of the basal keratinocytes. C Full thickness squamous cell atypia with scattered bizarre keratinocytes. D Full thickness squamous cell atypia with marked nuclear pleomorphism.

Genetics

The atypical keratinocytes of BD contain large numbers of aneuploid cells {241}. Increased expression and mutation of TP53 observed in lesions of BD suggest that loss of normal TP53 tumour suppressor activity may be an important mechanism of oncogenesis in BD {375,1075, 1946}. Allelic deletion of one or more 9q chromosome markers has been detected in occasional lesions of BD. However, no deletion of 9p markers was seen {1866}. There have been no clonal chromosomal abnormalities by cytogenetic analysis of cell cultures from BD {1003}.

Prognosis and predictive factors

Surgical excision with complete removal may cure BD. The origin of BD from pilar outer root sheath cells at the sebaceous gland level explains in part the high recurrence rate, following treatment with superficial curettage and desiccation, topical fluorouracil, and X-ray. Invasive adnexal carcinoma may develop in untreated plaques of BD of prolonged duration following expansile growth. The metastatic rate in these uncommon tumours was 18% and fatality was observed in 10% of cases in a large case series {1203}.

Bowenoid papulosis

Definition

Bowenoid papulosis is a clinicopathological entity characterized by the presence on the genitalia of solitary or multiple verruca-like papules or plaques with histology resembling full thickness epidermal dysplasia as seen in Bowen disease.

Synonyms

Multicentric pigmented Bowen disease, multifocal indolent pigmented penile papules

Epidemiology

Bowenoid papulosis occurs mainly in young individuals and although uncommon the incidence is increasing. There is a male predominance.

Etiology

The etiopathogenesis of this condition almost certainly favours linkage to human papillomavirus infection particularly oncogenic types 16, 18, 33,35 and 39. DNA sequences have been identified by various workers {908,1737,2113}. Consequently in females there is a higher incidence of abnormal cervical/vaginal smears both in affected patients and in partners of men with penile lesions. Whilst controversies regarding the biological potential of bowenoid papulosis exist, with the possibility of invasive malignancy, in most cases the clinical course is benign and some lesions regress.

Localization
Bowenoid papulosis was first described as a condition affecting the groin {1438}. It was later defined {1305,2447} as an entity involving the genitalia or perigenital areas. Isolated cases of extragenital bowenoid papulosis have been described {902,1147}.

Clinical features
The lesions are usually asymptomatic with variable clinical presentation: multiple generally small, round fleshy papules, isolated or confluent (2.0-20 mm), with a smooth papillomatous surface, sometimes with desquamation resembling lichenoid or psoriasiform dermatoses. The colour of lesions can vary from pink to reddish-purple to brown / black.

Histopathology
The histological features demonstrate epidermal atypia ranging from partial to full thickness atypia similar to in situ squamous cell carcinoma i.e. Bowen disease. On the genitalia changes may be termed vulvar intraepithelial neoplasia (VIN) III or penile intraepithelial neoplasia (PIN) III by some pathologists {570}. There is loss of architecture. The basement membrane is intact. Mitoses are frequent, sometimes with abnormal forms often in metaphase. Dyskeratotic cells are also seen. Typical koilocytes are uncommon {908}. The stratum corneum and granular cell layer often contain small inclusion - like bodies which are deeply basophilic, rounded and surrounded by a halo.

Differential diagnosis
The basophilic bodies, together with the numerous metaphase mitoses, are the features which suggest a diagnosis of bowenoid papulosis rather than Bowen disease itself.

Histogenesis
A study based on histomorphology and DNA ploidy analysis has suggested that bowenoid papulosis is a form of low-grade squamous cell carcinoma in situ {269}. Electron microscopy has shown structures resembling viral particles {1274,1790} within the granular layer.

Somatic genetics
Many of the atypical keratinocytes of bowenoid papulosis not unlike Bowen disease, contain large numbers of aneuploid cells. Increased expression and mutation of TP53 observed in lesions suggest that loss of normal TP53 tumour suppressor activity is likely to be an important mechanism of oncogenesis in bowenoid papulosis. To date, there have been no clonal chromosomal abnormalities by cytogenetic analysis of cell cultures from bowenoid papulosis.

Prognosis and predictive factors
Bowenoid papulosis appears in many cases to remain benign {1790} and spontaneous regression has occasionally occurred; however, close follow up is essential.

Actinic keratosis

C. James
R.I. Crawford
M. Martinka
R. Marks

Definition
A common intraepidermal neoplasm of sun-damaged skin characterized by variable atypia of keratinocytes.

Synonyms
Solar keratosis

Epidemiology
Actinic keratoses (AKs) usually present in older individuals. The fair-skinned, the freckled and those who do not tan easily are at increased risk. Lesions have developed in areas of vitiligo {2023, 2564}. The rate is higher in men because of greater sun exposure {1049}. In the Australian Caucasian population, AKs are discovered in 40-60% of individuals over 40 {789,1515}, rising to 80% in the seventh decade {1049}. Patients with Rothmund-Thompson, Cockayne and Bloom syndromes and xeroderma pigmentosum are at increased risk {791}.

Etiology
Both cumulative and intermittent sunlight exposure is implicated {790}. Ultraviolet B (UVB) is the most harmful, but a supplemental effect of ultraviolet A (UVA) is demonstrated {694}. AKs are increased after PUVA therapy {11}. UVB induces DNA thymidine dimer formation, which can target TP53, with impaired apoptosis

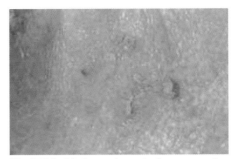

Fig. 1.24 Actinic keratosis on the face, presenting as a group of irregularly shaped small papules.

of damaged keratinocytes in cells with two TP53 mutations {1150,1396,1696, 2602}. Clonal proliferations of these cells form actinic keratoses and after further genetic damage, invasive SCC may develop. Ultraviolet light can act as an initiator and promoter of carcinogenesis {2602}. Epidermodysplasia verruciformis–associated HPV types have been discovered in AK's after renal transplantation {2354}.

Localization
Sun-exposed areas are involved: face, ears, balding scalp, dorsal hands, forearms and lateral neck {2218}.

Clinical features
Patients commonly present with multiple persistent, asymptomatic erythematous lesions. Most measure less than 1 cm and are hyperkeratotic. Atrophic lesions predominate on the face. Thickening and tenderness may indicate the development of invasive carcinoma.

Macroscopy
Most lesions are circumscribed <1cm scaly macules or slightly elevated papules or plaques, ranging from erythematous to grey-brown with adherent yellow-brown scale. Some are larger, more irregularly shaped and pigmented {1128}, whilst others, particularly on the dorsal hands and forearms, are hyperkeratotic or verrucous {244}. A keratin horn may be produced.

Histopathology
Six types of AK are described: hypertrophic, atrophic, bowenoid, acantholytic, pigmented and lichenoid {233,1446}. Most lesions reveal parakeratosis and hypogranulosis. Disordered keratinocyte maturation with cytologic atypia is present, including nuclear enlargement, hyperchromasia, pleomorphism, nucleolar prominence, mitotic activity, dyskeratosis and cytoplasmic pallor. Grading as Keratinocyte Intraepidermal Neoplasia (KIN I, II and III) in a manner similar to that used for the uterine cervix {506} has

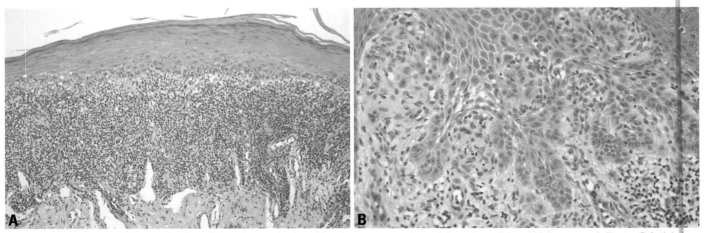

Fig. 1.25 Actinic keratosis. **A** There is focal parakeratosis, acanthosis and basal squamous atypia overlying a dense lichenoid inflammatory infiltrate. **B** Actinic keratosis. There are elongated rete ridges with squamous cell atypia and focal acantholysis.

the enzymes required for transcription or replication of viral DNA and therefore is entirely dependent on subverting cellular proteins for these functions. In particular, in HPV types 16 and 18, proteins E6 and E7 promote continued cell cycling of suprabasal epidermal cells by abrogation of the functions of TP53 and pRb, respectively. HPV genomes are thereby amplified to high levels during vegetative viral replication for assembly into infectious virions after encapsulation by L1 and L2 proteins in the granular layer and above. Virus assembly does not lyse keratinocytes, but rather the infectious virus is shed with desquamating cornified cells, and viral release is facilitated by disruption of the keratinocyte intracellular filamentous network by viral E4 proteins.

Host immune response {2246,2608}: Persistent papillomavirus infections are common, indicating that HPVs have evolved mechanisms to evade immune surveillance. There is no viraemic phase, low levels of viral proteins are expressed in the basal cell layer, and extensive virion production only occurs in the more immunologically privileged terminally differentiated layers. However, a successful immune response is eventually generated in most cases, since two thirds of cutaneous warts regress spontaneously within 2 years and multifocal lesions often regress concomitantly. Cell mediated immune responses appear to be primarily responsible.

Localization

Warts can occur on any skin or mucosal surface. Certain HPV subtypes cause specific kinds of warts and show special affinity for particular body locations. Subtypes causing common warts are found on the hands, fingers, and palms. Periungual subtypes are often seen in nail biters. Verruca plantaris is seen on the sole of the feet. Condylomata acuminata lesions (genital HPV infection) appear on the vulva, cervix, perineum, anus, or penis. Scrotal condylomata are very rare and only seen in 1% of HIV positive males.

Table 1.02
Correlation between cytopathological changes of verrucas and causal HPV types

Clinical manifestation	HPV types[a]	Epidermal changes[b]	Cytopathic effect (location)
Verruca vulgaris			
	2	Prominent	Eccentric nucleus; condensed heterogeneous keratohyaline granules (granular)
	4	Prominent; endophytic	Large, vacuolated keratinocytes with no keratohyaline granules and small, peripherally located, 'signet ring' nuclei (granular)
	7 (Butcher's wart)	Prominent	Central, small, shrunken nuclei within proliferating rete ridges (granular)
Palmo-plantar			
	1 (Myrmecia)	Prominent, endophytic	Vacuolated cells with large, eosinophilic keratohyaline granules forming ring-like and sickle-like figures. Basophilic nuclear inclusions (spinous, granular)
	60 (Ridged wart)	Acanthosis and mild papillomatosis; endophytic	Eosinophilic, homogeneous and solitary inclusions
	65 (Pigmented plantar wart)	Prominent; endophytic	Eosinophilic, homogeneous and solitary inclusions
	63	Prominent; endophytic	Intracytoplasmic, heavily stained keratohyaline material with filamentous inclusions that encase the vacuolated nucleus
Verruca plana	3	Subtle; no parakeratosis and basket-weave like appearance of stratum corneum	Central, pyknotic, strongly basophilic 'bird's eyes' nuclei (upper spinous and granular)
Epidermodysplasia verruciformis	5	Nests of large, clear cells; stratum corneum loose with basket-weave like appearance	Basophilic cytoplasm containing keratohyaline granules of various shapes and sizes; clear nucleoplasm (upper spinous and granular)
Condyloma acuminata	6,11	Marked acanthosis, some papillomatosis and hyperkeratosis	Less prominent vacuolisation of granular cells

[a] Most common associated HPV genotype
[b] Epidermal changes comprise papillomatosis, compact hyperkeratosis, focal parakeratosis, hypergranulosis, acanthosis.

Clinical features and correlation with viral genotyping

Cutaneous and mucosal HPV types form two distinct groups that infect skin or mucosa, although viral tropism is not absolute {605}. Clinical manifestations depend on the HPV type involved, the anatomical location and the immune status of the host {1282}.

Cutaneous infections: In general, classification of warts is based on morphology and anatomic localization and cutaneous warts have traditionally been classified as verruca vulgaris or common warts, palmoplantar warts, including superficial and deep types, verruca plana or plane warts and epidermodysplasia verruciformis (EV). Recent studies suggest that histological and clinical characteristics of warts are mainly determined by viral genotype, indicating that HPV typing may allow a more accurate classification. However, the use of highly sensitive PCR techniques for HPV detection and genotyping has highlighted the presence of a greater diversity of HPV types than was previously appreciated {975}. These individuals often harbour multiple HPV types, particularly epidermodysplasia-verruciformis (EV)-HPV types. These HPVs were previously thought to occur only in the context of the rare genodermatosis EV, characterized by infection with unusual, widespread, cutaneous warts and associated with increased risk of non-melanoma skin cancers harbouring EV-HPV types on ultraviolet radiation exposed sites {1492}. There is also mounting evidence that EV-HPV types play a cofactor role with UVR in NMSCs arising in immunosuppressed individuals {974}.

Mucosal infections: Over 25 HPV types are recognized to infect anogenital and aerodigestive mucosa {605}, and sub-clinical infections are more common than visible warts {1282}. Genital warts are generally caused by low-risk mucosal HPV types rather than the high-risk types associated with anogenital neoplasia {605}. Bowenoid papulosis (section 1.5.01) may clinically resemble genital warts, but histologically resembles squamous cell carcinoma in situ and contains high-risk HPV types. Giant condyloma acuminata (Buschke-Lowenstein tumour) may also resemble genital warts but is an anogenital verrucous carcinoma harbouring low-risk HPV types {2476}. Oral warts are also associated with HPV types 6 and 11 and focal epithelial hyperplasia (Heck disease) resembling gingival, buccal and labial flat warts or condylomata usually harbours HPV 13 or 32 {2476}.

Verruca vulgaris

Definition
Verruca vulgaris is a benign, squamous papillomatous lesion caused by infection with the human papilloma virus (HPV).

Synonym
Common wart.

Epidemiology
Verruca vulgaris occurs predominantly in children and adolescents, although adults are also frequently infected. They have been found in up to 20% of school students {1262}. Clinically detectable verrucae develop from a few weeks to 18 months after inoculation {1691}.

Etiology
Common warts are preferentially associated with HPV-2, but they may also be caused by other types such as HPV-1, HPV-4 and HPV-7. In children, HPV-6 and/or HPV-11 are rarely found. Other HPV types have rarely been implicated, usually in immunosuppressed individuals {106}.

Localization
Common warts may be solitary or multiple, and they are usually found on exposed parts, particularly the fingers and on the dorsum of the hands.

Clinical features
They are hard, rough-surfaced papules that range in diameter from about 0.2:1.5-2.0 cm. New warts may sometimes form at sites of trauma (Koebner phenomenon).

Histopathology
Common warts show marked hyperkeratosis and acanthosis. There are outgrowths of epidermis presenting as slender spires in filiform warts or blunter digitate processes in other variants. Columns of parakeratosis overlie the papillomatous projections. There may be haemorrhage into these columns. Hypergranulosis is present where the cells contain coarse clumps of keratohyaline granules. Koilocytes (large vacuolated cells with small pyknotic nuclei) are present in the upper malpighian layer and the granular layer. Small amounts of keratohyalin may be present in the cytoplasm of these cells. There is often some inward turning of the elongated rete ridges at the edges of the lesion. Tricholemmal differentiation and squamous eddies may be seen in old warts.

Dilated vessels are often found in the core of the papillomatous projections. A variable lymphocytic infiltrate is sometimes seen, and this may be lichenoid in presumptive regressing lesions.

Prognosis and predictive factors
Most warts are only a cosmetic problem. Rarely, Bowen disease or squamous cell carcinoma may develop in a common wart, usually in immunocompromised patients {1611}. Thrombosis of superficial vessels, haemorrhage and necrosis of the epidermis are rarely seen in regressing common warts.

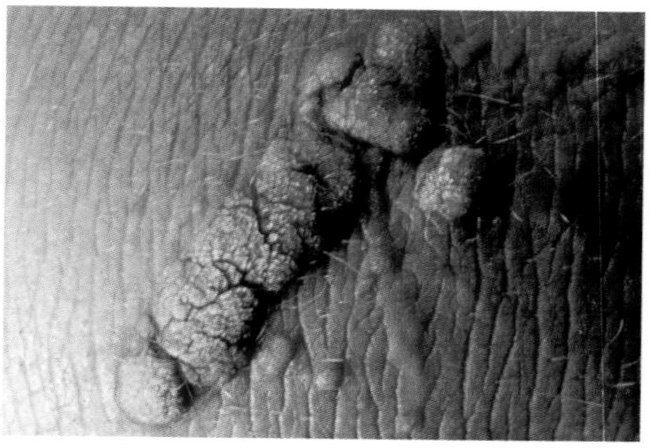

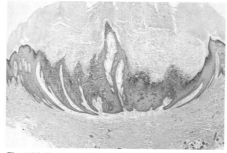

Fig. 1.29 Verruca vulgaris showing the Koebner phenomenon. Note the linear arrangement of the lesions as a consequence of scratching.

Fig. 1.30 Verruca vulgaris. There is hyperkeratosis, papillomatosis and inturning of the elongated rete ridges.

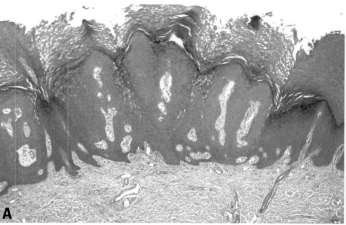
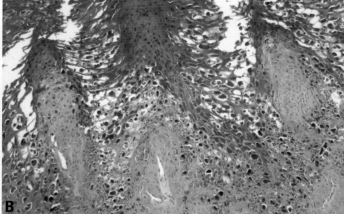

Fig. 1.31 Verruca plantaris. **A, B** Plantar wart. Note papillomatosis, acanthosis, hyperkeratosis, viral cytopathic changes.

Verruca plantaris

Definition
Verruca plantaris is a benign, human papillomavirus (HPV)-induced epithelial proliferation occurring on the sole of the foot. It is characterized by the formation of thick, hyperkeratotic lesions {505,648, 1214}.

Synonyms
Plantar wart, deep foot warts, myrmecia

Epidemiology
Plantar warts are most common in children and young adults; possibly because of immaturity of the immune system or sport-related repetitive microtrauma. They are most frequent over pressure points {505,648}. Particularly in children they may spontaneously regress within a few months, but in adults and immunocompromised patients they can persist for years. Rarely chronic lesions are associated with the development of verrucous carcinoma {594}.

Clinical features
Plantar warts are sharply defined, rounded lesions, with a rough keratotic surface, surrounded by a thickened horn. They tend to grow into the foot and are covered by black dots representing thrombosed capillaries {505,648,1214}. They do not retain the normal fingerprint lines of the feet, as calluses (corns) do. They often occur in multiples, and can be painful {1055,2390}. They are traditionally divided into the superficial warts (mosaic), which are ordinary verrucae, and deep warts (myrmecia). Several other variants have been recently described {1055,1214,1556}.

Histopathology
The mosaic–type shows acanthosis, papillomatosis, hyperkeratosis, vacuolated cells (koilocytes) in the upper Malpighian layer, vertical tiers of parakeratotic cells and clumped keratohyaline granules. Myrmecia are characterized by an endophytic proliferation of rete ridges covered by thickened keratin and promi-nent eosinophilic intracytoplasmic inclusions. The nuclei are retained in the stratum corneum and appear as basophilic round bodies surrounded by a clear halo {505,1055,1214}.

Regression of palmo-plantar warts is often associated with thrombosis of superficial vessels, haemorrhage and necrosis of the epidermis and a mixed inflammatory cell infiltrate.

Pathogenesis
HPV is the established cause. Correlations between the variety of wart and the HPV type are as follows:

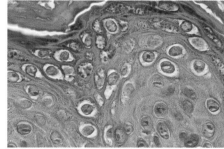

Fig. 1.34 Flat wart.

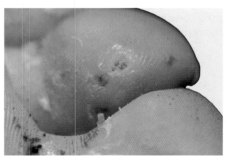

Fig. 1.32 Verruca plantaris on the volar surface of the toe. Clinically, the lesion was painful.

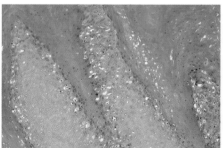

Fig. 1.33 Plantar wart (myrmecia type). Nuclei are retained in the stratum corneum as basophillic round bodies surrounded by a clear halo.

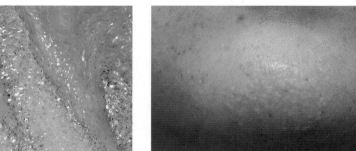

Fig. 1.35 Multiple flat warts on the chin of a young female.

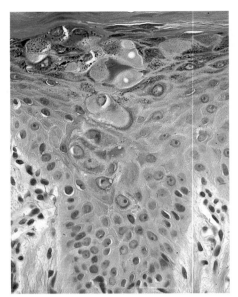

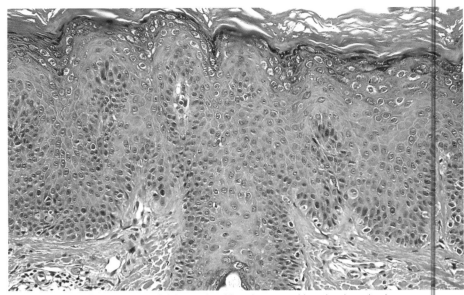

Fig. 1.36 Flat wart in a patient with epidermodysplasia.

Fig. 1.37 Flat wart. There are superficial vacuolated keratinocytes with perinuclear clearing.

Deep plantar wart (myrmecia) - HPV1, HPV63 {505,2390}.
Common and mosaic wart - HPV2, HPV4 {1055}
Endophytic common wart - HPV4 {1055}
Ridged and flat warts (associated with or without cyst, respectively) - HPV60 {505, 1055,1214,2390}
Large plantar wart - HPV66 {1556}

Verruca plana

Definition
Verrucae planae are benign, HPV-induced, slightly elevated, flat-topped, smooth papules.

Synonyms
Flat wart, verruca plana juvenilis.

Epidemiology
Verrucae planae are relatively common. Children, adolescents and young adults are most frequently affected.

Etiology
HPV types 3 and 10 are most commonly associated with verruca plana. Minor trauma, atopic dermatitis and immuno-suppression are possible predisposing factors {778,909,2262}.

Localization
Most lesions are located on the back of the hands and fingers, distal forearm, lower leg and face.

Clinical features
Flat warts generally are smaller than common warts and typically develop as small round to oval epidermal papules measuring 1-4 mm in diameter. Lesions are mostly skin-coloured with a smooth and flat surface, but may be hyperpigmented. The number ranges from one to several hundred and the distribution is asymmetric, sometimes linear (Koebner phenomenon).

Histopathology
Histology reveals a loose hyperkeratosis with basket-weave-pattern but little or no papillomatosis as in verruca vulgaris. There is plate-like epidermal hyperplasia of about twice the thickness of the surrounding normal epidermis with compressed papillae but dilatation and tortuosity of capillaries in the papillary dermis. Superficial epidermal layers show koilocytosis, vacuolated keratinocytes with perinuclear clearing around centrally located nuclei (so-called "birds-eye cells") and hypergranulosis.
Flat wart-like lesions can be encountered in patients with epidermodysplasia verruciformis. These lesions may show typical blue-grey cytoplasm {907,909,1491}.
Regression of plane warts is accompanied by superficial lymphocytic infiltrate in the dermis with exocytosis and single epidermal cell apoptosis {2476}.

Prognosis and predictive factors
Flat warts commonly persist for several years. Due to immunologic rejection in some long-standing cases, lesions have disappeared almost from one day to the next showing some local inflammation without leaving a scar. There are no reports regarding recurrences in such cases. In other cases warts lose evidence of viral cytopathic change and persist as localized verrucous epidermal hyperplasia {909}.

Acanthomas

D. Weedon
E. Haneke
M. Martinka
G.W. Elgart
R.J. Mortimore
C. Gross

R.M. Williamson
G.F. Kao
R.E. Wilentz
M. Morgan
S. Chimenti
L.L. Yu

Definition

Acanthomas are benign tumours of epidermal keratinocytes. The proliferating keratinocytes may show normal epidermoid keratinization or a wide range of aberrant keratinization, which includes epidermolytic hyperkeratosis (epidermolytic acanthoma), dyskeratosis with acantholysis (warty dyskeratoma) or acantholysis alone (acantholytic acanthoma). Seborrhoeic keratosis, melanoacanthoma, clear cell acanthoma, large cell acanthoma and keratoacanthoma all fulfil the criteria for an acanthoma.

Epidermolytic acanthoma

Definition

A benign tumour presenting as solitary or multiple discrete lesions and demonstrating the characteristic histologic features of epidermolytic hyperkeratosis {1628, 2151}.

Epidemiology

The reported age range is 3-72 years with a slight male predominance and various racial groups affected {515}.

Etiology

The etiology remains unknown but trauma {2033}, sun exposure {2298} and PUVA {1677} have been proposed as causes of disseminated epidermolytic acanthoma.

Localization

They can occur at any skin site and may involve oral or vaginal mucosa {515, 601,1869,2151}.

Clinical and macroscopic features

Epidermolytic acanthomas are generally asymptomatic, flat or elevated keratotic papules 2-12 mm in diameter {515,601, 1291,1628,1677,1712,1869,2033,2151, 2298}. Lesions may be solitary, multiple (localized to a region), or disseminated {515}.

Histopathology

Epidermolytic acanthoma is characterised by compact hyperkeratosis, perinuclear vacuolization of the cells of the stratum Malpighii sparing only the basal layer, indistinct reticulate cell boundaries and hypergranulosis with larger basophilic keratohyaline granules than normal and intracytoplasmic amorphous eosinophilic bodies i.e. epidermolytic hyperkeratosis {14}.

Genetics

Based on patterns of keratin expression determined by immunohistochemical techniques, a somatic mutation involving K1 and K10 genes has been postulated {515}.

Patients with disseminated disease may also have germline mutations, with offspring at risk for congenital ichthyosiform erythroderma/generalized epidermolytic hyperkeratosis.

Warty dyskeratoma

Definition

Warty dyskeratoma is a benign papulonodular lesion characterized by an endophytic proliferation of squamous epithelium typically occurring in relation to a folliculosebaceous unit and showing prominent acantholytic dyskeratosis.

Synonyms

Isolated dyskeratosis follicularis
Follicular dyskeratoma

Epidemiology

Warty dyskeratoma occurs mostly in middle aged to elderly adults {1166}.

Etiology

There are no known etiological factors. A recent study using PCR showed no evidence of HPV in 13 cases {1166}.

Localization

The head and neck region is most commonly involved {873,1166,2306,2321}. Cases arising in oral {869} and laryngeal {1185} mucosa and in a subungual {147} location have been reported. It has been suggested that lesions arising in sites devoid of hair follicles may be a separate entity {1166}.

Clinical features

Most lesions are solitary flesh coloured to

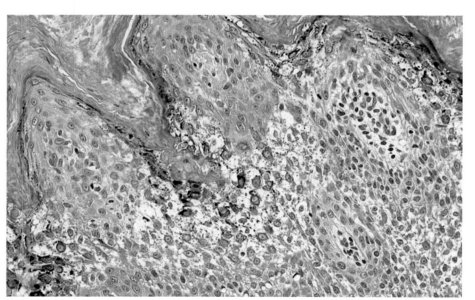

Fig. 1.38 Epidermolytic acanthoma. This lesion shows hypergranulosis and marked cytoplasmic vacuolization with clumps of eosinophilic material, sparing the basal layer.

brown papules, nodules or cysts with an umbilicated or pore-like centre or central keratin plug {873,1166}. Most are 1-10mm in size {873}. Occasionally the lesions are multiple {121,2306}.

Histopathology
Warty dyskeratoma is a well-demarcated endophytic lesion characterized by prominent acantholytic dyskeratosis. This results in suprabasal clefting with formation of villi which protrude into a lacuna. There is typically abundant keratin present within the centre of the proliferation forming a plug {829,873,1166, 2306}. Keratin pearls are commonly seen as are small cysts lined by infundibular type epithelium {1166}. Mitotic figures are commonly identified and may exceed 5 per HPF {1166}.

Three architectural variants have been described, namely cup-shaped, cystic and nodular and combinations of these may occur {1166}. There may be an epidermal collarette present and the surrounding epidermis may show papillomatosis, hypergranulosis and hyperplasia {1166}. A connection to folliculosebaceous structures is commonly demonstrable {873,1166}.

The stroma often shows a characteristic appearance with dense collagen or fibroblasts and focal intrastromal clefts. There may be an associated mixed inflammatory cell infiltrate {873,1166, 2321}.

Differential diagnosis
Comedonal Darier disease shows identical histological features and is differentiated on clinical grounds {623}.
Familial dyskeratotic comedones is a rare condition which tends to spare the scalp and face and shows less marked acantholysis and dyskeratosis than warty dyskeratoma {941}.

Histogenesis
It has been recently suggested that this lesion is a follicular adnexal neoplasm {1166}.

Acantholytic acanthoma

Definition
Acantholytic acanthoma is a rare benign epidermal tumour. The lesion displays a striking characteristic microscopic feature of acantholysis that bears resemblance to that seen in several vesiculobullous disorders {320,1566,1885,2476}.

Epidemiology
In the 31 cases reported by Brownstein {320}, the patients ranged in age from 32-87 years. The median age was 60 years; the male to female ratio was 2:1.

Etiology
Although it is known that immunosuppression increases the incidence of cutaneous neoplasms, the role of impaired immune surveillance resulting in acantholytic acanthoma is speculative {1885}.

Localization
Truncal skin, i.e., back, chest, or flank, is most commonly involved, followed by extremities, neck, groin, axilla, ear, scrotum and shoulder.

Clinical features
Acantholytic acanthoma is a solitary, keratotic, asymptomatic to occasionally pruritic papule or nodule. Multiple lesions have been recorded in a renal transplant patient {1885}.

Macroscopy
The scaly, flesh-coloured, hyperkeratotic growths range in size from 0.5-1.2 cm.

Histopathology
The tumour shows a well-defined area of papillomatous epidermal hyperplasia. There is hyperkeratosis with prominent acantholysis involving multiple levels of the epidermis. Suprabasal or subcorneal clefts with some dyskeratotic cells (corps ronds and grains) and occasional villi are noted. The upper dermis contains a variable perivascular lymphohistiocytic and occasional eosinophilic infiltrate.

Differential diagnosis
Acantholytic acanthoma must be distinguished from other acantholytic disorders and from various acanthomas. Pemphigus, Grover disease, and Hailey-Hailey disease are disorders with more extensive clinical papulovesicular eruptions.
Epidermolytic acanthoma shows epidermolytic hyperkeratosis, and no acantholysis is present. Clear cell acanthoma contains numerous pale cells, with abundant intracytoplasmic glycogen, which is absent in acantholytic acanthoma.

Solar lentigo

Definition
Solar lentigo simplex is characterized by a clinically flat epidermis with microscopic acanthosis and highly localized well-circumscribed pigment on sun exposed skin. It is discussed here because of its relationship to reticulated seborrhoeic keratosis, lichen planus-like keratosis and large cells acanthoma. Recent work suggests that solar lentigo is not a disorder of melanocytes.

Synonyms
Actinic lentigo, lentigo senilis, "ink spot" lentigo.

Epidemiology
They are common pigmented lesions most frequently seen on the sun-exposed skin of light skinned individuals who are middle aged to elderly.

Localization
These lesions are most common on the face, upper trunk and exttremities, particularly the forearm. They spare the palms and soles. There is relative sparing of sun-protected areas, but some lesions may occur in these sites.

Clinical features
Solar lentigos are well-circumscribed mainly flat (macular) localized collections of pigment. The lesions are common and are ubiquitous in light skinned individuals.
Individual lesions may be smooth-edged, but many have an irregular outline. Most appear entirely uniform in colour and range from light tan to brown to black.

Histopathology
Lesions are characterized by elongation of the rete ridges which are usually short and bulb like. Rete ridge hyperplasia is less conspicuous, and may be absent, in lesions of the face. As they evolve into the reticulated form of seborrhoeic keratosis, there is further elongation of the rete ridges which connect with adjacent processes forming netlike acanthosis. In addition, there is basal hyperpigmentation that may be quite heavy. There appears to be mild increase in basal melanocytes but this is accounted for by the increase in epidermal volume. This increase is usually not appreciated on

routine examination. Occasionally, lesions develop a heavy lichenoid inflammatory infiltrate: such lesions are called lichen-planus-like keratosis.

Differential diagnosis
The separation between seborrhoeic keratosis and lentigo is somewhat arbitrary, but most authors describe the epidermis as flat in lentigo simplex while the skin surface is clearly raised in seborrhoeic keratosis.

Prognosis
Solar lentigos may evolve into the reticulated form of seborrhoeic keratosis. Uncommonly, a lentigo maligna may arise in a solar lentigo of long standing. They appear to be a common precursor lesion of malignant melanoma in patients with xeroderma pigmentosum.

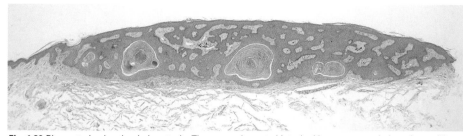

Fig. 1.39 Pigmented seborrhoeic keratosis. There are elongated interlocking retes consisting of a proliferation of bland and pigmented basaloid and squamous cells with formation of pseudo horn cysts

Sebborrhoeic keratosis

Definition
Seborrhoeic keratoses are benign hyperplastic tumours of epidermis which are more common in older individuals.

Synonyms
Seborrhoeic wart, senile wart, stucco keratosis, melanoacanthoma.

Epidemiology
Seborrhoeic keratoses are the most common of the cutaneous neoplasms and occur in the majority of elderly Caucasian patients. These lesions are by no means limited to Caucasians, but are present in numerous older individuals of any race. The lesions are unusual in children and even young adults are rarely affected. Identical histological features are seen in certain epidermal naevi.

There is no appreciable sex predilection. In part due to the very widespread incidence of the lesion, most cases are sporadic although several syndromes are associated with seborrhoeic keratosis. Recent studies support the long held belief that seborrhoeic keratosis is a clonal process in the skin {1679}.

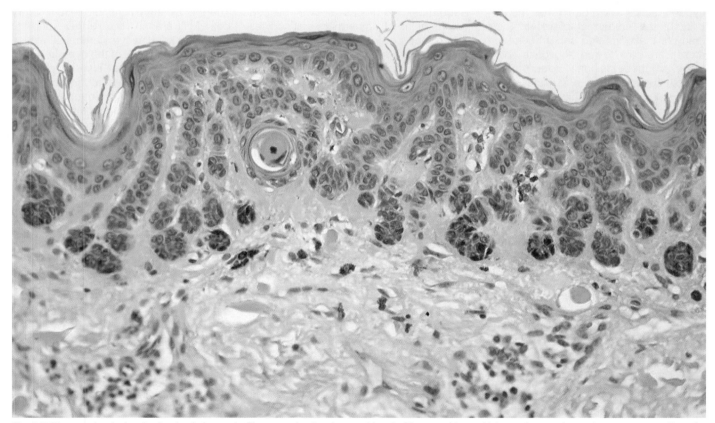

Fig. 1.40 Pigmented reticulated seborrhoeic keratosis. There are slender elongated interlocking rete ridges with hyperpigmentation and no squamous cell atypia, accompanied by focal pseudo horn cyst.

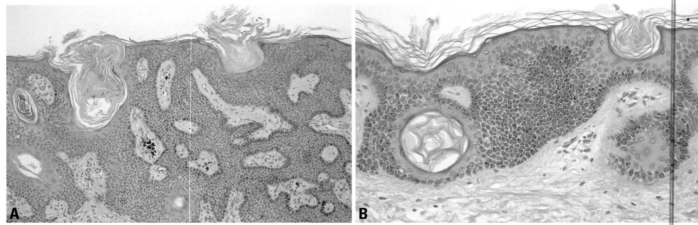

Fig. 1.41 Pigmented seborrhoeic keratosis. **A** and **B** There are elongated interlocking retes consisting of a proliferation of bland and pigmented basaloid and squamous cells with formation of pseudo horn cysts

Clinical features

Seborrhoeic keratoses are slightly raised, tan to brown or black papules. Sun-exposed skin is especially affected, but lesions may be present on any site of the skin except for palms or soles. They often have a "stuck on" appearance and may be easily removed. Irritated lesions often demonstrate a crust and prominent hyperkeratosis which diminishes the visibility of the epidermal pigment. Thus, many of these irritated seborrhoeic keratoses are pink to red and quite scaly. Many of these lesions appear more smooth-surfaced and are mistaken for basal cell carcinoma clinically.

While most seborrhoeic keratoses are uniform in colour, speckled examples are common. Pigmented seborrhoeic keratoses may be mistaken clinically for malignant melanoma. There is some correlation between the many described histological variants of seborrhoeic keratosis and the clinical appearance of the tumour.

Keratoses are generally very well circumscribed clinically. Usual lesions are oval in configuration, but linear or unusually shaped lesions are common.

Dermatosis papulosa nigra appears to be a form of multiple seborrhoeic keratoses of the face seen primarily in patients of African descent. This condition is not known to be associated with any type of internal malady {658}.

Leser-Trélat syndrome

This syndrome is the rapid onset of multiple pruritic seborrhoeic keratoses associated with malignancy. The tumours associated have primarily been of gastrointestinal origin, but lymphomas and leukaemias have also been reported. It should be emphasized that some authors dispute the syndrome entirely and favour a coincidental association due to the high frequency of seborrhoeic keratoses in elderly patients {955, 2110}.

Histopathology

Seborrhoeic keratoses are well-defined proliferations of epidermal keratinocytes which may be endophytic, exophytic or flat. There are seven major types of seborrhoeic keratosis:

Acanthotic (common) seborrhoeic keratosis

The acanthotic type is composed of broad columns or sheets of basaloid or squamoid cells with intervening horn cysts. There may be varying degrees of hyperkeratosis, papillomatosis and acanthosis.

Reticulated seborrhoeic keratosis

This common variant is often sampled histologically because clinical examples are frequently deeply pigmented. They form a net like or retiform pattern of acanthosis.

Pigmented seborrhoeic keratosis

Pimented seborrhoeic keratoses are in every way similar to usual seborrhoeic keratoses, but in addition demonstrate pronounced epidermal melanin pigment.

Clonal seborrhoeic keratosis

Clonal seborrhoeic keratosis is an unusual variant, which demonstrates whorled collections or nests of keratinocytes within the thickened epidermis. These foci of enlarged keratinocytes arranged in circular collections are suggestive of the epidermal collections seen in some cases of in situ squamous cell carcinoma, but lack the cytological atypia inherent in malignant neoplasms.

Irritated seborrhoeic keratosis

There is a heavy lichenoid inflammatory cell infiltrate in the upper dermis. Apoptotic keratinocytes are usually quite numerous. Features of the hyperkeratotic type (see below) may also be present. Sometimes there is a heavy inflammatory cell infiltrate, including neutrophils, which may not have lichenoid features. Squamous eddies are often present in the epidermis.

Hyperkeratotic seborrhoeic keratosis

This variant shows varying degrees of hyperkeratosis, papillomatosis and acanthosis. Some cases show inflammatory features similar to the irritated variant.

Flat seborrhoeic keratosis

There is mild hyperkeratosis, often mild basal pigmentation ('dirty feet') and only minimal acanthosis. There are no horn cysts. The cells contrast with those of the adjacent normal epidermis by being more compact.

Immunoprofile

All studies confirm the presence of keratins throughout the tumour. Some studies have also demonstrated the presence of carcinoembryonic antigen (CEA) {314,319,665}.

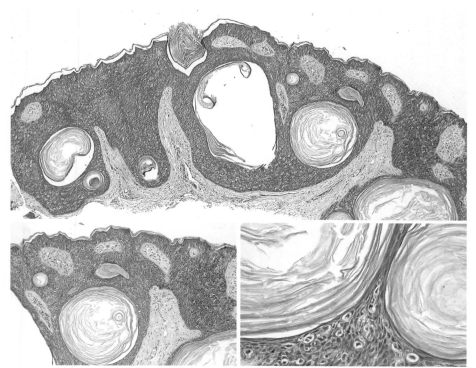

Fig. 1.42 Melanoacanthoma. There are elongated interlocking rete ridges consisting of a proliferation of bland basaloid and squamous cells with formation of pseudo horn cysts, intimately mixed with numerous melanocytes throughout the lesion.

Differential diagnosis

Dowling Degos disease has lesions indistinguishable from seborrhoeic keratosis except for their small size and the presence of a reticulated network of adjacent lesions.

The hyperkeratotic form may resemble a verruca vulgaris. Seborrhoeic keratoses lack parakeratotic columns overlying the digitate hyperkeratosis and there is no haemorrhage, dialated capillaries, koilocytosis or inward turning of the acanthotic downgrowths.

Precursor lesions

Some believe that the solar lentigo (lentigo senilis) is a precursor lesion of reticulated seborrhoeic keratosis. Others regard it as an early form of this lesion.

Prognosis and predictive factors

In a small number of cases Bowen disease coexists with seborrhoeic keratosis.

Melanoacanthoma

Definition

Melanoacanthoma of the skin is a benign mixed proliferation of keratinocytes and melanocytes. It is considered to be a variant of seborrhoeic keratosis.

Melanoacanthoma of the oral mucosa is an unrelated disorder.

Synonyms

Melanoacanthosis, deeply pigmented seborrhoeic keratosis.

Epidemiology

Most patients are adults beyond 40 years of age. Sex predominance is not known. There are no reliable frequency data.

Localization

Most melanoacanthomas are located on the trunk.

Clinical features

Clinically, the lesion resembles a darkly pigmented seborrhoeic keratosis. There are no characteristic symptoms. It may resemble a melanoma with dermatoscopy.

Histopathology

Melanoacanthoma has the same architecture as common seborrhoeic keratoses. However, they stand out by their abundant dendritic melanocytes in virtu-ally all layers of the lesion. The keratinocytes are rich in melanin granules.

Clear cell acanthoma

Definition

Clear cell acanthoma (CCA), is a benign epidermal neoplasm characterized by the presence of glycogen-rich clear/pale cells.

Synonyms

Degos acanthoma, pale cell acanthoma.

Localization

It is usually located on the lower extremities of middle-aged or elderly individuals. Other sites are the upper extremities, head and neck, trunk, buttocks and genital area.

Clinical features

It usually occurs as a solitary, slowly growing, dome-shaped papule, nodule or plaque. The lesion has sharp margins, sometimes with a keratotic scale, and a red or pink colour, giving the tumour a vascular appearance. Clinical variants include multiple, pigmented, giant, atypical, cystic and polypoid CCA {345}.

The clinical differential diagnosis may include pyogenic granuloma, irritated seborrhoeic keratosis, squamous and basal cell carcinoma, melanocytic naevus and nodular amelanotic melanoma.

Histopathology

There is a circumscribed, sharply demarcated epidermal proliferation with psoriasiform elongation of plump and interconnected rete ridges. The keratinocytes differ from those of the adjacent normal epidermis by their pale/clear cytoplasm containing a large amount of glycogen, best demonstrated with a periodic acid-Schiff reaction. The keratinocytes of the basal layer and the intraepidermal portion of the adnexae are not involved. Parakeratosis, infiltration of neutrophils, which may form a microabscess in the stratum corneum, and the absence of the granular layer are additional characteristic findings. Dilated capillaries and a scattered inflammatory infiltrate can be observed in the papillary dermis. The presence of melanophages in the papillary dermis and an increased number of melanocytes provide clues to the diagnosis of a pigmented CCA.

Histogenesis

The histogenesis of CCA is not yet completely clear. Initially considered a tumour of sweat gland or hair follicle origin, these sites were later excluded because of the different cytokeratin expression compared to CCA {1743}. Some investigators hypothesized that CCA is a benign epidermal tumour of unknown etiology, probably caused by a specific disturbance of keratinocyte differentiation. The expression of involucrin and epithelial membrane antigen further suggest that CCA is derived from surface epithelium. However, since CCA shows histopathologic findings and cytokeratin expression similar to those observed in psoriasis, others believe that it might represent an inflammatory disease rather than a neoplastic process {742}.

Large cell acanthoma

Definition

Large cell acanthoma, a benign lesion, is now considered to be a stage in the evolution of a solar lentigo to a reticulated seborrhoeic keratosis {1576,1959}. It was thought to represent a particular type of actinic keratosis {1875,2095}, Bowen disease {2038}, or a distinct entity {69,1871,2039}.

Epidemiology

Most patients are middle-aged to elderly persons. Sanchez Yus et al (1988) estimated that approximately 1-2.5 LCAs are diagnosed per 1000 skin biopsies whereas Scholl (1982) saw only 4 cases among > 1000 actinic keratoses and > 3200 seborrhoeic keratoses.

Etiology

Chronic sun exposure is the probable cause of LCA.

Localization

Most lesions tend to occur on the trunk and extremities.

Clinical features

The lesion resembles a solar lentigo, flat seborrhoeic keratosis or stucco keratosis. Most cases are lightly pigmented flat plaques or patches, usually less than 10 mm in diameter. Hyperkeratosis or even verrucous appearance has been described. In Black patients, LCA may present as darkly pigmented lesions

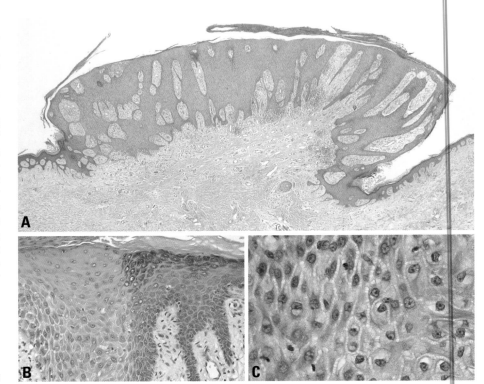

Fig. 1.43 Clear cell acanthoma. **A** There are well circumscribed interlocking columns of pale to clear keratinocytes with absent granular layer and no squamous cell atypia. **B** Note sharp demarcation between normal epidermis (right) and tumour (left). **C** High power view of tumour cells showing pale cytoplasm due to glycogen accumulation.

{2165}. Hypopigmentation is also seen {69}. Dermatoscopy may rule out melanoma.

Histopathology

Large cell acanthoma is a sharply delimited lesion standing out by its unique large keratinocytes that have about double the size both of their cytoplasm and nuclei compared to normal keratinocytes. Often, considerable numbers of melanocytes are present. Three variants have been described: a basic pattern with mild to moderate acanthosis, a verrucous pattern with papillomatosis and hyperkeratosis, and a flat-hyperkeratotic pattern {2039}. The granular layer is thick, there is usually orthohyperkeratosis and the rete ridges may be slightly bulbous.

The growth fraction is low {86,1576} although there is a considerable proportion of both aneuploid and hyperdiploid cells {86}.

Differential diagnosis

Flat seborrhoeic keratoses differ by the smaller size of the constituent cells. Solar keratoses show parakeratosis and greater nuclear pleomorphism.

Keratoacanthoma

Definition

Keratoacanthoma is a squamoproliferative tumour, mainly of hair-bearing skin. Although it has distinctive clinical and histological features, some regard it as a variant of squamous cell carcinoma {190,1701}.

ICD-O code   8071/1

Synonym

Well-differentiated squamous cell carcinoma (keratoacanthoma type).

Epidemiology

Most cases develop in older persons, particularly in the sixth and seventh decades. There is a male preponderance. Keratoacanthomas are more frequent in subtropical areas.

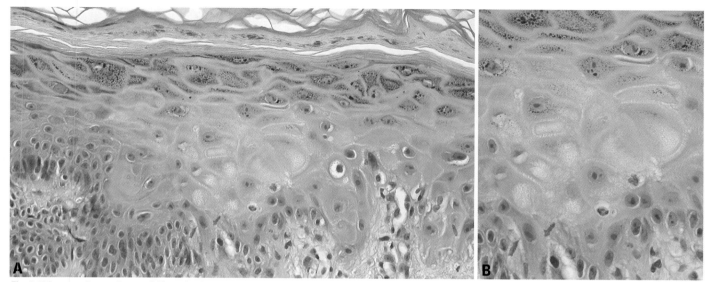

Fig. 1.44 Large cell acanthoma. A There is abrupt transition between normal epidermis (left) and large cell acanthoma (right). There is hyperkeratosis, hypergranulosis and markedly enlarged keratinocytes. B The tumour cells have enlarged nuclei without hyperchromasia and a low nuclear to cytoplasmic ratio.

Etiology

Exposure to excessive sunlight is the most frequently incriminated factor in their etiology. Viruses have also been implicated, particularly in immunosuppressed patients in whom DNA sequences of HPV have been detected in 20% of cases {2270}. Chemical carcinogens produce similar tumours in some animals, but their role in humans is speculative.

Localization

In temperate climates, up to 70% of lesions develop on the face. In subtropical areas, there is a much greater tendency for lesions to arise on the arms, dorsum of the hands and the lower extremities.

Clinical features

Keratoacanthomas are usually solitary,

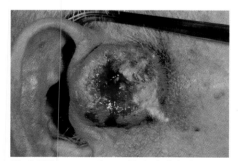

Fig. 1.45 Keratoacanthoma. Typical clinical appearance of exophytic tumour with central crateriform ulceration filled with keratin plug.

pink or flesh-coloured, dome-shaped nodules with a central keratin plug. They measure 1-2 cm in diameter. They tend to grow rapidly over 1-2 months with spontaneous involution after 3-6 months. Uncommonly, lesions persist for more than 12 months. Because local tissue destruction can occur during growth and involution, active treatment is usually advocated.

Several clinical variants occur:

Giant keratoacanthoma, a lesion greater than 2-3 cm in diameter.

Keratoacanthoma centrifugum marginatum, which undergoes progressive peripheral growth with coincident central healing {1740}.

Subungual keratoacanthoma, a destructive form that may produce pressure erosion of the distal phalanx. They usually fail to regress spontaneously {146}.

Multiple keratoacanthomas, which may be eruptive (Grzybowski type), self-healing (the Ferguson Smith type, which is autosomal dominant in inheritance and caused by an abnormality on chromosome 9q22-q31), and a mixed eruptive and self-healing type (Witten and Zak type).

Multiple lesions can also occur in immunosuppressed patients {625}, in the Muir-Torre syndrome (see below) and at sites of trauma {1789}.

Macroscopy

They are usually pale nodules with a central keratin plug.

Histopathology

Keratoacanthomas are exoendophytic, squamoproliferative nodules with a central, keratin plug. Fully developed lesions show lipping (buttressing) of the edges of the lesion which overlap the central keratin-filled crater, giving it a symmetrical appearance. Blunt downgrowths of squamous epithelium extend into the dermis with an irregular lower border to the tumour. The cells at the periphery of the squamous islands are basaloid in type. As they mature, they become large squamous cells with a distinctive pale eosinophilic cytoplasm. Mitoses may be seen, but atypical mitoses and stromal infiltration suggest a squamous cell carcinoma. SCCs are acknowledged to occur in less than 1% of keratoacanthomas found in subtropical regions. In one series, the reported incidence of a supervening squamous cell carcinoma was approximately one-quarter of all keratoacanthomas {2040}.

A mixed inflammatory cell infiltrate, often including eosinophils and neutrophils may be present in the stroma. Neutrophils may extend into the epithelial nests, producing small microabscesses. Hyperplasia of sweat duct epithelium may be present in some cases.

Perineural invasion is an incidental and infrequent finding, often in facial lesions. It does not usually affect the prognosis or behaviour of the lesions, although local recurrence has been reported in such cases. Several cases with intravenous

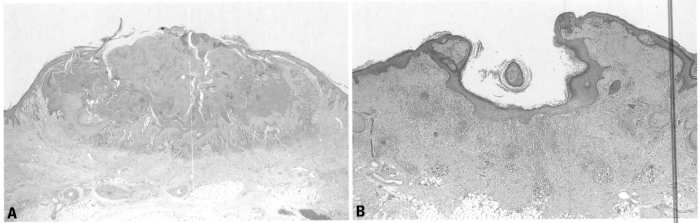

Fig. 1.46 A A low-power view of keratoacanthoma demonstrating a central crateriform lesion filled with a keratotic plug and flanked by epidermal buttresses and consisting of tongues and lobules of squamous cells pushing into the deep dermis. **B** Regressed keratoacanthoma. The crateriform architecture remains but the tumour cells are replaced by flattened epidermal keratinocytes, accompanied by dermal fibrous scarring, a lichenoid inflammatory infiltrate and focal foreign body giant cell reaction to keratin in the dermis.

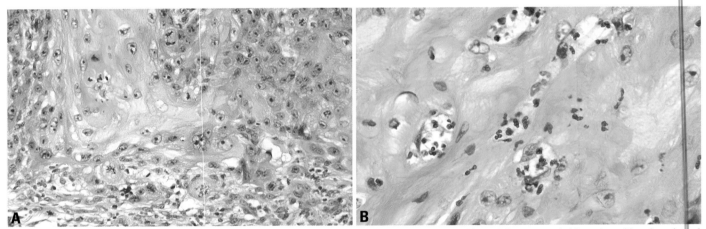

Fig. 1.47 Keratoacanthoma. **A** The tumour cells have abundant pale eosinophilic cytoplasm and pleomorphic nuclei, accompanied by a dermal lymphocytic and eosinophilic infiltrate. **B** Focal neutrophilic aggregates in tumour nests are characteristic of keratoacanthoma.

growth and a favourable outcome have been recorded {842}.

Regressing keratoacanthomas are shallower lesions with a large keratin plug and buttressing at the margins. There is progressive dermal fibrosis and disappearance of tumour nests in the dermis. Foreign body giant cells may be present around residual keratin fragments. (PCNA / MIB-1 labelled proliferating cells are found in the periphery of the squamous nests in keratoacanthoma, in contrast to a more diffuse pattern in squamous cell carcinoma. Expression of TP53 is found in both tumours. Subungual keratoacanthomas have characteristic dyskeratotic cells, some showing dystrophic calcification, towards the centre of the tumour nests. This variant has fewer neutrophils and eosinophils.

The differential diagnosis from squamous cell carcinoma may be difficult or impossible in superficial shave and punch biopsies. Features favouring keratoacanthoma include the flask-like configuration with a central keratin plug, the pattern of keratinization, the large central squamous cells, the lack of anaplasia and a sharp outline between tumour nests and the stroma {555,2477}.

Histogenesis

The great majority of keratoacanthomas develop on hair-bearing skin {474} and are presumed to be derived from follicular keratinocytes, perhaps with a programmed life span. Those rare tumours that arise on glabrous skin and mucous membranes presumably derive from epithelial keratinocytes.

Genetics

A genetic defect has been reported in patients with the Ferguson Smith type of "multiple self-healing epitheliomas" (keratoacanthomas). The Muir Torre syndrome, in which sebaceous tumours develop in association with visceral tumours, usually gastrointestinal cancers, and often with keratoacanthomas, epidermal cysts and colonic polyps, is inherited as an autosomal dominant trait. Mutations have been found in some cases in one of the DNA mismatch repair genes MLH1 and MSH2.

Prognosis and predictive factors

Most lesions regress spontaneously over several months {260}. This regression may, in part, be immunologically mediated {1782}. Even lesions with perineural and intravenous invasion have a favourable outcome. Keratoacanthomas can recur in up to 8% of cases. This is more likely with lesions on the fingers, hands, lips and ears. Trauma may be responsible for recurrent lesions in some cases. Rare cases that have developed metastasis have been reported {1038}. Possible explanations include misdiagnosis of the original lesion, the development of a supervening squamous cell carcinoma not recognized in the original material, genuine 'rogue' variants or transformation of the initial lesion into a squamous cell carcinoma in immunosuppressed patients {2476}.

Lichen planus-like keratosis

Definition
Lichen planus-like keratosis (LPLK) is a benign lesion of the skin that represents the attempted immunologic regression of a solar lentigo, seborrhoeic keratosis, large cell acanthoma or other epidermal proliferative lesion {1569,2150}.

Synonyms
Benign lichenoid keratosis.

Epidemiology
LPLK is a relatively common lesion. Most patients are middle-aged to elderly. There is a female predominance.

Etiology
The cause of the lesion is not exactly known. However, chronic sunlight exposure appears to be an important factor.

Localization
Most LPLKs are located on the upper trunk and upper extremities.

Clinical features
Clinically, LPLK presents as a flat, irregularly hyperkeratotic plaque with often irregular borders. It may be irregularly pigmented or pale in colour. The lesion resembles a basal cell carcinoma, Bowen disease, actinic keratosis or flat seborrhoeic keratosis. Itching and some pain may occur {1373}. Dermatoscopy can rule out melanocytic lesions.

Histopathology
LPLK is characterized by a lichenoid lymphocytic infiltrate leading to basal vacuolar change and numerous apoptotic cells. There is hypergranulosis and hyperkeratosis, frequently with parakeratotic foci. Actinic elastosis is often present {785}. Features of solar lentigo, large cell acanthoma or early seborrhoeic keratosis may be present at the margins. The inflammatory infiltrate often extends around the superficial vascular plexus.

Differential diagnosis
Lichenoid solar keratosis shows atypia of epidermal keratinocytes. In lichen planus, the inflammatory cells do not usually extend around the superficial vascular plexus. Furthermore parakeratosis, plasma cells and/or eosinophils may be present in LPLK. Similar changes may be seen in lichenoid drug eruptions. Clinical information may be required to separate these entities.

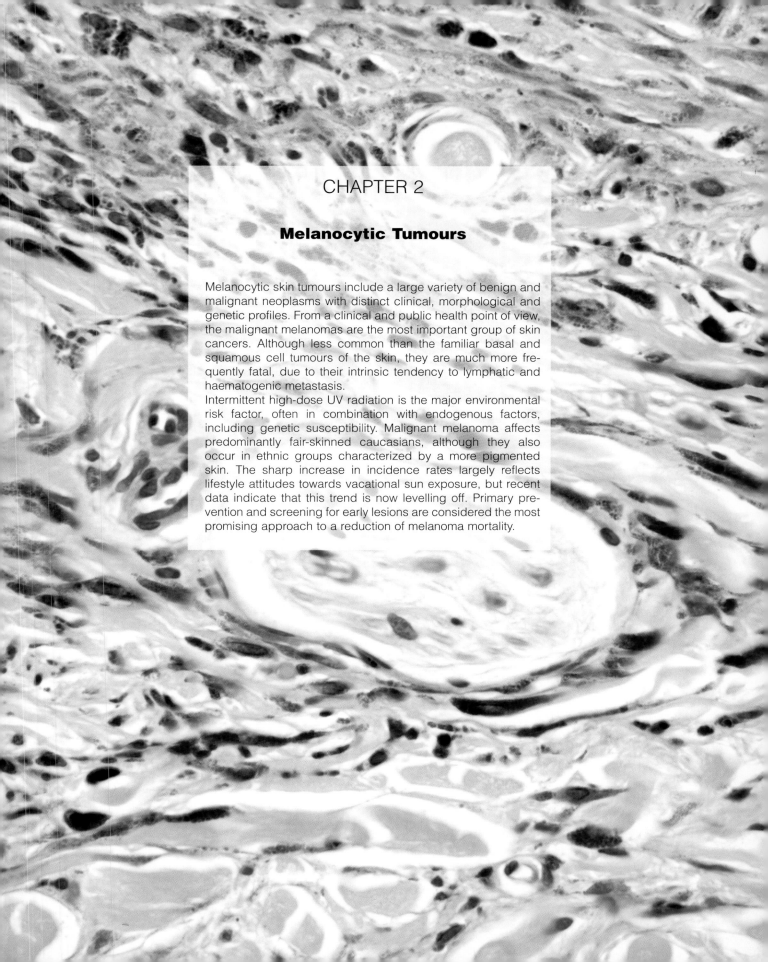

CHAPTER 2

Melanocytic Tumours

Melanocytic skin tumours include a large variety of benign and malignant neoplasms with distinct clinical, morphological and genetic profiles. From a clinical and public health point of view, the malignant melanomas are the most important group of skin cancers. Although less common than the familiar basal and squamous cell tumours of the skin, they are much more frequently fatal, due to their intrinsic tendency to lymphatic and haematogenic metastasis.

Intermittent high-dose UV radiation is the major environmental risk factor, often in combination with endogenous factors, including genetic susceptibility. Malignant melanoma affects predominantly fair-skinned caucasians, although they also occur in ethnic groups characterized by a more pigmented skin. The sharp increase in incidence rates largely reflects lifestyle attitudes towards vacational sun exposure, but recent data indicate that this trend is now levelling off. Primary prevention and screening for early lesions are considered the most promising approach to a reduction of melanoma mortality.

WHO histological classification of melanocytic tumours

Malignant melanoma	8720/3	Dermal melanocytic lesions	
Superficial spreading melanoma	8743/3	Mongolian spot	
Nodular melanoma	8721/3	Naevus of Ito and Ota	
Lentigo maligna	8742/2	Blue naevus	8780/0
Acral-lentiginous melanoma	8744/3	Cellular blue naevus	8790/0
Desmoplastic melanoma	8745/3	Combined naevus	
Melanoma arising from blue naevus	8780/3	Melanotic macules, simple lentigo and lentiginous naevus	
Melanoma arising in a giant congenital naevus	8761/3	Dysplastic naevus	8727/0
Melanoma of childhood		Site-specific naevi	
Naevoid melanoma	8720/3	Acral	
Persistent melanoma	8720/3	Genital	
		Meyerson naevus	
Benign melanocytic tumours		Persistent (recurrent) melanocytic naevus	
Congenital melanocytic naevi		Spitz naevus	8770/0
Superficial type	8761/0	Pigmented spindle cell naevus (Reed)	8770/0
Proliferative nodules in congenital melanocytic naevi	8762/1	Halo naevus	8723/0

---

[1] Morphology code of the International Classification of Diseases for Oncology (ICD-O) {786} and the Systematized Nomenclature of Medicine (http://snomed.org). Behaviour is coded /0 for benign tumours, /3 for malignant tumours, /2 for non-invasive tumours, and /1 for borderline or uncertain behaviour.

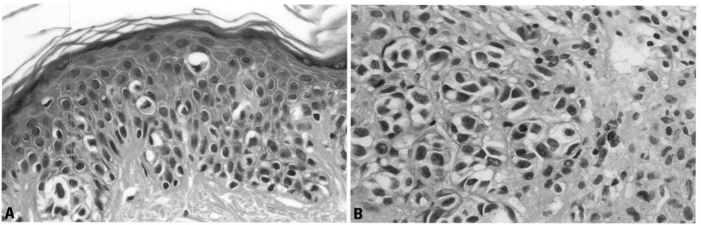

Fig. 2.14 Superficial spreading melanoma. **A** Single cells and small nests are irregualrly arranged along the junction. Toward the centre a large melanocyte is present in mid-spinous layer. A Langerhans cell is in nearly the same position toward the edge but is much smaller. **B** The invasive portion of the melanoma, showing nuclear pleomorphism. At the base there is a lymphocytic infiltrate.

other and may merge. There is often a lack of maturation, manifested by a failure of nests, cells, nuclei or nucleoli to become smaller towards the base of the lesion. Pigment is often irregularly distributed. Mitoses, sometimes atypical, are often seen whereas necrotic melanocytes are rarely identified. A lymphocytic infiltrate may be present at the base of the neoplasm or may infiltrate among its cells (so-called tumour infiltrating lymphocytes or TILS). Melanoma may undergo regression, which clinically and grossly most often involves a portion of the lesion, or occasionally its entirety. Histologically this regression may be complete or partial within a given area. Complete regression of a portion of a melanoma ("segmental regression") is manifested by absence of melanocytes in the affected area. In partial regression, there is a strikingly diminished number of melanocytes compared to the remainder

of the lesion. In both forms there is fibrosis of the papillary dermis, vascular proliferation and ectasia, and variably dense infiltrates of lymphocytes and melanophages. The epidermis may show loss of rete ridges. The type of regression described above affects the radial growth phase. Occasionally, a vertical growth phase may undergo regression, and sometimes the regressed portion may be replaced by a large mass of melanophages, representing a phenomenon called "tumoural melanosis".

Immunoprofile
There are no specific differences in the immunophenotype of SSM and other forms of melanoma.

Somatic genetics
SSM has a high incidence of mutations in the BRAF oncogene on chromosome 7q34 {1493}. The most common chromo-

somal aberrations in SSM are losses of chromosomes 9, 10, 6q, 8p and gains of chromosomes 1q, 6p, 7, 8q and 20 {173} Melanomas with increased copies of chromosome 7 that show mutations of B-raf selectively increase the copy number of the mutated allele suggesting that the mutation precedes the chromosomal aberration {1493} The minimal deleted region on chromosome 9 includes the CDKN2A locus on 9p21 as can be seen by high-resolution comparative genomic hybridization (CGH) {876}

Prognosis and predictive factors
The prognosis of SSM does not differ significantly from other forms of melanoma (see Introduction).

Nodular melanoma

R. Bergman
S. Brückner-Tuderman
J. Hercogova
B.C. Bastian

Definition
Nodular melanoma (NM) is a subtype of malignant melanoma (MM) exclusively in vertical growth phase.

ICD-O code   8721/3

Epidemiology
In most parts of the world, NM is the second most common subtype of MM, and accounts for 10 to 15% of all melanomas in Caucasian people {163,436}. NM appears on the average, in older individuals than the common superficial spreading MM (SSM) {436,493}.

Etiology
Most of the skin characteristics and risk factors associated with the development of NM are similar to those of SSM {1364}, including fair or red hair, blue eyes, fair skin, tendency to develop freckles and sunburns, excessive exposure to ultraviolet radiation, numerous common naevi, giant congenital naevi, atypical (dysplastic) naevi, melanoma in a first degree relative, familial atypical mole-melanoma syndrome, immunosuppression, xeroderma pigmentosum and prior melanoma {624,2304}.

Localization
NM may occur in any location, but as for SSM, it is more common on the trunk, head and neck, and lower legs {163}.

Clinical features
NMs typically present as a rapidly expanding papule, nodule or plaque. They are occasionally polypoidal and even pedunculated. They are usually well circumscribed and symmetric and frequently reach a size of approximately 1 cm before diagnosis. The skin markings are often obliterated with frequent ulceration and crust. The colour is often black or blue, although a subset of NM is amelanotic. The amelanotic variety frequently has a subtle blush or peripheral rim of pigment {163,436}.

Macroscopy
As in the clinical features.

Tumour spread and staging
The tumour spreads first to the local lymph nodes and then to internal organs. The staging system devised by the American Joint Committee on Cancer includes aspects of the primary tumour, the status of lymph nodes, and the presence and location of any metastases (TNM staging) {130}.

Histopathology
Scanning magnification discloses a raised, dome-shaped, or polypoid tumour, often, but not always, exhibiting some asymmetry. The overlying epidermis may be thin, effaced or ulcerated. Melanoma cells may be present in the overlying epidermis but not beyond the margins of the dermal component (some allow an extension up to 3 adjacent epidermal rete ridges beyond the dermal component). The dermal component is typified by a cohesive nodule or small nests of tumour cells that have a "pushing" or "expansile" pattern of growth. The tumour cells most frequently are epithelioid, but other cell types, including spindle cells, small epithelioid cells resembling naevus cells, and giant mononuclear or multinucleate forms, may predominate or be admixed with other cell types. The cell population usually appears monomorphous but closer examination reveals frequent cellular enlargement, nuclear enlargement, variation in nuclear size and shape, hyperchromatism, and prominent nucleoli.

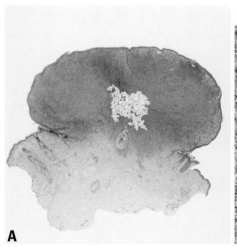
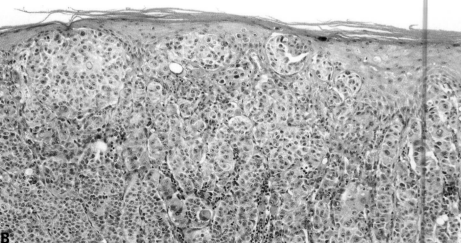

Fig. 2.15 Nodular melanoma. **A** On scanning magnification the tumour has a polypoid configuration with slight asymmetry. Cohesive nodules of tumour cells fill the dermis. **B** Superficial portion of the tumour. Epithelioid melanoma cells are present as single units and in nests that vary in size and shape along the dermoepidermal junction and above it. Similar nests are present in the upper dermis along with numerous melanophages and lymphocytic infiltrates. Some of the epithelioid melanoma cells contain fine melanin granules.

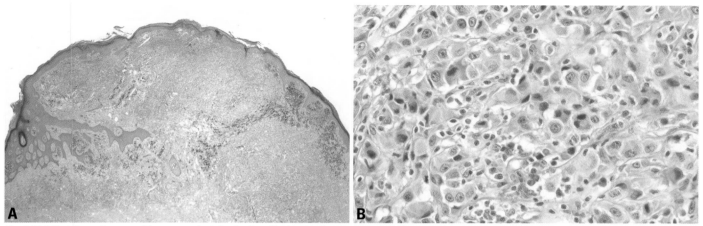

Fig. 2.16 A Nodular melanoma with asymmetrical distribution of lesional cells, lymphocytic infiltrates and melanophages. **B** The tumour is composed of melanocytes with large, pleomorphic, vesicular nuclei, some in mitosis.

High nuclear-to-cytoplasmic ratios are often noted. The tumour cells fail to "mature" with progressive descent into the dermis. The cytoplasm of the epithelioid cells often has eosinophilic granular qualities. It may contain melanin granules that vary in size, or appear fine and "dusty". There is absence of melanin in the amelanotic tumours. The surrounding stroma may demonstrate variable mononuclear cell infiltrates, fibroplasia, telangiectasia, and melanophages {154,163}.

Immunoprofile
S-100 protein, HMB-45, Melan A (MART-1), MAGE-1, NKI/C-3, tyrosinase, melanoma cell adhesion molecule (Mel-CAM) MUC18 and microphthalmia transcription factor (MITF), are expressed by most melanomas {732,1500,1855}. Melanoma cells also express bcl-2 protein, neuron specific enolase and vimentin {626,1861,2131}. Antigens which may demonstrate higher rates of expression in melanoma cells than in naevus cells include Ki-67 (MIB-1), proliferating nuclear antigen (PCNA), p53, cyclin D1, and p21 WAF1(9). The loss of expression of CDKN2A (cyclin dependant kinase inhibitor), and the increased expression of ß3 integrin, have been associated with vertical growth phase and more invasive forms of melanomas {1029,1500,1904,2277,2278,2406}.

Electron microscopy
The demonstration of stage II melanosomes is the hallmark of melanoma diagnosis. They are rarely found in other tumours. Other frequent findings are nuclear pseudoinclusions, prominent nucleoli and cytoplasmic intermediate filaments corresponding morphologically to vimentin filaments. In a minority of melanomas poorly developed intercellular junctions may be present {1016}.

Precursor lesions and histogenesis
It is more common for NM to begin de novo than to arise in a pre-existing naevus {163}. One hypothesis holds that NM represents a final common pathway of very rapid tumour progression from a brief intraepidermal proliferative phase of SSM, lentigo maligna, or acral lentiginous MM {154,163}.

Somatic genetics
Comparative genomic hybridization and mutation analyses have revealed marked differences between melanomas depending on the anatomic site and sun-exposure patterns {173,1493}. These studies did not find unique genetic features in nodular melanomas that justify regarding them as a unique type, supporting the 'common pathway' hypothesis {154,163}.

Genetic susceptibility
The proportion of melanomas that have a familial basis ranges from 6% to 14%. Approximately 20% of all individuals with a family history of melanoma have mutations in CDKN2A which maps to chromosome 9p21. In very few families CDK4 mapping to chromosome 12q14 has been found to be mutated {1851}.

Prognosis and predictive factors
In the T (tumour) category, tumour thickness increased mitotic rate and ulceration are the most powerful predictors of survival, and the level of invasion has a significant impact only within the subgroup of thin (≤1 mm) melanomas {131}. Other adverse prognostic factors include increased tumour vascularity, vascular invasion, microscopic satellites, male gender, increased age, and anatomic location on the head, neck and trunk {122,1528,2597}. In the N (nodes) category the following three independent factors have been identified: the number of metastatic nodes, whether nodal metastases were clinically occult or clinically apparent, and the presence or absence of primary tumour ulceration. In the M (metastases) category, nonvisceral metastases are associated with a better survival compared with visceral metastases {131}.

Lentigo maligna

P. Heenan
A. Spatz
R. Cerio
B.C. Bastian

Definition

Lentigo maligna (LM) is a form of melanoma in situ that occurs on the sun-exposed skin of elderly people, mainly on the face but also, less often, at extrafacial sites including the neck, upper back and forearm. It is characterized histologically by linear and nested proliferation of atypical melanocytes along the dermo-epidermal junction and down the walls of hair follicles and sweat ducts. The melanocytic lesion is associated with severe actinic damage, manifested by epidermal atrophy and solar elastosis. When dermal invasion by atypical melanocytes occurs in association with (LM), the term lentigo maligna melanoma (LMM) is used.

ICD-O code   8742/2

Synonyms and historical annotation

LM has also been known as Hutchinson melanotic freckle, after Hutchinson first

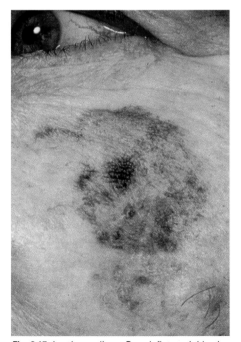

Fig. 2.17 Lentigo maligna. Broad, flat, variably pigmented lesion with a very irregular, ill-defined border on the cheek of a 78-year-old patient.

described it as "senile freckle" in 1892 {1090} and subsequently as "lentigo-melanosis" {1089}. Dubreuilh {652} described these lesions as "mélanose circonscrite précancéreuse" which subsequently came into common use as melanosis circumscripta precancerosa until the classification of Clark {492} in 1967 introduced the category of melanoma commencing in lentigo maligna (Hutchinson's melanotic freckle). That classification was widely but not universally accepted; the World Health Organization (WHO) classification of 1974 classified superficial spreading melanoma and melanoma arising in Hutchinson melanotic freckle (lentigo maligna melanoma) in one category {2337}. The World Health Organization (WHO) classification of 1996 separated melanoma in-situ into superficial spreading or pagetoid type and lentigo maligna melanoma, whilst acknowledging that there may be no essential biological difference between some or perhaps all categories of melanoma {999}.

Etiology

The strong association between LM and its occurrence in the severely sun-damaged skin of elderly people has been widely accepted as evidence that LM and LMM represent a distinctive form of melanoma, resembling etiologically the non-melanocytic skin cancers, and suggesting that LM arises in response to accumulated sun exposure, in contrast with the more common forms of melanoma that appear to be related to intermittent sun exposure {1048}. It has also been suggested, however, that differences in body site distribution between the commonly accepted different types of melanoma, through their interaction with amount and pattern of sun exposure, can explain virtually all the observed pathological and epidemiological differences between LM and the more common types of melanoma that occur in widespread anatomical distribution {16,996}. Recent studies have found that LM remains the main histologic type

of melanoma in situ on the head and neck and that patients with LM are less likely than patients with melanomas of the trunk to have more than 60 naevi whereas they had a stronger association with the number of solar keratoses {2508}.

Pathogenesis

According to some authorities, the term LM encompasses a phase regarded as a melanoma precursor in which there is proliferation of melanocytes in severely sun damaged skin in intermittent pattern without the confluent growth, pagetoid spread and nesting of atypical melanocytes that, according to this concept, represent malignant melanoma in-situ of LM type, whereas the lesions with less severe, intermittent junctional proliferation are termed atypical melanocytic hyperplasia {759} or, preferably, atypical lentiginous melanocytic proliferation.

Localization

Head and neck are by far the most common sites in both sexes. Extrafacial LMM differs in its site distribution between women and men {549}. A study in Scotland showed that extrafacial LMM in men occurred mainly on the trunk whereas in women 80% occurred on the limbs, mainly the lower leg. The mean age of patients with extrafacial LMM was significantly lower than that of patients with head and neck LM, suggesting that the association between LMM and sunlight may not be related only to the cumulative effects of solar exposure.

Clinical features

LM may be recognized as a small lesion, usually as a mottled light brown macule with irregular margins on the face of a fair skinned elderly patient with evidence of severe solar skin damage, only a few millimetres in diameter, but usually greater than 10 mm. The classical lesions are broad, flat zones of varied pigmentation with an irregular border. With increasing size of the lesion, variation in pigment and irregularity of the border also become more pronounced, nodules may develop within the lesion and the borders may become difficult or impossible to define where zones of pallor or mottled pigmentation merge imperceptibly with the surrounding skin.

Histopathology

LM is characterized by a predominantly junctional proliferation of atypical melanocytes, frequently extending down the walls of hair follicles and sweat ducts, in association with epidermal atrophy and severe solar elastosis. Although the junctional proliferation may form a confluent linear pattern in some areas, elsewhere the atypical melanocytes may be distributed as single units separated by basal cells. Irregular junctional nests of atypical melanocytes are frequently present, as are multinucleate giant cells including those of starburst type {512}. Marked pleomorphism is a feature of the atypical melanocytes which show cytoplasmic retraction artefact and nuclei of stellate, ovoid and crescentic forms, some of them pressed against the cell wall, with a variable chromatin pattern and clear or variably pigmented cytoplasm. Pagetoid foci of atypical epithelioid melanocytes present an appearance indistinguishable from melanoma in situ of so-called superficial spreading type.

A lymphocytic infiltrate and focal fibroplasia are frequently present in the papillary dermis underlying LM, with severe solar elastosis and telangiectasia. Regression, shown by fibrosis, hypervascularity, melanophages and a patchy lymphocytic infiltrate, is a common feature and should prompt a careful search for invasion by atypical melanocytes. The presence of regression at a lateral margin of excision should be emphasized in the report as an indication for re-excision, even when the margins appear clear of atypical melanocytes.

In LMM, dermal invasion occurs in association with LM. The invasive component may consist of atypical melanocytic spindle cells more frequently than is seen in the other common forms of cutaneous melanoma, but epithelioid, small naevoid and tumour giant cells may also be present in varied proportions. The cells of these various types may occur in cohesive groups, strands or as single cells in a diffuse pattern, often associated with lymphocytes and melanophages. The

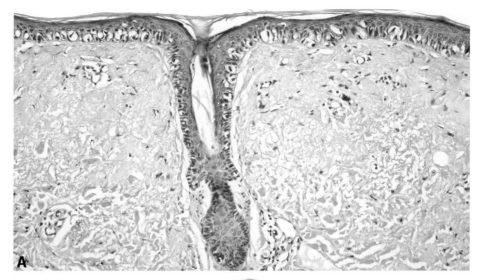

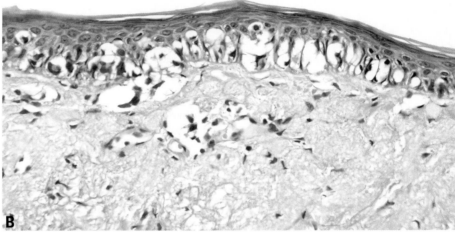

Fig. 2.18 Lentigo maligna. **A** Atypical melanocytes, mainly epithelioid cells with clear cytoplasm, are arranged in confluent pattern along the dermo-epidermal junction and extending down the wall of a central hair follicle. A few single atypical melanocytes are also present above the basal layer. The epidermis is atrophic overlying severe elastosis. **B** Severe nuclear pleomorphism and scattered multinucleate giant cells are present in the junctional proliferation and down the walls of adnexal structures including a sweat duct.

degree of pigmentation varies, including cells with abundant clear cytoplasm adjacent to cells in which the morphologic detail may be obscured by coarse melanin granules.

The invasive component in LMM may be desmoplastic and/or neurotropic with very subtle, diffuse invasion that predisposes to incomplete excision and true local recurrence. Dermal invasion may also originate from atypical melanocytes in the walls of hair follicles and sweat ducts, thus creating a problem in measurement of tumour thickness because it is inappropriate to measure tumour thickness from the granular layer of the epidermis in this instance.

The degree of pigmentation in LM may vary markedly between different examples of the tumour and within one tumour. Zones of amelanosis at the periphery of the lesion may lead to failure by the pathologist to detect atypical cells at the margin of excision, thus leading to persistent growth and "local recurrence" of the tumour.

Differential diagnosis

In cases of extensive amelanosis (amelanotic LM) {60}, the distinction between in-situ squamous cell carcinoma or extra-mammary Paget disease may be difficult in routine sections, necessitating the use of special stains to demonstrate epithe-

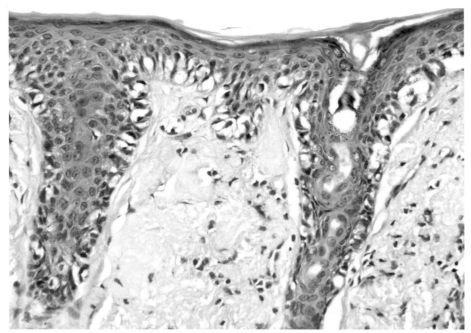

Fig. 2.19 Lentigo maligna. Focal pagetoid growth is present in addition to junctional proliferation including small nests of atypical melanocytes.

lial mucin in extra-mammary Paget disease, and immunostaining, including the use of antibodies to cytokeratins, melan-A and S-100 protein and, as further aids to the diagnosis of Paget disease, carcinoembryonic antigen, and BerEP4.

The distinction between LM and benign forms of junctional melanocytic proliferation is made on the basis of the characteristic cytologic atypia, confluent growth of atypical cells along the junction with frequent extension down the walls of adnexal structures and, commonly, extension of growth above the basal layer in pagetoid pattern.

Histogenesis

LM develops from epidermal melanocytes, most likely due to the cumulative DNA damage resulting from long-term sun exposure {1048}. A recent study of the differential expression of proliferation- and apoptosis-related markers in lentigo maligna and the keratinocytes in solar keratosis has found that the epidermis in LM shows overall low proliferation and a low apoptotic tendency, perhaps aiding aberrant melanocyte proliferation in the early stages of melanoma development {718}.

Somatic genetics

A recent study has shown an association between DNA repair-deficiency and a high level of *TP53* mutations in melanomas of xeroderma pigmentosum patients {2231}. The LMM found in xeroderma pigmentosum patients of the XP complementation group, group XP-C, were associated with an accumulation of unrepaired DNA lesions. Lentigo maligna melanomas have been found to rarely show mutations in BRAF {1493}. Comparative genomic hybridization shows more common losses involving chromosome 13 and less common losses of chromosome 10, when compared to other melanoma types {173}.

Prognosis and predictive factors

Complete excision of lentigo maligna, as a form of melanoma in situ and, therefore, incapable of metastasis, is curative. Prognosis for LMM has been a contentious issue. For many years, it was commonly believed that the prognosis for melanomas of LMM type is better than for other types of melanoma. Most evidence, however, suggests that for melanomas classified as different types according to their histological features, their differences in survival correspond to differences in tumour thickness rather than to their differences in histologic type {20,1296}.

Acral-lentiginous melanoma

Y. Tokura
B.C. Bastian
L. Duncan

Definition

Acral-lentiginous melanoma (ALM) is a distinct variant of cutaneous melanoma, which occurs on the palms, soles, and subungual sites, and has a characteristic histologic picture. Following the three other major clinicopathological subtypes of melanoma, i.e. superficial spreading melanoma, lentigo maligna melanoma, and nodular melanoma, ALM was proposed as the fourth subtype by Reed in 1976 {1905}. In this article, we also use the term acral melanoma and define it as a melanoma located on the non-hair bearing skin of the palms and soles or under the nails. The reason for this usage is described below.

ICD-O code   8744/3

Synonyms

Historically, this type of melanoma has been designated as ALM {1905}, acral melanoma {494}, palmar-plantar-subungal-mucosal melanoma (P-S-M melanoma) {2129}, or unclassified plantar melanoma {100}. Although often considered to be interchangeable, ALM and acral melanoma embody distinct concepts that must be distinguished from each other. ALM is a histologic designation that shows similarities to lentigo maligna melanoma, while acral melanoma is an anatomic designation that refers to melanoma located on the acral sites. Acral melanoma, thus, encompasses both ALM and such subtypes as superficial spreading melanoma and nodular melanoma that may develop in acral locations. Occasionally, the terms acral melanoma and acral lentiginous melanoma are used interchangeably, since the majority of cases of acral melanoma are ALM {1071,1592,1905} and the histological distinction between ALM and superficial spreading melanoma is not always possible {2220}. Even if acral melanoma is an anatomic nomenclature, its use is different among articles. We define it as a melanoma located on the non-hair bearing skin of the palms and soles or under the nails because of presentation of the genetic data. Although P-S-M melanoma was described on the basis of clinical and histologic similarities between the tumours on these sites, the acral melanomas and mucosal ones are recommended to be treated separately, because of their different clinical behaviours {494}.

Epidemiology

Racial differences are quite pronounced in the incidence and predilection sites of melanomas. This is particularly true for acral melanoma wherein acral melanoma comprises 2% and 80% of cutaneous melanomas in Caucasian and dark-skinned patients respectively. In a German study approximately 7% of patients with cutaneous melanoma had

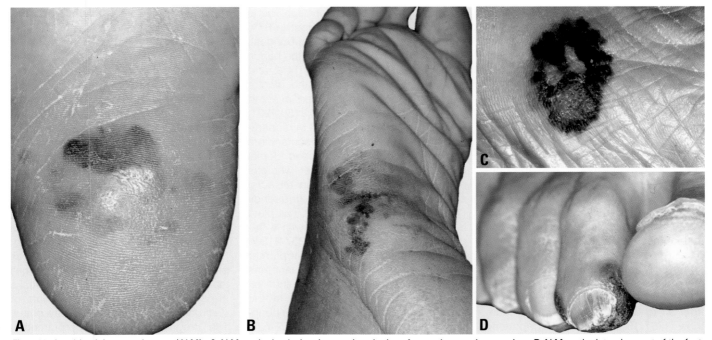

Fig. 2.20 Acral-lentiginous melanoma (ALM). **A** ALM on the heel, showing varying shades of tan to brown pigmentation. **B** ALM on the lateral aspect of the foot, showing irregularly bordered pigmentation with a slightly ulcerated lesion. **C** ALM on the sole, showing an irregularly pigmented macule with notched borders. **D** ALM on the second toe, showing subungual pigmented lesion extending to adjacent skin.

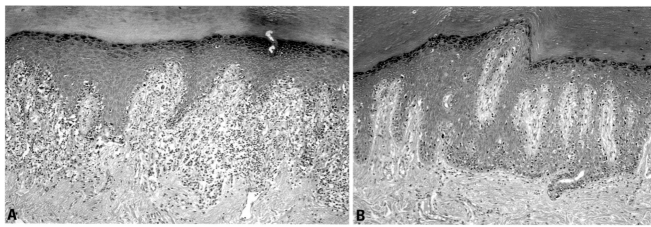

Fig. 2.21 Acral-lentiginous melanoma. **A** ALM, showing marked acanthosis, elongation of the rete ridges, broadened horny layer, and large, atypical melanocytes with large, often bizarre nuclei and nucleoli, and cytoplasm filled with melanin granules. **B** ALM, showing lentiginous proliferation of atypical melanocytes at the border of the tumour.

tumours located on acral sites {1337}. Whereas 77% of cutaneous melanoma in Japanese patients occurs on acral sites {2130}. In African and African-Americans, the highest incidence of cutaneous melanoma has been reported on relatively non-pigmented areas, such as the soles, nail plates, and mucous membranes {1417}. Thus, ALM is the most common type of melanoma in dark-skinned peoples and Asians {1268, 2129}. Nevertheless the absolute incidence of acral melanoma in dark-skinned African and light-skinned Caucasian populations in North America is similar, suggesting that the observed racial difference may relate to a decreased incidence of non-acral melanoma in African American populations {2268}. Compared with the escalating incidence that typifies other melanoma subtypes, the incidence of ALM has remained static {661}.

Overall, ALM occurs in an older patient population than does superficial spreading or nodular melanoma, and, in populations where ALM is common, this tumour more often afflicts men than women. Overall, the age distribution of ALM is similar to that of lentigo maligna melanoma, peaking in the seventh decade of life, whereas superficial spreading melanoma and nodular melanoma peak in the sixth decade {1337}. The mean age of ALM ranges from 55 to 68 years in European countries {767,1337,2123}. In Japanese patients, there is a peak in the sixth decade in both males and females. In Japan, Korea, and Taiwan, men are

affected twice as often as women {1220, 1268,1428,2130}. On the other hand in western countries, there is less of a male predominance in patients with ALM {1337,2220}.

Localization

The term acral has been used differently throughout the literature. Most publications use acral for the non-hair bearing, i.e. glabrous skin of the palms and soles, and the nail bed, whereas others also include the dorsal aspect of the hands and feet under this term. In a German study, using the latter definition, acral melanoma occurred on the feet in 87% cases (plantar sites, 57%; subungual, 5%; and dorsum, 9%) and on the hands in 23% (palm, 1%; subungal, 14%; and dorsum, 9%) {1337}. Thus, the plantar sites were greatly more often affected than the palmar sites {1337,2130,2201, 2220,2296}. In contrast to ALM, superficial spreading melanoma occurs more commonly on the sun-exposed dorsal aspects of the hands and feet, whereas nodular melanoma occurs on all acral sites with relatively equal frequency {1337}. In addition to the sole, nail plate is an especially frequent site with a frequency of 16-19% in ALM {1337,2130}. In contrast to the palmar/plantar melanomas, subungual melanomas occur more often on the hands than on the feet {745,1221,2130,2315}. In the Japanese series, the number of subungual melanomas on the fingers is 62-72% and on the toes 28-38%, with an 82% incidence on the thumbs and great toes {1221,2130}. The high percentage of

occurrence on the thumbs and great toes may suggest a role for trauma in the etiology of subungual melanoma {2130}. Since sun exposure obviously plays little role in palmoplantar sites, the causative role of ultraviolet light is presumed to be negligible in ALM.

Clinical features

Acral melanomas in the early stages appear as a pigmented macule similar to lentigo maligna. Acral melanomas commonly exhibit clinical evidence of a biphasic growth pattern, with a more rapid evolution from an entirely flat clinical lesion to a lesion containing an elevated focus than is observed in the other types of melanoma. The radial growth phase of ALM is characterized by a macular pigmented lesion with highly irregular, notched borders and varying shades of pigmentation. Within a background pigmented macule, acral melanomas often develop a clinically apparent vertical growth phase. This is manifest as an elevated papule or nodule, sometimes with a verrucous surface, and corresponds to the histological vertical growth phase of malignant melanocytes. Ulceration is more often seen in ALM than in other types of melanoma.

Subungual melanomas often begin as brown to black discolouration of the nail that frequently become bands or streaks of pigmentation. Thickening, splitting, or destruction of the nail plate may occur. The irregular macular hyperpigmentation, coloured tan to dark brown, is also recognized around the nail plate {2130}. In one study, 17% of the patients noticed the pre-existence of some pigmented skin lesions, and 21% related a history of trauma {2130}. Pigmented streaks are not uncommon in patients with deeply pigmented skin, nevertheless, a history of a new or recently changing pigmented lesion should prompt the consideration of a biopsy for histological evaluation of the lesion. In this case, reflection of the proximal nail fold to enable biopsy of the nail bed may be necessary for definitive diagnosis.

Unfortunately, clinical misdiagnosis is not uncommon in patients with ALM {409, 767,1327,1592,2222}. Therefore, awareness of atypical presentations of ALM that may contribute to misdiagnosis or diagnostic delay assumes particular importance. ALM lesions are frequently treated or followed for considerable time under the clinical diagnosis of wart, callus, fungal disorder, subungual haematoma, keratoacanthoma, nonhealing ulcer, foreign body, naevus, ingrown toenail, etc {2222}.

Histopathology

The histology of ALM is characteristic but not distinct. In the radial growth phase, the lesions are characterized by marked acanthosis, expanded cornified layer, elongation of the rete ridges, and lentiginous proliferation of atypical melanocytes along the basal epidermis at the border of the tumour {1337,1767}. The intraepidermal component of acral melanoma includes large, atypical melanocytes with large, often bizarre nuclei and nucleoli, and cytoplasm filled with melanin granules {2130}. These melanocytes in the basal layer often exhibit long, elaborate dendritic processes {2130}.

Atypical melanocytes can extend along the sweat ducts into the deep dermis.

In the vertical growth phase, tumour nodules often contain predominantly spindle-shaped cells and are associated with a desmoplastic reaction {2130}. The junctional component of thicker tumours often shows nesting of tumour cells and upward migration to the cornified layer {1337}.

Immunoprofile

As in the other types of melanomas, immunohistochemical stainings for S-100 protein, HMB-45, and MART-1 (also known as Melan-A) are of great diagnostic value in ALM. S-100 protein (positive cases, 95%) is a more sensitive marker than either HMB-45 (80%) or MART-1 (70%) {1268}. However, S-100 protein-negative ALM has been reported {83}. The intensity of HMB-45 but not of S-100 protein is correlated well with the melanin content. HMB-45-negative cases are all amelanotic, but amelanotic cases are not all negative for HMB-45 {1268}. The melanoma cells also express vimentin {1268}. Focal staining for CAM5.2 or epithelial membrane protein may occasionally be found {1268}.

Somatic genetics

Comparative genomic hybridization (CGH) of melanomas on acral non-hair bearing skin showed distinct differences to melanomas on non-acral skin {171}. A study of 15 acral melanomas and 15 superficial spreading melanomas from non-acral sites showed that all (100%) acral cases had gene amplifications, whereas amplifications were found in two of the superficial spreading melanomas (13%). The most common amplified region is chromosome 11q13 which occurred in 50% of these types of melanoma. A recent study has shown that cyclin D1 is one of several candidate genes in this region. This conclusion was based on the observation that amplification of the cyclin D1 gene was always accompanied with overexpression of the cyclin D1 protein, and that inhibition of cyclin D1 expression in vitro and in xenograft models led to apoptosis or tumour shrinkage {2072}.

FISH studies on primary lesions of acral melanoma showed that the amplifications arise early in acral melanoma and can already be detected at the in situ stage {171}. The *in situ* portion of acral melanoma may extend beyond what is recognizable histopathologically. FISH detected gene amplifications were identified in single basal melanocytes immediately adjacent to the in situ component of acral melanoma; they were equidistantly spaced and looked histopathologically inconspicuous {171}. Based on the observation that these "field cells" were found at the histopathologically uninvolved excision margins of an acral melanoma that recurred multiple times the authors propose that field cells may be a form of minimal residual melanoma that leads to persistence if not removed. More recent studies using array CGH have confirmed the frequent gene ampli-

fications in acral melanoma preferentially involving chromosome 11q13. In addition, the studies revealed that all melanomas showed these features, independent of their histological growth pattern, as long as they were located on glabrous, i.e. non-hair bearing skin of the palms and soles or subungual sites (Bastian et al, to be published). In addition, melanomas involving these anatomic sites also had a significantly lower mutation rate of the BRAF oncogene (6/39, 15%) than melanomas on the trunk (23/43, 53%) {1493}. The molecular genetic analyses therefore suggest that melanomas of the palms of soles and subungual sites represent a genetically distinct form of melanoma, independent of their histological growth pattern.

Prognosis and predictive factors

In general, the prognosis of invasive acral melanoma is poor. This can partly be explained by the above described diagnostic delay and increased tumour thickness at the time of diagnosis. However, there are some studies suggesting that acral melanomas may undergo a more aggressive course independent of tumours thickness {151,308, 661,1337}. In a study from Germany, 63 out of 64 patients (98.5%) with melanoma of the sole subsequently developed metastases {775}; a corresponding figure from Japan in 1983 was 35% {2130}. The same hospital recorded that the 5-year survival rate of subungal melanoma increased from 53% in 1969-82 to 83% in 1983-93 {1221}, presumably because of early awareness of lesions and development of treatment {2012}. However, others have reported that ALM is not a significant prognostic indicator {661,2201}, and adjustment for histologic and clinical stage renders the prognostic importance of anatomic location insignificant {151, 308}. These conflicting results can in part be explained by the different definitions used for acral melanomas in the studies. Future studies using refined criteria including genetic information are necessary to assess the prognosis of this melanoma type.

Desmoplastic melanoma and desmoplastic neurotropic melanoma

S.W. McCarthy
K.A. Crotty
R.A. Scolyer

Definition

Desmoplastic melanoma (DM) is a spindle cell melanoma in which the malignant cells are separated by collagen fibres or fibrous stroma. It displays variable cytological atypia, cellularity and stromal fibrosis and more often than not has an accompanying junctional component. Neurotropism is a common associated feature (in at least 30% of cases) and when it occurs such tumours are termed desmoplastic neurotropic melanomas (DNM). The neurotropism may be perineural or intraneural and often extends beyond the desmoplastic component. DM may also present as a recurrence or occasionally as a metastasis from other types of melanoma.

ICD-O code   8745/3

Historical annotations

DM was first described by Conley et al. in 1971 {526} as a clinically inconspicuous superficial melanocytic lesion, mainly on the head and neck, with an atypical junctional component, preceding the development of a bulky dermal and subcutaneous tumour. The latter was composed of atypical melanocytes and spindle cells often with elongated nuclei and a dense collagenous ground substance. Many others subsequently highlighted the frequent neurotropism of DMs.

Epidemiology

Desmoplastic melanomas represent between 1-4% of melanomas. In a large series from the Sydney Melanoma Unit

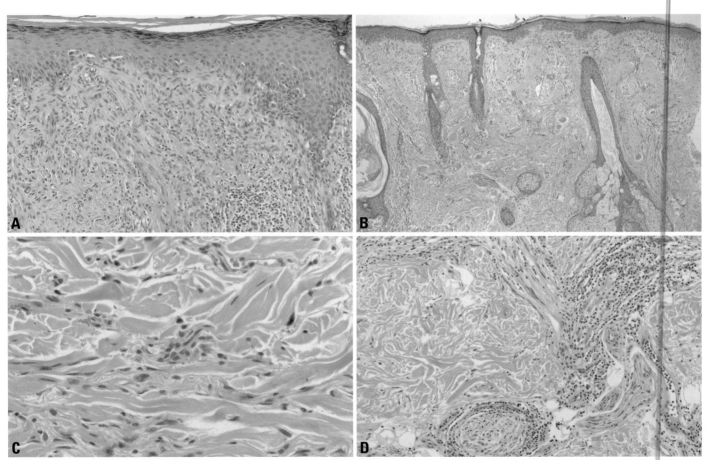

Fig. 2.22 Desmoplastic neurotropic melanoma. **A** Male, 73 yrs, cheek. A few atypical enlarged melanocytes are present in the junctional zone. The fibrohistiocytic pattern is accompanied by scattered lymphocytes, some in clusters. Mitoses are hard to find. **B** Female, 24 yrs, lip. There are "neural transforming" areas with thick neuroid bundles in the upper dermis. Note occasional atypical junctional melanocytes, a few subepidermal spindle cells and scattered lymphocytes. **C** Male, 73 yrs, cheek. Malignant spindle cells with elongated nuclei appear to be within and between collagen bundles. **D** Female, 24 yrs, lip. "Neural transforming" areas with neuroid bundle (top of picture) containing atypical elongated spindle nuclei. Intraneural and perineural involvement of a small nerve is also present. There is a prominent infiltrate of lymphocytes.

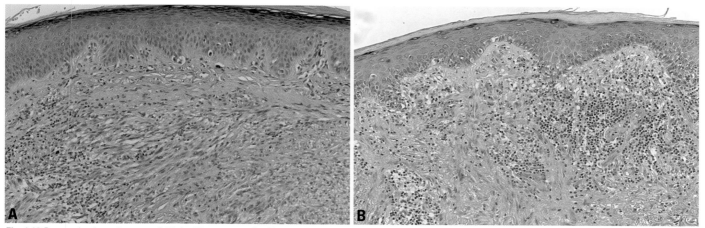

Fig. 2.23 Desmoplastic melanoma. **A** Male, 57 yrs, upper lip. Abnormal junctional melanocytes, spindling dermal melanocytes and a patchy lymphocytic infiltrate. **B** Female, 76 yrs, forearm. Abnormal junctional melanocytes and dermal spindle cells with patchy lymphocytes.

(SMU) the median age at diagnosis was 61.5 years (range 24-91) {1867,1868}. As in other histogenetic types of melanoma, males are more often affected (M:F = 1.75:1) {358A,1867,1868}.

Etiology
The etiology is unknown, but the majority occurs in sun-exposed skin. Some have occurred in irradiated areas {1125}.

Localization
DM may be found in many sites but most commonly involves the head and neck region (37%), including ear, nose and lip {1077}. Males predominate except on the lower limbs. The vulva is a rare site for DM {1664}.

Clinical features
Most present as a painless indurated plaque but some begin as a small papule or nodule {2501}. Almost half lack pigmentation {1867}. Pale lesions are often mistaken for basal cell carcinoma, dermatofibroma or a scar. Pigment is usually due to an associated lentigo maligna

(LM)/Hutchinson melanotic freckle (HMF) or superficial spreading melanoma.
Unusual presentations include a young age {439,1077}, an erythematous nodule {1326} and alopecia {563}.

Macroscopy
Ulceration is uncommon although it was found in 17% of the SMU cases {1868}.

Tumour spread and staging
The tumours usually infiltrate deeply into the reticular dermis but local spread may involve subcutaneous tissue, deep fascia including periosteum and pericranium, bone and salivary gland. Neurotropic foci may be found well beyond the main tumour. In the SMU series, neurotropism was found only in tumours exceeding 1.5 mm in thickness and Clark level 4 or 5 {1867,1868}. Initial metastases from DM may involve regional lymph nodes or distant sites.

Histopathology
In DM the spindle-shaped melanocytes, which often resemble fibroblasts and are

usually non-pigmented, are found in and between mature collagen bundles. The latter may be thickened and/or associated with a mild to marked stromal fibrosis. The distribution of spindle cells is usually haphazard but occasionally they form parallel bundles or storiform areas. The spindle cells often extend into the subcutis diffusely or in fibrous bands and may involve deep fascia, especially pericranium. The overlying epidermis may be thinned or thickened. Characteristically there are accompanying small islands of lymphocytes and plasma cells within and/or at the edge of the tumour. The cytological atypia of the spindle cells usually varies from mild to moderate. However, even in cases with mild atypia, there are usually a few larger or more elongated hyperchromatic nuclei. The cytoplasm of the spindle cells is often poorly defined. In examples where the spindle cells are small, well scattered and associated with solar elastosis, the lymphoid islands may be the main clue to the diagnosis. Paucicellular variants are easily missed on punch and shave biop-

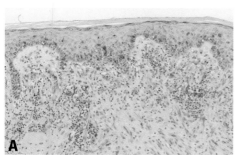
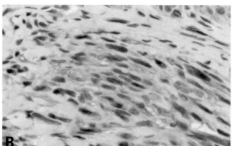
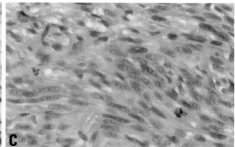

Fig. 2.24 Desmoplastic melanoma. **A** The spindle cells stain poorly with S100 unlike the Langerhans cells and interdigitating cells. **B** Variable S-100 positive nuclear and cytoplasmic staining. **C** Crowded abnormal spindle cells and atypical mitoses.

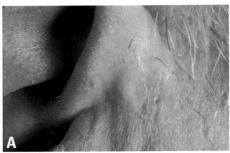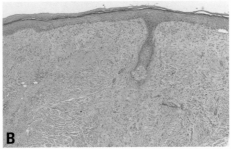

Fig. 2.25 Desmoplastic melanoma. **A** Firm, skin-coloured plaque. **B** Male, 68 yrs, scalp. This punch biopsy was initially diagnosed as a scar. Only an occasional spindle cell was S-100 positive and no abnormal junctional melanocytes were found. A larger desmoplastic melanoma was removed from the same site 6 months later. Clues to the diagnosis are the small foci of lymphocytes and permeation of the band of dermal elastosis by spindle cells.

sies. Junctional change is sometimes minimal or absent {1125}. Occasionally there is an associated banal naevus. Vascular invasion is rare. Even rarer cases show heterotopic bone and cartilage {1644}.

The median Breslow thickness in the SMU series was 2.5 mm (0.2-18 mm) {1867,1868}. The thickness and extent of invasion is usually best determined in S-100 stains. The mitotic rate is variable but is often low. Abnormal mitoses are common in the more cellular tumours.

The neurotropism is characterized by the presence of one or more foci in which the spindle cells extend in a circumferential fashion around nerves in the dermis or deeper and/or thickened nerves containing abnormal cells within their nerve sheath. Spindle cells may also form structures resembling nerves ("neural transforming"). Neurotropism may be present in melanomas without desmoplasia.

Melanomas of any histogenetic type may have desmoplastic areas. The proportion of desmoplasia in a melanoma necessary for the diagnosis of DM has been ill-defined in several studies, but proposals for diagnostic criteria have been made {358A,985A,1546A}.

Metastases in lymph nodes may be epithelioid cells, or spindle cells with or without desmoplasia.

Immunoprofile

The spindle cells are positive with S-100 although only a few nuclei are positive in some otherwise typical cases. HMB45 is usually negative except for any foci of epithelioid cells {2476}. NSE, NKI/C-3 and smooth muscle actin {1929} may be positive. Melan A (MART-1) is usually negative. Microphthalmia transcription factor (MTF) is not a sensitive or specific marker {356,885,1294}. Type IV collagen and laminin are frequently expressed in DM {1857}. Vimentin is usually positive although positive staining does not usually assist in diagnosis.

Differential diagnosis

The differential diagnosis includes desmoplastic naevus {958}, which like DM may have perineural extension but lacks asymmetry, mitotic activity, marked nuclear atypia and lymphoid infiltrates. Well established desmoplastic Spitz naevi may have many HMB45 negative spindle cells but these naevi are usually symmetrical with epidermal thickening, include at least a few plump cells and have rare or absent mitoses. Sclerosing cellular blue naevi, which are most frequent on the scalp, also lack mitoses and are more or less diffusely HMB45 positive. Immature scars, especially in re-excision specimens, may focally resemble DM as they may have some S-100 positive spindle cells {476,1951}, foci of lymphocytes and mitoses.

Other differential diagnoses include dermatofibroma/fibrous histiocytoma, fibrosarcoma, "malignant fibrous histiocytoma", malignant peripheral nerve sheath tumour and leiomyosarcoma. These tumours can usually be separated by morphology and appropriate immunohistochemistry.

Histogenesis

It is most likely that the desmoplastic cells are derived from melanocytes that have undergone adaptive fibroplasia. Some authors have suggested that the desmoplasia occurs because of a fibroblastic stromal response and neurofibrosarcomatous differentiation of the tumour cells {2476}. Ultrastructurally, premelanosomes and melanosomes are rare and the spindle cells have the features of fibroblasts. There is abundant rough endoplasmic reticulum and sometimes intracytoplasmic collagen and macular desmosomes {2476}.

Somatic genetics

Chromosomal aberrations and gene mutations have been found in sporadic and familial melanoma {799}. Allelic loss at the neurofibromatosis type 1 (NF1) gene locus is frequent in DM {931}. Basic fibroblast growth factor (bFGF) and other fibrocytokines are often present in the nuclei of DMs {1335}. Loss of heterozygosity of matrix interacting protein 1 (MXI1) is frequent {1893}. No BRAF mutations were found in 12 desmoplastic melanomas {596}, consistent with the finding that melanomas on chronically sun-exposed skin only rarely have BRAF mutations {358B,596,1493}.

Prognosis and predictive factors

Recurrences are common especially after incomplete excision {526}, marginal excision <10 mm or if neurotropism is present {1867,1868}. The conflicting results regarding the risk of regional node field metastases and prognosis of DM patients may be due to a heterogeneity of tumours classified as DM and failure to account for tumour thickness {2115A}. Regional nodal metastases appear to be very uncommon in paucicellular DMs with prominent fibrosis and are associated with longer survival {358A, 932A, 985A}. Otherwise, disease-free survival rates are similar to other melanomas of comparable thickness {126}. Neurotropism, HMB45 positivity, high mitotic rate, male gender, thickness, ulceration and site all appear to affect survival which overall is 79% at 5 years {1868}. Of patients with a recurrence, 78.2% experienced it within 2 years.

Wide local excision is the treatment of choice {99A}. Radiation therapy has been effective in some cases {71,1125}.

Melanoma arising from blue naevus

L. Requena
J. A. Carlson

Definition
A melanoma that arises in association with dermal melanocytosis, most frequently cellular blue naevus.

Synonyms
"Malignant blue naevus" or "blue naevus-like melanoma" are terms used to describe melanomas arising in association with a cellular blue naevus or those primary melanomas that resemble blue naevi and lack an in situ component.

ICD-O   8780/3

Epidemiology
Melanoma associated with blue naevus is an exceedingly rare tumour with over 165 reported cases. It affects predominantly Caucasians and all age groups with the majority of cases occurring between 20 and 60 years, with a mean age at diagnosis of 44 years {2066, 2332}. Slightly more females than males have been reported (82 females; 76 males). Occasionally, dark-skinned patients develop melanoma in association with a blue naevus {548,1352,1629}.

Localization
In decreasing order, the sites most frequently affected are the scalp (33%), orbit and face (32%), trunk- mostly back and buttocks (19%), extremities (7%) and hands or feet (7%). Involvement of the vulva and vagina have also been reported {422,2233}.

Clinical features
Most melanomas associated with blue naevus (93%) develop in a pre-existing dermal melanocytosis that was congenital (35%), acquired during infancy or childhood (15%) or identified during their adult years (43%). These associated lesions were cellular blue naevi (52%), common blue naevus (16%), naevus of Ota (14%), naevus of Ito (1%) {2066, 2414}, or ocular melanocytosis {542, 1127,2332,2431}. On average, these melanocytoses were present for 24 years before melanoma developed, with a range of 3 months (infant with congenital facial blue naevus {2066}) to 78 years (naevus of Ito {2414}). For congenital and childhood onset melanocytoses, melanoma developed after a mean duration of 34 years (range 3 months to 78 years) whereas for adult onset common or cellular blue naevi, melanoma developed on average after 14 years (range 1 – 56 years). The majority (83%) of affected patients described recent, often rapid, growth or presented with proptosis in the case of orbital melanomas within a year of diagnosis. Other symptoms include colour change or ulceration, and in the case of orbital melanomas, diplopia and blurred vision. The melanoma is typically a large black nodule with mean diameter of 2.1 cm (range 0.5–8.0 cm). In some cases, satellitosis due to cutaneous metastatic deposits appear around the primary nodule {64,276,364,856,1018, 1588,1981,2066}. However, this feature

can also represent the well-known phenomenon of satellitosis associated with the common and cellular blue naevus (agminated blue naevus) {616,1059, 1195,2008}. Similarly, cellular blue naevus can also present with regional lymph node deposits {143,1357,2261}. In the former cases, histopathologic examination of the satellite lesions reveals features of benign blue naevus and the lesions present benign biological behaviour with no development of distant lesions.

Etiology
The etiology of melanoma associated with blue naevus is unknown, but the presence of longstanding dermal melanocytosis is likely a risk factor. Ocular and oculodermal melanocytosis (naevus of Ota) is strongly associated with uveal melanoma {2192,2193} and has been reported with meningeal melanocytoma (blue naevus) of the brain {1877} and primary melanomas of the central nervous system {253,569,1104, 1713,1930,2046}. Based on this association and numerous reports of melanoma of the face, orbit or brain associated with oculodermal melanocytosis patients presenting with naevus of Ota should be considered at lifetime risk for melanoma of the skin, orbit or central nervous system, a risk that may be similar in nature to that identified for large congenital melanocytic naevi with melanoma and neurocutaneous melanocytosis {254}. Additional associa-

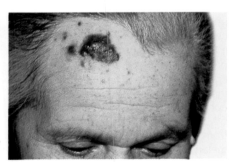

Fig. 2.26 Melanoma arising from blue naevus. Note the presence of satellitosis (Courtesy of Dr. H. Kerl).

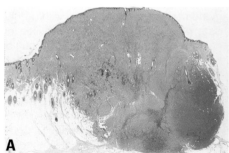
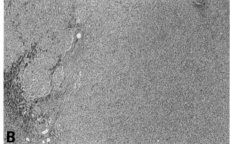

Fig. 2.27 Melanoma arising from blue naevus. **A** Scanning magnification showing a blue naevus with a nodule of malignant melanoma in deeper areas. **B** In deeper areas the nodule of malignant melanoma was composed of sheets of cells destroying pre-existing structures of the dermis.

Melanoma arising from blue naevus   79

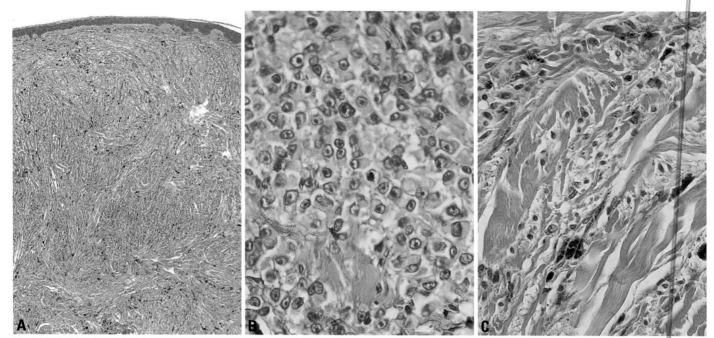

Fig. 2.28 **A** Superficial areas showing stereotypical histopathologic features of a common blue naevus. **B** Higher magnification demonstrated that neoplastic melanocytes of the melanoma showed epithelioid appearance and marked atypia, with large eosinophilic cytoplasm, pleomorphic nuclei and prominent nucleoli. **C** Neoplastic melanocytes of the blue naevus showed small monomorphous nuclei. Note the striking collagenization of the dermis and the abundant number of melanophages.

tions of unknown influence include subacute cutaneous lupus erythematosus, leukoderma, Becker's naevus and prostate adenocarcinoma in one patient {1629}, papillary thyroid carcinoma {94}, acute lymphocytic leukaemia {2119}, psoriasis {238}, and oral contraceptives {1404}. Phototherapy has been associated with cellular blue naevus development {810}.

Histopathology
By definition, a melanoma that develops in a pre-existing blue naevus is a dermal melanoma without the features of melanoma in situ involving the dermo-epidermal junction or adnexal epithelium. In fact, 82% of all reported cases described an adjacent common and/or cellular blue naevus. The absence of an identifiable benign naevus component in some reports may be the result of replacement of it by the melanoma or incomplete sampling of the benign element. Although these cases could represent de novo melanomas, a subtle, hypocellular dermal melanocytosis as seen in naevi of Ota and Ito, and Mongolian spots may not have been observed. Reports of orbital, facial and shoulder melanomas associated with

naevi of Ota and Ito, and ocular melanocytoses attest to this latter possibility of under-reporting {542,660,1783, 2332,2414}.

At scanning magnification, two histopathologic patterns are evident. One is represented by the benign component of the blue naevus, which may range from very focal to comprising the main bulk of the neoplasm. Often this benign component is represented by a cellular blue naevus and less frequently the lesion contains a common blue naevus. Most cases, however, show a combination of the so-called cellular and common blue naevi, making this distinction useless. The areas of cellular blue naevus consist of solid aggregations of closely arranged monomorphous ovoid cells with abundant pale cytoplasm containing little or no melanin and round vesicular nuclei with inconspicuous nucleoli. In contrast, the areas of common blue naevus are made up of elongated spindled bipolar melanocytes, with long branching dendritic processes most of them filled with abundant granules of melanin. Melanophages and sclerotic bundles of collagen are also frequently observed between the fascicles of dendritic melanocytes.

Although the malignant component may involve the superficial dermis and ulcerate the epidermis, more often it appears as a deep-seated expansile asymmetric nodule involving the reticular dermis and subcutaneous fat. Usually, there is an abrupt transition from the benign blue naevus component to the nodule of melanoma. The nodule or nodules of melanoma show both architectural and cytological features of malignancy. The melanomatous component consists of sheets of cells that involve diffusely the deep dermis destroying the pre-existing structures with pushing margins and sharp demarcation between the neoplasm and adjacent dermis or subcutaneous tissue. Neoplastic melanocytes appear as large spindled to epithelioid cells with abundant cytoplasm and pleomorphic and hyperchromatic nuclei, with prominent nucleoli and frequent mitotic figures. Usually they contain little or no melanin. Without the associated benign component, these dermal nodules would be histopathologically indistinguishable from typical nodular or metastatic melanoma. Necrosis of individual cells as well as necrosis en masse may be also seen in the melanoma component, although this finding seems to be less frequent than in melanomas arising de novo ("malignant blue naevus") {973}. A perivascular inflammatory infiltrate, mostly composed of lymphocytes, which is usually lacking in blue naevus, is often seen around the melanoma arising in blue naevus.

Melanoma arising in the setting of blue naevus should be differentiated from the so-called atypical cellular blue naevus {118,2371}. These lesions show clinicopathologic features intermediate between typical cellular blue naevus and malignant melanoma associated with blue naevus. The lesions show architectural atypia, characterized by asymmetry and infiltrative margins, as well as cytologic atypia, which consist of hypercellularity, nuclear pleomorphism, hyperchromasia, mitotic figures and necrosis. However, follow-up data of patients with atypical cellular blue naevus demonstrated that no patient experienced either a local recurrence or lymph node or visceral metastasis.

Melanoma associated with blue naevus should be also distinguished from *large plaque-type or giant cellular blue naevus* with subcutaneous cellular nodules {358, 1059}. Large pigmented plaques of childhood onset that show slow enlargement during adolescence and subsequent nodule formation clinically characterize this rare plaque variant of cellular blue naevus. Histopathologically, they exhibit multifocal dermal and subcutaneous proliferations of fusiform and dendritic pigmented melanocytes, with highly cellular nodules located in deeper areas of the plaque. The follow-up of patients with large plaque-type blue naevus with subcutaneous cellular nodules indicates that these lesions behave in a benign fashion.

Metastatic melanoma mimicking blue naevus can also be confused with melanoma associated with a blue naevus {354,2517}. These blue-naevus-like metastases occurred in the same anatomic region as the primary tumour or near the skin scar of a dissected lymph node metastasis and were histopathologically characterized by atypical epithelioid melanocytes, mitotic figures, and an associated inflammatory cell infiltrate at the periphery of the lesions. In contrast with melanoma arising in a pre-existing blue naevus, metastatic melanoma to the skin simulating blue naevus lacks the benign blue naevus component.

Animal type melanoma (epithelioid melanocytoma) is a rare variant of primary cutaneous melanoma that may also mimic melanoma associated with blue naevus {567,1917}. Sheets and nodules of heavily pigmented epithelioid melanocytes that tend to aggregate along hair follicles and involve the entire thickness of the dermis with extension into the subcutaneous tissue histopathologically characterize animal-type melanoma. Epithelioid melanocytes in deeper areas show abundant, heavily pigmented cytoplasm and pleomorphic nuclei with prominent eosinophilic nucleoli and mitotic figures. Histopathologic features of melanoma in situ at the dermo-epidermal junction are few or absent, and neoplastic cells do not show evidence of maturation from superficial to deeper dermal areas. The overall architectural and cytologic features of animal-type melanoma closely resemble those of melanoma associated with blue naevus, but animal-type melanoma lacks the benign component of blue naevus or history of a pre-existing melanocytosis.

Metastatic spread
Melanoma associated with blue naevus is an aggressive tumour with frequent metastatic disease to regional lymph nodes (31% of reported cases) and distant sites (42%). Sites of metastasis, in decreasing order of frequency, include liver (36%), lung (22%), brain (16%), skin (13%), bone (9%), and in less than 6% of reported cases, spleen, heart, kidney, pancreas, adrenal, thyroid and parotid glands, ovary, and gastrointestinal tract. Melanuria and generalized melanosis have also been described in its terminal stage {2185}. Metastases can appear as late as 20 years after diagnosis {813}, but the median and mean time of discovery is 1.75 and 3.6 years after diagnosis.
Metastasis to lymph nodes should be differentiated from the presence of blue naevus cells in the capsule of the node {181,392,405,1357,1358}. This well-known pseudo-metastasizing phenomenon seems to be the result of migration arrest during embryogenesis and is characterized by monomorphous melanocytes of blue naevus involving only the capsule and the marginal sinuses of the lymph node. In authentic metastases, nests of atypical melanocytes replace most of the parenchyma of the node, effacing its architecture.

Immunoprofile
Immunohistochemical studies in lesions of melanoma associated with blue naevus have demonstrated a strongly positive reaction of the neoplastic cells, both of the benign and malignant components, for vimentin, S-100 protein, HMB-45 and NKI/C-3 {280,1708,1996}. However, the number of silver positive nucleolar organizer regions (AgNOR score) {813,1826} and growth fraction as measured by proliferating cell nuclear antigen (PCNA) and Ki-67 (MIB-1) are significantly lower in the benign component of blue naevus than in the nodule of melanoma {1708,1826}.

Electron microscopy
Although some authors have interpreted the neoplastic cells of melanoma associated with blue naevus as being related with Schwann cells {1588}, electron microscopic studies have demonstrated the presence of melanosomes in the cells, as well as the lack of cytoplasmic enclosures of unmyelinated axons, which rule out the possibility of Schwann cell differentiation. Although the melanosomes in many cells of the malignant component are devoid of melanin {1014}, incubation with dopa demonstrates that they are strongly dopa-positive {1625}, thus confirming their melanocytic nature.

Somatic genetics
Results of DNA flow cytometry studies in melanoma associated with a blue naevus are variable revealing diploid cell populations in 4 cases {1574,1826} and aneuploid populations in 2 cases {1826}. A molecular analysis failed to demonstrate loss of heterozygosity on microdissected samples in one case of melanoma associated with blue naevus, using a panel of eight genes (MTS1, MXI1, CMM1, p53, NF1, L-myc, hOGG1, and MCC), many of which are commonly associated with conventional melanomas {94}. These findings suggest that melanoma associated with blue naevus may represent a distinct entity with a different molecular pathway to tumourigenesis than that of conventional melanomas. However, in a comparative genomic hybridization study comparing common blue naevi, cellular blue naevi, and atypical cellular blue naevi with melanoma associated with a blue naevus, melanomas associated with blue naevus showed chromosomal abnormalities similar to that of con-

ventional melanoma whereas cellular and atypical cellular blue naevi exhibit infrequent numerical chromosome aberrations similar in character to that identified in proliferative nodules found in congenital melanocytic naevi {1490}.

Prognosis and predictive factors
Some authors have proposed that melanoma associated with blue naevus is a low-grade malignancy {1574}. However, the literature review does not support this opinion. For instance, in a series of 12 cases, metastases developed in 10, and 8 died of metastatic disease {527}, and in another series of 10 cases, 4 patients developed metastases and 3 of them died of disease {883}. Of the 160 cases reported with follow-up data, 34% of patients have died due to locally invasive or metastatic melanoma 20 months median, 41 months mean time from diagnosis (range 2–240 months). Therefore, melanoma arising in blue naevus is a highly aggressive tumour with poor prognosis similar to that of thick (>4.00 mm), AJCC stage IIB conventional melanomas {392}. Indeed, the Breslow thickness for this melanoma variant typically is much greater than 4 mm with a mean tumour thickness of 10 mm (range 2.8–45mm) {64,640,813,883,1844}. Possible prognostic factors indicative of a poor outcome include the presence of congenital melanocytosis, mixed melanoma cell type (both spindle and epithelioid

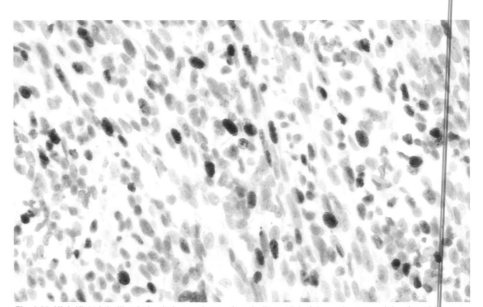

Fig. 2.29 High Ki-67 labelling index in hyperchromatic spindle nuclei of the melanoma arising from blue naevus. The benign portion of the lesion (not shown) had a very low labelling index.

melanocytes), older age, high mean mitotic count (>4/40 high power field), and lymphocyte count (>100 per 20 high power field) {2332}. These prognostic factors were identified in a study of primary orbital melanoma where 90% of the patients had an associated blue naevus and 47.5% had congenital melanocytosis (naevus of Ota or ocular melanocytosis). The role of sentinel lymph node dissection and postoperative adjuvant therapy remains to be determined. Sentinel lymph node dissection in the staging of melanoma associated with a blue naevus is advocated by some authors {2173} and one patient with metastatic disease to the lymph nodes was alive and without evidence of disease two years after surgery followed by therapy with interferon {640}.

Melanoma arising in giant congenital naevi

H. Kerl
C. Clemente
P.E. North

I Sanchez-Carpintero
M.C. Mihm
B.C. Bastian

Definition
A proliferation of malignant melanocytes arising either in the epidermal component or the dermal component of a giant congenital naevus associated with risk of metastasis and death.

ICD-O code   8761/3

Synonyms
Malignant melanoma arising in a garment naevus; malignant melanoma arising in a bathing trunk naevus; malignant melanoma arising in a giant hairy naevus.

Epidemiology
About 1% of all infants have some kind of a congenital pigmented skin lesion {568}. The giant congenital naevus (GCN) is estimated to occur in around 1 per 20,000 infants {67,411,1306}. The risk of malignant transformation of a GCN has been estimated at from 5-20% but more recent studies based on statistical analyses suggest a figure of 6%. The GCN is a direct precursor of melanoma {1197, 1207,1927,2218}. There is a bimodal distribution to the occurrence of melanoma in GCN. Most develop in childhood before the age of 10 {1508} with a second peak of incidence in adult life.

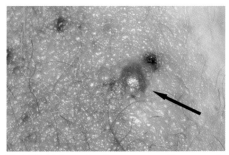

Fig. 2.30 Malignant melanoma presenting as a reddish brown nodule in the midst of the congenital naevus.

Sites of involvement
Malignant melanoma can occur anywhere in a giant congenital naevus. The lesion most commonly arises in lesions on the trunk but can appear in any area even in congenital naevi of the meninges {568,1306,1927}.

Clinical features
The definition of GCN varies and includes a naevus with a diameter larger than 20 cm. Frequently large areas of the body (more than 2% of the body surface) are covered in a garment-like fashion {1306,1927}. The trunk and head and neck are the most common sites for these naevic lesions. The melanoma, very rarely present at birth, usually

appears as a rather rapidly growing asymmetrical nodule or plaque of blue-black, reddish or even rarely flesh colouration {568,1009}. Melanoma can occasionally present as a cystic lesion. Therefore, any GCN that develops an apparent subcutaneous cyst must be biopsied. Melanoma is only one of many benign and malignant tumours that may occur in GCN {1009,1928}.

Macroscopy
The lesion usually appears either as a firm nodule, or as a boggy discoloured area, usually dark brown or black in the midst of the naevus. If the lesion arises in the dermis, the tumour can sometimes only be seen on cut surface as a separate nonencapsulated nodule amidst the otherwise tan or pale tan coloured naevus in the dermis or subcutis.

Histopathology
Histologically, the tumours are often asymmetrical and sharply demarcated from the adjacent congenital naevus. If superficial, there is effacement of the rete ridges of the epidermis and often ulceration. The intraepidermal component usually is composed of epithelioid cells with pigmentation. Pagetoid spread is commonly noted. The tumour cells of the dermal component usually form expansile

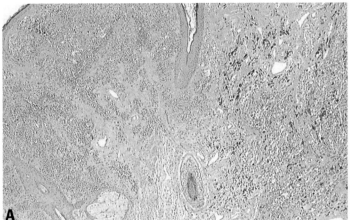
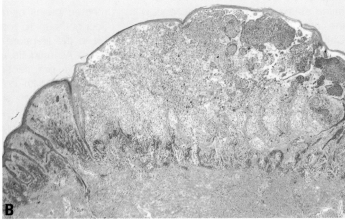

Fig. 2.31 Melanoma arising from large congenital naevus. **A** The melanoma is clearly separate from the naevus cells that are on the left. **B** A protuberant nodule shows the small dark naevus cells to the left and at the base of the melanoma that is composed of nests with dyscohesion.

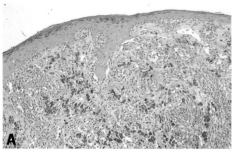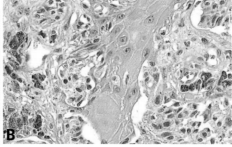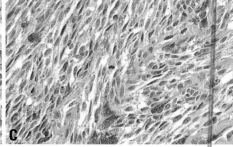

Fig. 2.32 Melanoma arising from large congenital naevus. **A** There is a distinctive proliferation of malignant melanocytes invading the dermis. Note thinning of the rete ridges with a proliferation of malignant melanocytes invading the dermis as spindle cells with an admixed population of melanophages. **B** Reveals epithelioid cells in nests invading the epidermis giving rise to spindle cells in the dermis. **C** The malignant spindle cells show nuclear hyperchromasia and mitoses.

nodules. They exhibit fully transformed malignant characteristics with very irregular chromatin patterns and prominent nucleoli. There is variable pigmentation. Both single cell and zonal necrosis may be observed. The melanoma cells as they abut or infiltrate as cords into the adjacent naevus show no evidence of maturation but maintain their fully malignant characteristics. Mitoses are common and atypical forms are usually present. A lymphocytic host response is often noted. Occasionally, a desmoplastic host

response may be observed as well as focal mucinosis. In our experience, the vertical growth phase dermal nodules may exhibit prominent areas of different cell types with different degrees of pigmentation {568,703,1197,1928}.

Histologically, the presence of a residual dermal naevic component with congenital features may be quite difficult to find, particularly, if present in the wall of a vessel.The differential diagnosis includes the proliferative nodules that also arise in large congenital naevi.

Somatic genetics

Comparative genomic hybridization shows that melanomas arising in congenital naevi show similar chromosomal aberrations as melanoma arising independently {175}. By contrast, the proliferative nodules arising in early life do not show chromosomal aberration supporting the view that they are benign {175}.

Childhood melanoma

R.L. Barnhill

Definition

Melanomas developing in individuals prior to the onset of puberty are childhood melanomas and thereafter they are designated as melanomas in adolescents with the age limitation of 18 to 20 years. Childhood melanomas can be further subcategorized as 1) congenital melanoma (onset in utero to birth), 2) infantile melanoma (birth to one-year of age), and 3) childhood melanoma (one year to onset of puberty).

Epidemiology

The incidence of melanoma is exceptionally rare in prepubertal individuals (estimated incidence approximately 0.4% among all melanomas) {269A, 1487A} and uncommon under the age of 20 years (incidence approximately 2%) {123A}. The incidence of melanoma has doubled

in patients aged 15 to 19 years over the past decade but has remained unchanged in younger individuals {204A,1037A}. Less than 80 well documented cases of melanoma in children younger than 10 years have been recorded in the literature over a period of 30 years. As in adults, childhood melanomas have a predilection for Caucasians. Individuals with congenital naevi especially large varieties, atypical naevi, family history of melanoma, xeroderma pigmentosum, and immunosuppression are at increased risk for childhood melanoma.

Localization

Melanomas developing in patients up to 16 years of age most commonly involve the trunk (50%), followed by the lower extremities (20%), head and neck (15%), and upper limbs (15%).

Clinical features

Melanomas in individuals under the age of 20, particularly in adolescents, show fairly similar clinical features as compared to melanomas in adults {123A, 1916A}. However, melanomas in prepubertal individuals are so rare that they are usually unsuspected. Features suggesting melanoma in a pigmented lesion such as a congenital naevus are rapid increase in size, bleeding, development of a palpable nodule (e.g., in a giant congenital naevus), colour change of a nodular lesion, surface changes such as ulceration, and loss of clearly defined margins. Recognition of melanoma appearing de novo requires a high index of clinical suspicion, especially for amelanotic lesions. Utilizing the conventional ABCDE criteria (Asymme-try, ill-defined Borders, irregular Colour, and large

Blue naevi

E. Calonje
K. Blessing
E. Glusac
G. Strutton

Common blue naevus

Definition
Common blue naevus (BN) is a benign, usually intradermal melanocytic lesion characterized by pigmented dendritic spindle-shaped melanocytes and, more rarely, epithelioid melanocytes. The melanocytes are usually separated by thickened collagen bundles.

ICD-O code   8780/0

Epidemiology
BN is relatively frequent, has predilection for females and presents mainly in young adults between the second and fourth decades. Although most tumours are acquired, congenital examples have been documented {1872}. Familial cases may be seen and usually present with multiple lesions {258,1292}.

Localization
The anatomical distribution is wide but most lesions occur on the distal upper limbs (particularly the dorsum of the hand), followed by the lower limbs, scalp, face and buttocks. Lesions have also been documented in the vagina {1002,2356}, cervix {2393}, prostate {1414}, oral cavity (mainly the hard palate) {327,328} and the capsule of lymph nodes without a primary cutaneous lesion {695,858,1497}.

Clinical features
The most common presentation consists of a single asymptomatic, relatively well-circumscribed, dome-shaped blue or blue-black papule less than 1 cm in diameter. The characteristic blue colour is produced by the Tyndall effect. Tumours may rarely present as a plaque {1025,2494}. Eruptive lesions have rarely been documented. Exceptional clinical presentations include a speckled variant {1044}, hypopigmented lesions {278}, an example with satellite lesions {1195} and a case with widespread lesions. Localized hypertrichosis has been described in a single case {57}.

Histopathology
BN and cellular blue naevus show a wide histological spectrum, frequently overlapping with other melanocytic lesions including deep penetrating naevus and pigmented Spitz naevus {1637}.
BN is typically located in the reticular dermis and only exceptionally extends into the papillary dermis or subcutis. The epidermis appears unremarkable, except in the rare so-called compound blue naevus, in which dendritic junctional melanocytes are identified {733, 1190}. Low-power examination reveals a generally symmetric but often ill-defined tumour of variable cellularity. Concentration around adnexa without adnexal destruction is typical. Poorly cellular lesions often display prominent sclerotic stroma making the diagnosis difficult. Lesions with very poor pigmentation are rarely encountered {234,402}. Tumour cells are bland and spindle-shaped or dendritic and usually contain abundant cytoplasmic coarse melanin pigment. Nuclei are small, and an inconspicuous basophilic nucleolus is sometimes present. Numerous melanophages are a relatively constant feature in the vicinity of tumour cells. Extension of tumour cells into nerves and, less frequently, blood vessel walls, may be found. Mitotic figures are exceptional. Rarely, a blue naevus may coexist with a trichoepithelioma {48}.
In some instances, metastatic melanoma may mimic common blue naevus {354}.
Blue naevus may co-exist with other types of naevus (see combined naevus).

Immunoprofile
Tumour cells are usually diffusely positive for melanocytic markers including S-100, HMB45, melan A and microphthalmia transcription factor (MITF-1). Unlike the case in most other benign melanocytic naevi and in melanomas, HMB45 strongly stains the entire lesion in blue naevi.

Somatic genetics
Mutations in the BRAF gene appear to be rare in BN. Chromosomal aberrations are uncommon {1490}.

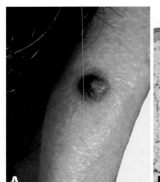
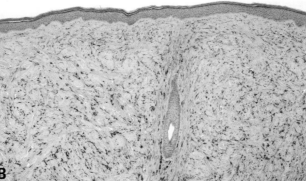
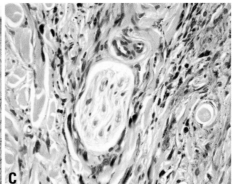

Fig. 2.44 Common blue naevus. **A** Typical clinical appearance of a common blue naevus. **B** A more cellular example with hyalinization of dermal collagen. **C** Melanocytes often extend into the perineurium of dermal nerves.

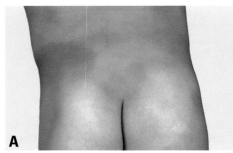 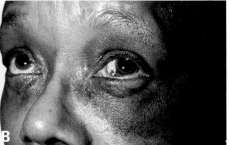 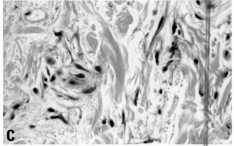

Fig. 2.45 A Mongolian spot. Typical prominent macular blue/grey discolouration on lower back and buttocks. **B** Naevus of Ota with involvement of the periorbital skin and conjunctiva. The blue cast is typical. **C** Naevus of Ota. Bipolar, deeply pigmented melanocytes in the reticular dermis.

Prognosis and predictive factors

BN is benign, and malignant transformation is exceptional {883} (see chapter Melanoma arising from blue naevus). Simple excision is curative and local recurrence is very rare {973}.

Mongolian spot

Definition

Mongolian spot (MS) is a form of dermal melanocytosis presenting on the lower back and characterized by scattered pigmented dendritic melanocytes in the reticular dermis.

Epidemiology

MS presents at birth and has marked predilection for Black and Oriental patients with the same sex incidence {1260,1261}. The incidence in Caucasian children is approximately 9.5% {543}.

Localization

Most lesions occur on the lower posterior trunk with predilection for the sacro-gluteal region. Lesions identical to MS and naevus of Ito or naevus of Ota may present rarely in other anatomical sites.

Clinical features

MS is characterized by a macular area of blue-green or blue-grey discolouration varying in size from a few to 10 or more cm. Lesions fade gradually, usually disappearing completely when patients reach adolescence.

Association with cleft lip {1096} and the mucopolysaccharidoses, including Hurler and Hunter syndromes) {880, 2063} has been documented. Lesions with the clinical and histological features of MS may rarely present at other body sites.

Histopathology

The epidermis and superficial dermis appear unremarkable. Low-power examination reveals a mild increase in cellularity in the deep reticular dermis, consisting of few variably pigmented dendritic melanocytes, which are usually oriented parallel to the epidermis. Melanophages are occasionally seen.

Naevus of Ito and Naevus of Ota

Definition

Naevus of Ito (NI) and naevus of Ota (NO) are dermal melanocytoses with identical histological features, which differ in their characteristic clinical presentation. NI typically presents in the shoulder region, following the distribution of the lateral brachial and posterior supraclavicular nerves. NO involves the skin and mucosal surfaces (including the conjunctiva), following the distribution of the ophthalmic and maxillary branches of the trigeminal nerve.

Synonyms

Naevus Ota: Oculodermal melanocytosis, Naevus fuscoceruleus ophthalmomaxillaris.

Epidemiology

Both NI and NO are relatively rare, affect mainly patients of Oriental or African origin and have some predilection for females {1027,1307,1626,2243}. Presentation is mainly at birth (up to 50%) or during childhood and adolescence. Adult onset is very rare {447}.

Localization

NI typically involves the supraclavicular, deltoid and less commonly, the scapular area. NO usually involves the sclera, conjunctiva, and skin around the eye and zygomatic and temporal areas. Rarely the nasal and oral mucosa, optic tract and the leptomeninges are involved. Lesions identical to naevus of Ito or naevus of Ota may present rarely in other anatomical sites. A limited form resembling naevus of Ota presenting in the zygomatic area is called naevus of Sun.

Clinical features

Lesions are usually large, macular, ill defined and have a blue or blue-grey colour. A speckled appearance is seen rarely. There is no tendency for spontaneous regression. Bilateral involvement has been documented rarely {1026}. Co-existence between NI and NO is a rare occurrence {615,1026}. Glaucoma is a rare complication of NO {1434}.

Histopathology

The histology of NI and NO is indistinguishable. The epidermis appears unremarkable but may show increased melanin in basal cells and a mild increase in the number of basal melanocytes. In the superficial and mid-dermis there are scattered dendritic or spindle-shaped, often bipolar deeply pigmented melanocytes. Melanophages are rare.

Prognosis and predictive factors

Malignant transformation is exceptional and more common in NO {1783,2194, 2345,2414}. In the latter setting it may occur in the skin, eye or meninges.

Cellular blue naevus

Definition

Cellular blue naevus (CBN) is an acquired dermal/subcutaneous pigmented tumour with prominent cellularity and an expansile growth pattern.

ICD-O code   8790/0

Epidemiology

CBN tends to present between the second and fourth decades of life with female predilection, and it is more common in Caucasians. Congenital cases are exceptional {1095}.

Localization

The anatomical distribution is wide, but CBN have predilection for the buttocks and sacral region (50% of cases), followed by the scalp, face, distal limbs and other sites on the trunk {1957,2336}. Lesions may also rarely occur on the eyes, cervix, vagina, breast and spermatic cord {266,1957,2336}. Aggregates of tumour cells have been reported in the capsules of regional lymph nodes draining an area where an otherwise typical benign cellular blue naevus is present {287,1957,2261,2336}. This phenomenon is regarded as a benign occurrence rather than an ominous finding.

Clinical features

Tumours are usually large, varying from 1 to several centimetres, and the colour varies from light blue-brown to dark blue. Lesions are asymptomatic and grow very slowly, presenting as a non-ulcerated firm nodule {1957,2336}. Exceptional cases present as a large plaque {358}. Rare tumours arising in the scalp have been described with invasion of the underlying bone {1596} and even the brain {854}.

The epithelioid variant of blue naevus is very rare and has mainly been described in patients with Carney complex who

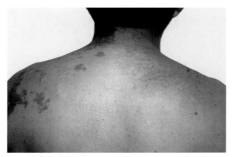

Fig. 2.46 Cellular blue naevi on the upper back.

usually present with multiple lesions {396,399}. Sporadic lesions are usually solitary and may occur in genital skin {1117,1646,1736}.

Macroscopy

The cut surface of a CBN characteristically shows a dark brown to black, well-defined dermal and subcutaneous tumour. In some cases there are areas of haemorrhage and cystic degeneration.

Histopathology

Low-power examination reveals a fairly characteristic picture with a dumbbell-shaped multinodular tumour occupying the reticular dermis and often extending into subcutaneous tissue. A junctional component is not usually found. Areas of pigmentation alternate with poorly pigmented areas and, in a minority of cases, pigment is very scanty {2595}. Cellular areas tend to be more prominent towards the centre of the tumour, and the cellularity may be most marked where the neoplasm protrudes into the subcutis. The

cellular areas may alternate with sclerotic or hypocellular areas. In most cases there are focal areas representing or simulating a common blue naevus. High power examination reveals bundles of oval or spindle-shaped cells with pale cytoplasm, alternating with bundles of deeply pigmented spindle-shaped cells. In addition, dendritic melanocytes and/or round, somewhat epithelioid melanocytes may be seen. Cytoplasmic melanin is coarse and granular, and nuclei are regular and vesicular, with a single small inconspicuous basophilic nucleolus. Maturation with depth is not a feature. A frequent finding however, is the focal presence of elongated slender melanocytes resembling Schwann cells, indicative of neurotization as seen in ordinary naevi. Some tumours exhibit a focal alveolar growth pattern {1597} and desmoplasia is occasionally prominent {1599}. Degenerative changes including haemorrhage, cystic change and fibrosis, are seen in some cases. Focal mild or prominent myxoid oedematous change may also be a feature {1598}, and balloon cell change has been documented {1806}.

Occasional cases display a number of unusual features including mitotic figures (1/10 HPFs), focal necrosis, and/or nuclear pleomorphism or hyperchromatism. Such cases show some overlap with the malignant variant of CBN and have been described as atypical CBN {118,2371}.

The epithelioid blue naevus is composed of large round epithelioid and short spindle-shaped deeply pigmented melano-

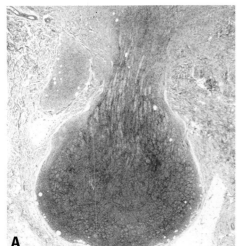
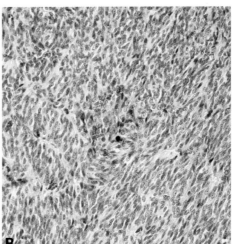
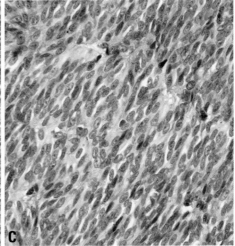

Fig. 2.47 Cellular blue naevus. **A** Typical low-power appearance with a dumb-bell architecture. **B** Bundles of bland spindle-shaped melanocytes alternating with focally pigmented cells. Scattered melanophages are also seen. **C** Typical small vesicular nuclei with a small basophilic nucleolus.

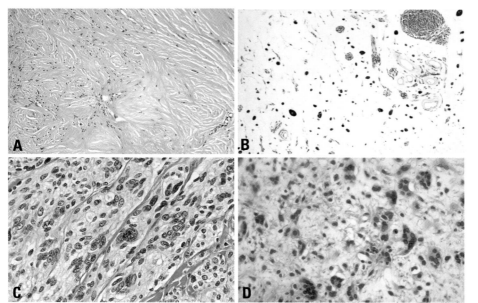

Fig. 2.48 Hypopigmented cellular blue naevus. **A** In some cases, melanin is almost completely absent. **B** Myxoid change may be prominent in some cases. **C** One of the melanocytes is much larger than the others. Some refer to such cases as 'atypical cellular blue naevus'. **D** Large melanocytes are present, some are multinucleated.

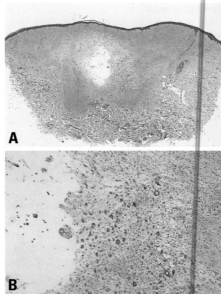

Fig. 2.49 Cellular blue naevus. **A** This lesion has a central focus of cystic change. **B** The edge of the cystic area.

cytes. Some examples of this variant of BN probably represent combined naevi {903}.

Immunoprofile
Tumour cells in CBN are positive for S-100, melan-A and HMB45. In tumours with prominent desmoplasia, and in those with neurotization, staining for melan-A and HMB45 tends to be patchy. CD34 has been reported to be positive in tumour cells in a group of congenital CBN {2204}.

Genetics
Similar to other naevi, cellular blue naevi do not show chromosomal aberrations when analysed by CGH. In a small series of atypical cellular blue naevi, three out of eight cases showed single chromosomal losses with chromosome 3p being affected in two of these cases {1490}.

Prognosis and predictive factors
Although limited case series have characterized these lesions as benign, some cases with atypical features have resulted in recurrences or death from systemic metastasis. They may therefore be regarded as having uncertain malignant potential and treated with complete excision if possible and perhaps longterm follow-up. Malignant transformation in CBN is very rare {64,883}.

Deep penetrating naevus

Definition
Deep penetrating naevus (DPN) is a distinctive deeply pigmented lesion showing overlapping features with blue naevus and Spitz naevus.

Synonym
Some cases have been described under the heading of plexiform spindle cell naevus {164}.

Epidemiology
DPN is an acquired lesion presenting mainly between the second and third decades of life with no sex predilection {1953,2127}.

Localization
DPN has a wide anatomical distribution with predilection for the face, upper trunk and proximal limbs {164,537,1575,1953, 2127}.

Clinical features
The tumour presents as a solitary, well-circumscribed blue or dark brown/black dome-shaped papule or nodule usually less than 1 cm in diameter.

Histopathology
Low power examination typically reveals a compound wedge-shaped deeply pig-

mented dermal and, very rarely, superficial subcutaneous tumour. The base of the lesion parallels the epidermis. The junctional component, which is usually present and may be subtle, consists of small round nests of ordinary naevus cells. In fact, in most cases, a superficial dermal component, representing an ordinary naevus, may be found and therefore these lesions may be regarded as combined naevi {1953}. Much less commonly, focal changes mimicking a Spitz naevus or a blue naevus are found {1953, 2127}. Tumour cells are arranged in nests or bundles and have a short spindle-shaped or, less commonly, round morphology. The cytoplasm contains

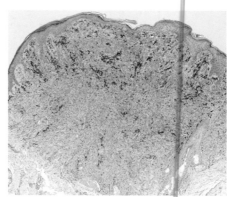

Fig. 2.50 Deep penetrating naevus with a typical wedge-shaped architecture.

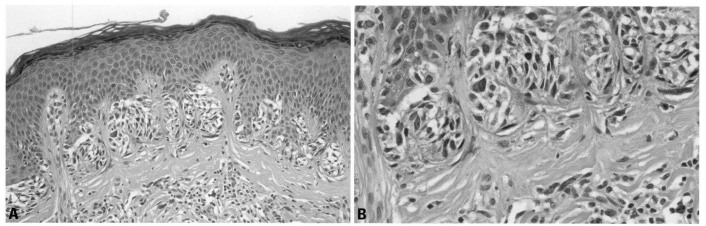

Fig. 2.57 Dysplastic naevus. **A** The naevus cell nests are confined predominantly to the tips of the rete pegs. **B** Note the cytological atypia with nuclear hyperchromasia.

as in no case are the atypical cytologic features as frankly atypical as seen in fully developed melanoma.

Immunoprofile

Mild to moderate staining of dysplastic naevi is observed using antibody to HMB45 antigen. This antibody also often stains intradermal melanocytes within melanomas but not as strongly in common melanocytic naevi {2214}. S-100 is a protein found in the central nervous system that is also present in melanocytes, including melanoma. S-100 protein is found at the dermo-epidermal junction and at all levels of the dermis in dysplastic naevi {1792}. However, S-100 staining is non-specific as it is seen in common naevi, dysplastic naevi as well as malignant melanoma.

Growth fraction / MIB-1 index

Some authors assert that the presence of the proliferation marker Ki-67 in dysplastic naevi indicates that these lesions are precursors to melanoma {760}. The percentage of cells that expressed Ki-67 was an independent prognostic factor {1308}. Kanter et al. found that percentages of MIB-1 immunoreactivity in the intradermal portion of the lesions was negligible for benign congenital and acquired naevi, as well as in dysplastic naevi compared to melanomas which exhibited a markedly increased proliferative activity, especially vertical phase melanomas {1201}. At the current time, it is not recommended that proliferation markers be used as a reliable method for distinguishing between naevi and melanoma.

Electron microscopy

The melanosomes in epidermal melanocytes in dyslastic naevi are abnormal, with incompletely developed lamellae and uneven melanization {2476}. Abnormal spherical and partially melanized melanosomes similar to those observed in superficial spreading melanoma have been observed by electron microscopy {672,1363}. Based on these transmission electron microscopy findings, one group suggested that dysplastic naevi lie on a continuum between naevi and superficial spreading melanoma. No correlation has been shown prospectively between ultrastructural findings and progression or predilection to the development of MM.

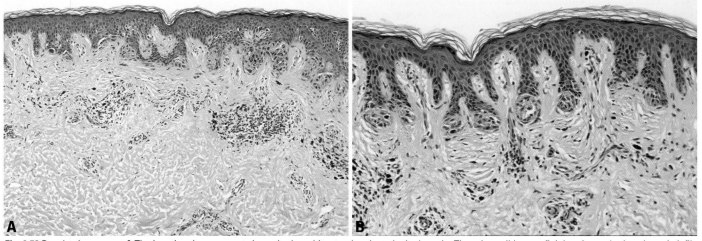

Fig. 2.58 Dysplastic naevus. **A** The junctional component shows both architectural and cytological atypia. There is a mild, superficial perivascular lymphocytic infiltrate. **B** Mild atypia of the junctional nests and dermal papillary fibroplasia. These is some melanin incontinence.

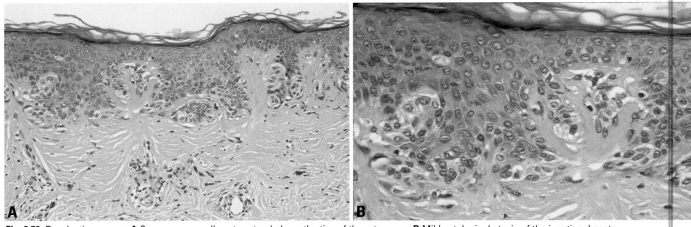

Fig. 2.59 Dysplastic naevus. **A** Some naevus cell nests extend above the tips of the rete pegs. **B** Mild cytological atypia of the junctional nests.

Variants

Toussaint and Kamino observed histopathologic changes of "dysplastic" naevi in other types of naevi. They also noted that some dysplastic naevi demonstrated features of other varieties of naevi. 2,164 cases of compound melanocytic naevi that fulfilled the histopathologic criteria for the diagnosis of compound dysplastic naevus were reviewed. 87.6% had the histopathologic characteristics of dysplastic naevus, 8.3% showed a dermal component with a congenital pattern, 3.1% demonstrated epidermal and dermal characteristics of Spitz naevus, 0.3% had features of a combined blue naevus, 0.6% had a halo phenomenon and 0.1% showed intradermal naevus. The authors advocate describing dysplastic melanocytic naevi by categorizing them into six groups: 1) dysplastic naevus; 2) dysplastic naevus with a congenital pattern; 3) dysplastic Spitz naevus; 4) dysplastic combined blue naevus; 5) dysplastic halo naevus; and 6) dysplastic neuronaevus {2370}.

Differential diagnosis

The clinical differential diagnosis of dysplastic naevi includes congenital melanocytic naevi, pigmented basal cell carcinoma, Spitz naevus, common acquired melanocytic naevi, melanoma in situ, and superficial spreading malignant melanoma. The histologic differential diagnosis includes melanoma, recurrent naevus, halo naevus, congenital naevus, a growing naevus in a child and Spitz naevus.

Grading

Some authors emphasize cytologic crite-ria for grading dysplastic naevi {1925}. In 1993, Duncan et al. advocated grading dysplatic naevi into groups based on cytology. Dysplastic naevi with slight, moderate and severe cytologic atypia were differentiated. However, concordance between experienced dermatopathologists ranged from 35% to 58%. Because of lack of reproducibility, DeWit et al. did not recommend grading atypia in dysplastic naevi {612}. An analysis of 12 histologic parameters in 123 dysplastic naevi failed to identify parameters useful in differentiating mild from moderate dysplasia {1854}. Despite these considerations, melanoma risk has been associated with the degree of atypia in dysplastic nevi {102}.

Somatic genetics
Cytogenetics and CGH

Jaspers et al. performed cytogenetic investigations on lymphocytes and fibroblasts from 25 individuals with dysplastic naevus syndrome and compared the results with a a control population of clinically normal relatives and unrelated individuals. In five DNS patients, increased frequencies of cells with random chromosomal rearrangements including translocations and inversions were observed. These abnormalities were absent in the control population {1134}.
Caporaso analyzed the karyotypes of 163 family members from 13 melanoma-prone families to investigate whether chromosomal instability contributes to familial melanoma. Cutaneous malignant melanoma and dysplastic naevi syndrome patients each had increased structural and numerical abnormalities compared with pooled controls {377}.

However, the criteria used to define lesions as "dysplastic" naevi were subjective from the outset so the validity of such studies remains in question.
Park and Vortmeyer examined the frequency of p16 and p53 deletion in nine dysplastic naevi and 13 benign intradermal naevi with five microsatellite markers. Hemizygous deletion was detected in seven of nine dysplastic naevi at one or more loci for p16. No loss of heterozygosity was detected in any of the benign intradermal naevi {1775}.

Molecular genetic alterations

Greene performed an extensive review of the genetics of malignant melanoma and dysplastic naevi in 1998. Many studies demonstrate an autosomal dominant mode of inheritance and speculate pleiotropic manifestations of a proposed melanoma gene on chromosome 1 (1p36). CDKN2A, a tumour suppressor gene localized on chromosome 9, is also reported to be a melanoma gene. The relationship of melanoma to mutation of CDKN2A has been confirmed {895}. Hussein evaluated skin tissue samples of melanoma, dysplastic naevi and benign melanocytic naevi for microsatellite instability. Microsatellites are short single sequence motifs repetitively scattered throughout the human genome. The variation in microsatellite pattern length between tumourous and matching non-tumourous tissues is referred to as microsatellite instability. Microsatellite instability has been associated with other familial and sporadic tumours. Hussein's results demonstrated MSI at 1p and 9p chromosomal regions in dysplastic naevi and malignant melanoma but not in benign naevi lending further support to others that have speculated on the presence of "melanoma genes" involving the short arm of chromosomes 1 (1p36) and 9 (9p21) {1087}. In 2002, Tucker provided 25-year prospective data regarding 33 families with familial melanoma and dysplastic naevi. Seventeen members were found to have mutations in CDKN2A. Tucker found that the majority of clinically diagnosed dysplastic naevi remained stable or regressed over time. The majority of melanomas detected over the course of the study arose from naevi although some arose de novo {2384}.

Genetic susceptibility

As discussed above, Clark originally described dysplastic naevi in relation to a familial syndrome called the B-K mole syndrome {496}. Most dermatologists agree that family members of patients with dysplastic naevi need evaluation {2373}. Familial dysplastic naevi and melanomas have rarely been reported with other systemic malignancies involving the central nervous and digestive system {129,213}.

Prognosis and predictive factors

The incidence of melanoma developing in a given dysplastic naevus has been estimated at 1:3000 per year. Therefore, dysplastic naevi should not be considered as high risk precursors of melanoma, but rather as markers that allow identification of individuals at increased risk for melanoma.

Number of dysplastic naevi and family history

Patients with greater numbers of naevi, dysplastic or otherwise, are at greater risk for melanoma {2386}. Dermatologists acknowledge patients with multiple dysplastic naevi, especially if there is a personal or family history, are at greater risk for developing melanoma {2373}. If patients are from "melanoma-prone families" and have clinically dysplastic naevi, as defined by criteria that include lesional diameter, their individual risk for developing a melanoma is several hundred times that of the general population, with a risk for lifetime incidence of melanoma approaching 100% {744,846}. The significance of a single histologically dysplastic naevus in this context has not been determined. One study evaluated patients with an established diagnosis of melanoma (n=716) compared with normal controls (n=1014) and found that one clinically dysplastic naevus was associated with a 2-fold risk, while 10 or more conferred a 12-fold risk of melanoma {2386}. In the same study, patients who bore 100 or more clinically non-dysplastic naevi had a relative risk of 3.4. Approximately 50% of dysplastic naevi patients with a family history of MM may have multiple primary melanomas {1320}.

Histopathological criteria

There is evidence that histological atypia does correlate with melanoma risk. A recent study of more than 20,000 naevi divided them microscopically into mild, moderate, or severe categories of dysplasia. A personal history of melanoma was present in 5.7 of the patients with mild, 8.1 with moderate and 19.7 with severe atypia. It was concluded that the risk of melanoma was greater for persons who tend to make naevi with high-grade histological atypia {102}.

Genetic predictive factors

Currently, there are no commercially available genetic tests that would be predictive of dysplastic naevi progression to melanoma.

Site-specific and Meyerson naevi

H. Kamino
D. Weedon

In some anatomic sites, naevi may have atypical histological features. This chapter discusses three clinicopathologic entities: acral, genital and Meyerson naevi, but other site-specific features have been described, including naevi occuring in flexures, umbilicus, ear and scalp.

Acral naevus

Definition
Acral naevi (AN) are benign melanocytic proliferations from the palms and soles.

Synonyms
AN or "naevi on volar skin" include histologic subtypes termed "Melanocytic Acral Naevus with Intraepidermal Ascent of Cells (MANIAC)" {1545} and "atypical or acral lentiginous naevus" {501,1511}.

Epidemiology
Clinical studies which are unable to distinguish lentigines from true naevi, record discrete pigmented volar lesions in less than 1{1763} to 92% {1416} of subjects, with most studies suggesting a range of 3–41% of the population {63,519,574, 1338,2223,2418}. In a histologically confirmed study, 3.9% of Caucasians had AN {1473}. Darker patients tend to have a greater percentage {519,1763} and higher total of naevi on acral surfaces {63,519,1553,2418}, though this is not always found {574,1416}. Pigmented acral lesions are generally more common in the second and third decades {63,1338,1415,2418}.

Localization
Plantar naevi are probably more common than palmar naevi {63,574,1473,2418}. AN may occur on both pressure-bearing and pressure-spared surfaces {45,63, 1415}.

Clinical features
AN are usually less than 8 mm with a light to dark brown striated macular component. Congenital AN can be particularly

difficult to clinically distinguish from melanoma {289,1511,2013,2017,2018}. On epiluminesence microscopy (ELM) dermatoscopy), the pigmentation of AN is accentuated in dermal glyphic furrows and occasionally around eccrine ostia, thereby creating reproducible patterns {45,1232,2014,2015}. In acral melanomas the pigment is distributed along the dermatoglyphic ridges {45}.

Etiology
The origin of AN is hypothesized to involve repeated trauma {701,2181, 2182}, foci of "unstable" melanocytes {1416} and racially-correlated variations in melanosome aggregation {1612}.

Histopathology
Distinction of acral naevi from melanoma can be difficult because both may be asymmetric, poorly circumscribed and have intraepidermal ascent of cells {292, 701,984,1545,2181,2182}. Suprabasal melanocytes in AN are relatively more columnar, circumscript and less voluminous than in melanomas {1246}. Signoretti et al. have shown that symmetry, circumscription, the columnar organization of ascending melanocytes and organization of the junctional component are all influenced by the histologic plane of section; to wit, naevi sectioned perpendicular to dermal glyphics are more likely to have benign attributes {2017, 2018}. Subsequently, severe melanocytic atypia and a dense lymphocytic infiltrate

have been found the most reliable features indicative of melanoma {493,707}.

Genital naevus

Definition
Melanocytic naevi on the perineum and genitalia, hereafter "genital naevi (GN)", include different naevic types distinguished and united by unusual, variably present junctional features.

Synonyms
A subgroup of GN with "unusual histologic features" {480,782} or "atypism" {1608} have been dubbed "atypical melanocytic naevus of the genital type (AMNGT) {495}".

Epidemiology
About 10% of men and women have pigmented genital lesions {574,784,1955}, but many are lentigines {784,1955}. Histologically confirmed GN occur in 2% of women {267,480,1955}.
AMNGT comprise a minority of all GN {267,480,1955}. They typically present by the twenties {1608} and, in contrast to vulvar melanoma, are seen exclusively in premenopausal women {1608,2015}. Dysplastic naevi may also occur on the genitalia but they are usually observed in people with dysplastic naevi elsewhere on their bodies {267,1608}. Vulvar naevi were said to have increased premalignant potential {1763}, though recent data

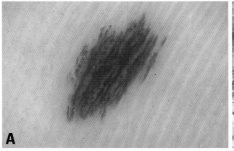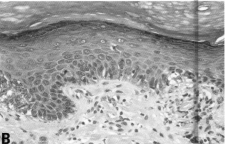

Fig. 2.60 Acral naevus. **A** Epiluminescence microscopy of an acral naevus demonstrating linear hyperpigmentation within the furrows of dermal glyphics. **B** Intraepidermal melanocytes with short dendrites are seen along and above the basal layer.

tubules peripherally. P53 is positive in less than 25% of the neoplastic cells. There is a low proliferative index, as Ki-67 is positive in less than 5% of the neoplastic cells. CK20, c-erb-2, and CD34 are negative {2207}.

Differential diagnosis
The principal differential diagnoses are with superficial biopsies of columnar trichoblastoma (desmoplastic trichoepithelioma) or morpheiform basal cell carcinoma (trichoblastic carcinoma), all of which are CK7 negative. Syringoma is a possible consideration in some cases. Rare examples of metastatic carcinoma to the skin can also mimic it.

Genetics
There is a single report of a 6q deletion {2538}. There is also a report of 2 microcystic adnexal carcinomas, one of which was diploid, and the other, aneuploid, when examined with DNA image cytometry {2437}.

Prognosis
Treatment is surgical, with microscopic control of margins if possible {9}. Radiotherapy has proven successful rarely, but some reported cases have taken on an even more virulent biology after such treatment.

Malignant mixed tumour

Definition
Malignant mixed tumour (MMT) is an exceedingly rare cutaneous adnexal carcinoma with a significant risk for aggressive behaviour and a propensity for metastasis. MMT is regarded as the malignant counterpart of benign mixed tumour {1919} albeit histological diagnosis is foremost based on the biphasic nature of the neoplasm rather than an admixture of benign mixed tumour remnants with carcinomatous tissue {2515}.

ICD-O code   8940/3

Synonyms
Malignant apocrine mixed tumour. Malignant chondroid syringoma.

Epidemiology
MMT represents an exceedingly rare cutaneous adnexal neoplasm which occurs in a wide age range (15 months

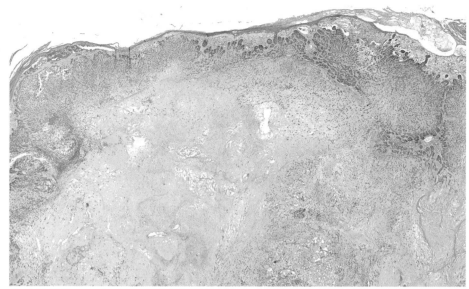

Fig. 3.05 Malignant mixed tumour. Lobulated biphasic tumour consisting of epithelial and mucinous-mesenchymal components. The former predominate at the periphery, while the latter predominate at the center.

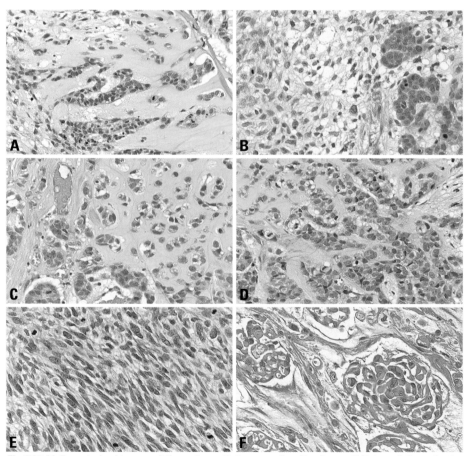

Fig. 3.06 Malignant mixed tumour. **A** Hyperchromatic tumour cells with mitoses. **B** Note variations of cytological differentiation and pleomorphism. **C** Focal zone of tubule formation. **D** Highly pleomorphic tumour lobules with mitoses at the periphery of the tumour. **E** Note the pseudo-sarcomatous pattern with hyperchromatic spindle cells and many mitoses. **F** Nests of plasmacytoid tumour cells amidst a myxoid stroma. Plasmacytoid epithelial differentiation is a hallmark of myoepithelial differentiation.

to 89 years; average 50 years) and is twice more common in women than in men {177,1919}.

Localization
In marked contrast to its benign counterpart MMT shows a predilection for the trunk and the extremities, foremost the hands and feet {177,961,1593,1903, 1919,2177,2377}.

Clinical features
MMT shares most clinical characteristics with its benign counterpart, albeit tumours of the former are much larger at the time of presentation (2-15 cm in diameter). Rarely, rapid growth, ulceration, or pain in a previously indolent skin tumour indicate carcinomatous growth. Most MMT, however, present in a rather bland way with a long history prior to excision. These tumours are well circumscribed and may appear cystic. They are not painful, not ulcerated, and show no distinctive clinical appearance.

Macroscopy
Grossly, most MMT are firm, circumscribed, asymmetrical cutaneous or subcutaneous tumours with a diameter of up to 15 cm. The tumour cut surface may reveal gelatinous material in variable amount {1919}. Because of the infiltrative tumour growth enucleation is not possible.

Histopathology
MMT originates within the dermis or superficial subcutis, and presents as a large, asymmetrical, poorly circumscribed, lobulated biphasic tumour with infiltrative tumour margins and adjacent satellite tumour nodules. Juxtaposed areas of benign and malignant mixed tumour may rarely occur, but are not a prerequisite for the diagnosis of MMT. MMT is composed of both epithelial and mesenchymal components, with epithelial components predominating at the periphery and mesenchymal chondromyxoid elements being more abundant toward the centre {2100}. The chondromyxoid tumour stroma is PAS-negative and consists of hyaluronic acid and sulphated acid mucopolysaccharides {1112}. Stroma ossification is rare {961, 2177}. Epithelial tumour aggregations present as confluent cords and nests of variable size and shape, with interspersed zones of tubule formation.

Tubular structures may be either of the elongated apocrine type lined by at least two layers of epithelial cells, with luminal cells exhibiting signs of apocrine secretion and abluminal cells showing plasmacytoid / myoepithelial differentiation, or – more rarely – of the eccrine type showing small round structures lined by a single layer of atypical epithelial cells {961, 1919}. Often, however, MMT consists only of solid aggregations devoid of tubules {928, 1919, 2471}. Epithelial tumour cells may either have a deceptively bland appearance {1112,2100} or show distinctive atypia and pleomorphism of nuclei with a high nuclear-cytoplasmic ratio and numerous mitotic figures {1919}. Zones of necrosis are common. Characteristic epithelial tumour cells are cuboidal with distinctive polygonal or plasmacytoid features {961, 1919}. The latter is considered an indicator of the myoepithelial/apocrine origin of the neoplasm and may be seen as a clue to the diagnosis of MMT {1919}.

Immunoprofile
Tumour cells may show a myoepithelial immunophenotype with coexpression of S100 and cytokeratin {177,976,1839, 2471} and actin expression in a minority of cells {1488}. Spindle cells within the myxoid stroma are vimentin-positive {2117}.

Electron microscopy
Tumour cells exhibit ultrastructural features of myoepithelia with desmosomes and abundant intracytoplasmic filaments {177,1839,2471}. However, ultrastructural studies so far have not presented convincing evidence of either apocrine or eccrine differentiation of MMT {1919}.

Variants
MMT may exhibit deceptively bland cytological features {1112,2100} albeit associated with distinctive architectural criteria of malignancy, e.g. asymmetry, poor circumscription, infiltrative tumour margins, and satellite nodules.
The recently described malignant mixed tumour of soft tissue {1062} shows overlapping histologic criteria with MMT of the skin. The former is considered to be part of the morphological spectrum of myoepithelial tumours of soft tissue.

Differential diagnosis
Extraskeletal myxoid chondrosarcoma

consists of non-cohesive elongated tumour nests without ductal or tubular structures. Tumour cells are cytokeratin negative. Mucinous carcinoma and myxopapillary ependymoma show distinct PAS positivity of the extracellular myxoid stroma. Cutaneous myoepithelial carcinoma favours monophasic differentiation with a very discrete myxoid stroma {1585}. MMT and cutaneous myoepithelial carcinoma may fall along a spectrum of tumours with overlapping histologic appearances {1585}.

Histogenesis
MMT probably does not originate in association with its benign counterpart, but develops de novo {1919}. A myoepithelial origin of MMT appears to be most plausible {177,1585,2100}, and MMT may be included in the spectrum of cutaneous myoepithelial neoplasms {1585}.

Prognosis and predictive factors
MMT proliferates in an invasive and destructive fashion, with a high rate of local recurrences and metastases (>50%) into regional lymph nodes, lung, and bone {177,1593}. Death ensues in >25% {177}. However, in >30% MMT neither recurred nor metastasized ("atypical mixed tumour of the skin") {177}. In general, MMT is characterized by its prolonged course {2467}. It is remarkable that non-metastasizing MMTs showed the same histological spectrum as those of proven malignancy {1919}, ranging from bland cytological appearance {961} to marked nuclear pleomorphism and a high mitotic count {2377}. Complete excision before metastasis results in tumour-free survival {1919}.

Porocarcinoma

Definition
Eccrine porocarcinoma is a malignant tumour related to the sweat gland duct, showing both intraepidermal and dermal components.

ICD-O code   8409/3

Synonyms and historical annotation
Epidermotropic eccrine carcinoma, malignant eccrine poroma, malignant hidroacanthoma simplex, malignant intraepidermal eccrine poroma, poroepithelioma. The tumour was first described

Prognosis
Syringomas are benign. Association with or progression towards carcinoma has not been described.

Poroma

Definition
Poromas are benign adnexal neoplasms with terminal ductal differentiation. Although historically considered a neoplasm of eccrine differentiation, poromas can show either eccrine or apocrine lineage.

ICD-O code   8409/0

Synonyms
Eccrine poroma, hidroacanthoma simplex, dermal duct tumour, syringoacanthoma

Epidemiology
Poromas usually present as solitary tumours on acral sites, although they can be seen in virtually any cutaneous location. Most poromas arise in middle age with no sex predilection. Uncommonly, multiple poromas are seen, either limited to palms and soles or in a widespread distribution, for which the term poromatosis has been applied.

Clinical features
Poromas typically manifest as dome-shaped cutaneous papules, nodules or plaques, generally measuring less than 1 cm in diameter. Some lesions are highly vascular and may show a tendency to bleed, particularly on acral sites. Uncommonly, poromas are pigmented. Rapid growth has been reported during pregnancy {920}. Multiple poromas have developed after electron beam therapy for mycosis fungoides {1348} and occur-

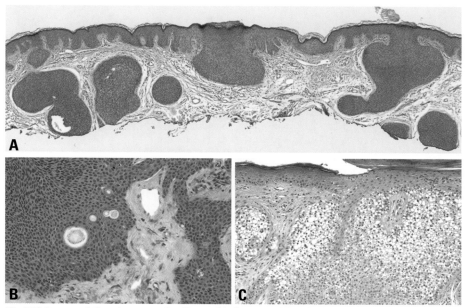
Fig. 3.25 Poroma. **A** Broad tongues of uniform epithelium extend into the dermis from the undersurface of the epidermis. **B** Pigmented poroma illustrating ductal structures and fibrovascular stroma. **C** Clear cell change may be prominent in some poromas.

rence in areas of chronic radiation dermatitis has been reported {1802}. Occurrence of poroma within a naevus sebaceous has been documented {1133}.

Histopathology
Poromas are well-circumscribed tumours composed of a proliferation of uniform basaloid, cuboidal cells punctuated by focal ducts and occasional cysts. The epithelial cells of poromas typically extend from the lower epidermis into the dermis in broad columns. The epithelium of poromas is sharply demarcated from adjacent keratinocytes. Nuclei are small and regular, and cytoplasm is modest in amount. The cytoplasm often contains glycogen. Most poromas contain ductal structures lined by PAS positive diastase-resistant cuticles. Small areas of necrosis as well as mitoses are seen in otherwise banal poromas, and are of no prognostic significance. Foci of sebaceous differentiation may be observed. The stroma surrounding poromas is often richly vascular, and may contain granulation tissue.
Architecturally, poromas show a spectrum of change from predominately intraepidermal lesions (hidroacanthoma simplex) to primarily dermal-based neoplasms (dermal duct tumour). Another rare variant has been termed syringoacanthoma, representing a clonal pattern

of poroma within an acanthotic epidermis with prominent surface keratinization.

Differential diagnosis
Histologically the differential diagnosis includes seborrheic keratosis, which typically shows keratinization with horn cysts, a more sharply demarcated lower border, and absence of ductal structures. Basal cell carcinoma may sometimes be considered histologically, but shows more obvious peripheral palisading, nuclear variability, and little or no glycogen.

Histogenesis
Poromas may show evidence of either eccrine or apocrine differentiation {970}. Immunohistochemical studies reveal that poroma cells express a cytokeratin phenotype similar to basal cells of the eccrine ducts in some cases {2466}. The absence of myoepithelial cells also suggests differentiation toward the excretory (ductal) component of sweat glands. Occurrence of poromas within folliculosebaceous lesions such as naevus sebaceous, and presence of sebocytes within poroma, implicates origin from apocrine glands in some cases {662, 970}.

Genetics
Some cases of poromatosis have been

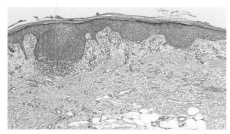
Fig. 3.26 Intraepidermal variant of poroma. There are discrete nests of bland basaloid and cuboidal cells within the epidermis, associated with acrosyringium.

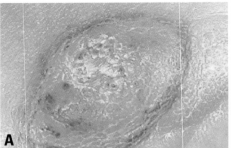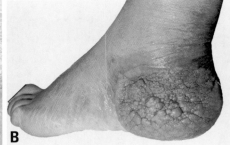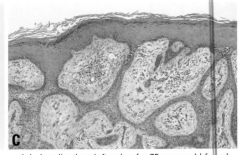

Fig. 3.27 Syringofibroadenoma. **A** Clinical features of the verrucous, solitary type of syringofibroadenoma; a nodule localized on left sole of a 75-years old female, lasting for three years. **B** Eccrine syringofibroadenoma (Mascaro). Presents in many cases as a verrucous plaque. **C** Eccrine syringofibroadenoma (Mascaro). There are branching cords of small keratinocytes attached in multiple foci to the undersurface of the epidermis.

associated with hidrotic ectodermal dysplasia {2519}. Rare cases of poroma have occurred in the setting of naevoid basal cell carcinoma syndrome {904}. Studies of p53 protein have shown high expression in some poromas as well as in some porocarcinomas, but staining is not correlated with duration of tumours {43}. Therefore, while p53 mutation may be involved in progression of some poromas to porocarcinoma, other oncogenes or factors are also likely to play a role in malignant transformation of poromas.

Prognosis

Poromas are benign and simple excision is curative.

Syringofibroadenoma

Definition

Syringofibroadenoma is a rare benign eccrine tumour with anastomosing strands and fibrovascular stroma, first described by Mascaro {1529}. Multiple lesions of syringofibroadenoma are referred to as eccrine syringofibroadenomatosis {456,2189}.

ICD-O code   8392/0

Synonyms

Eccrine syringofibroadenoma {663}, eccrine syringofibroadenomatous hyperplasia {1721}, eccrine syringofibroadenomatosis {456,2189}, acrosyringeal adenomatosis {950}.

Epidemiology

Syringofibroadenoma is rare, with about 75 reported cases. It occurs primarily in older adults.

Localization

Most of syringofibroadenomas arise on acral areas {498,685,769,2248,2313, 2344,2399}.

Clinical features

The most common clinical presentation is solitary, often verrucous papules or nodules {1529,2248,2313}. Unusual presentations include large plaques, linear lesions, and disseminated tumours {1259,2189,2248}.

Etiology

Occasionally, syringofibroadenoma can be associated with other entities, both inflammatory and neoplastic, including bullous pemphigoid {1720,1721}, lichen planus {780}, ulcers {1092,2399}, squamous cell carcinoma {1399}, sebaceous naevus {1719}, and chronic lymphoedema {806}. Based on the latter association and the presence of fibrous stroma, some authors consider syringofibroadenoma as a hyperplasia rather than a neoplasia {779,780,806,1092,1399,1719, 1720}. It may be associated with Schöpf-Schultz-Passarge syndrome {2189}, an autosomal dominant syndrome with palmoplantar keratoderma, hypodontia, and eyelid hidrocystomas, whose genetic aberration has been localized to chromosome 13q {1259}.

Histopathology

Syringofibroadenoma is characterized by multiple anastomosing cords and strands of monomorphous cuboidal cells {26,1529}. The epithelial cords extend usually into the mid-dermis, and are embedded in a loose fibrovascular stroma. Rarely, a clear cell variant has been observed {781,2415}.

Immunoprofile

Light microscopy usually leads to a specific diagnosis. The tumour cells are usually positive for both keratin 6 and 19 as well as filaggrin {1108,1304,1742,1745, 2314}.

Prognosis and predictive factors

Syringofibroadenoma is a benign condition, and solitary lesions are cured by complete excision, while the treatment of multiple lesions is dependent on the size and location. Cases of syringofibroadenoma with foci of atypical squamous cells have also been described {255, 1215}.

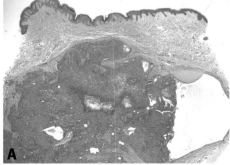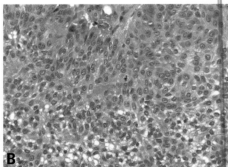

Fig. 3.28 Hidradenoma. **A** There is a multinodular solid and cystic proliferation of monomorphous adnexal keratinocytes. **B** Areas with cytoplasmic pallor are common ('clear cell hidradenoma').

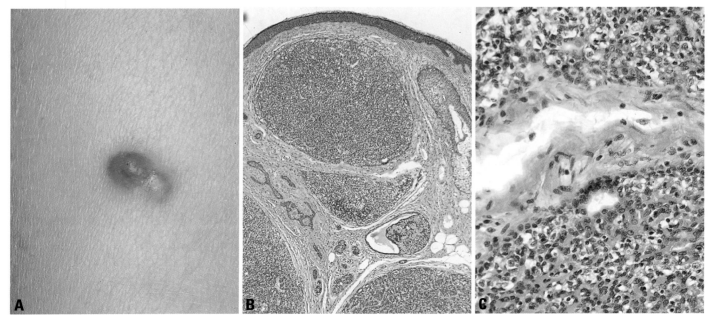

Fig. 3.29 Spiradenoma. **A** A pigmented and painful nodule on the posterior aspect of the arm. **B** These aggregations of neoplastic cells show round shape and smooth borders. **C** At higher magnification, numerous lymphocytes are seen scattered within the nodules of neoplastic epithelial cells. There are two distinct populations of neoplastic epithelial cells, dark and pale. Dark cells are small, basaloid cells with hyperchromatic nuclei and pale cells are larger with vesicular nuclei and ample pale cytoplasm.

Hidradenoma

Definition
Hidradenoma is a benign adnexal neoplasm, closely related to poroma, that displays a limited degree of ductal differentiation. While historically considered eccrine, recent evidence suggests that hidradenoma can be either apocrine or eccrine {825,1543}.

ICD-O code   8402/0

Synonyms
Clear cell hidradenoma, nodular hidradenoma, poroid hidradenoma, acrospiroma, solid-cystic hidradenoma {825,980,1374}.

Epidemiology
Hidradenomas are sporadic with no sex predilection. Most develop in adults, but childhood onset has been documented {715,1652}. Hidradenoma can also arise as a secondary neoplasm with naevus sebaceous.

Localization
Hidradenomas commonly develop on the scalp, trunk, and proximal extremities, and rarely on the hands and feet. Eyelid lesions have also been noted {911}.

Clinical features
Hidradenomas lack any distinctive clinical features, presenting as skin-coloured to red-brown nodules.

Histopathology
Hidradenoma is a mostly dermal neoplasm with a nodular, circumscribed pattern at scanning magnification. Sometimes an epidermal attachment can be identified. The intervening stroma is often sclerotic and may be highly vascularized, with ectatic vascular channels. Hidradenoma is composed of several types of cells:
Clear or pale cells, which contain abundant glycogen, and show distinct cell membranes {578}. The number of clear cells varies from lesion to lesion. When these cells predominate, the name clear-cell hidradenoma is appropriate {2544}.
Squamoid cells are polygonal with a central vesicular nucleus and eosinophilic cytoplasm, and often are arranged in whorls {1774}.
Mucinous cells are the least common component. They are large cells with fine basophilic granular cytoplasm. Cuboidal or columnar cells line the tubules and show evidence of apocrine differentiation {1427}.
Transition between different types of cells is frequent. The cells are arranged in sheets, punctuated by ducts and glandular areas which may show apocrine differentiation. Hybrid lesions including compact poroid cells with prominent ductal differentiation have been referred to as poroid hidradenomas.

Prognosis
Complete excision is curative.

Spiradenoma

Definition
Spiradenoma is a benign dermal neoplasm that can show either eccrine or apocrine differentiation, and significant morphologic overlap with cylindroma.

Historical annotation
Chandeluz, in 1882, probably first described this tumour {765}. Unna first coined the term spiradenoma. In 1956 Kersting and Helwig published the classic paper on spiradenoma in 136 patients {1250}. Additional series of spiradenoma have since been published {12,1496}.

ICD-O code   8403/0

Localization
Most spiradenomas appear on the face

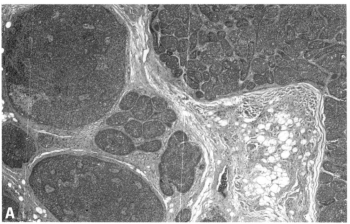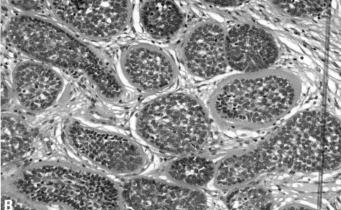

Fig. 3.30 Cylindroma. **A** There is a puzzle-like array of basaloid cells with relatively sharp circumscription of individual nodules. The larger nodules on the left show trabecular internal structure, suggesting overlap with spiradenoma. **B** The nests are outlined by a thick rim of PAS-positive and diastase-resistant basement membrane material.

and upper trunk, but they can also affect other sites.

Clinical features

Usually, spiradenoma appears as a solitary, well-circumscribed, firm nodule, measuring usually less than 1 cm, but giant variants {546} and multiple lesions have also been described {1725}. Unusual cases show multiple spiradenomas arranged in a zosteriform linear pattern {926,2162}. Spiradenoma appears in adult life, although there are also reports of congenital cases {2091}, and in one patient spiradenoma developed within a naevus sebaceous of Jadassohn {2154}. Pain is one of the main clinical characteristics of spiradenoma {926, 2091,2154}. The mechanism of pain or tenderness in spiradenoma is not clear.

Histopathology

At low power magnification, spiradenoma appears as a solid neoplasm composed of a single or few nodules of basaloid cells. These aggregations are round with smooth borders and involve the full thickness of the dermis, sometimes extending into the subcutaneous fat. Often, the intervening stroma is oedematous with ectatic vessels {546}. Dilated vessels rimmed by sclerosis have been interpreted as "ancient" changes due to long-standing lesions {2229}.

Another characteristic finding is the presence of abundant lymphocytes scattered within the tumour nodules. At higher magnification, two distinct populations of neoplastic epithelial cells can be seen, dark and pale. Dark cells are small,

basaloid cells with hyperchromatic nuclei located at the periphery, whereas pale cells, which are larger with vesicular nuclei and ample pale cytoplasm, tend to be near the centre of the clusters.

Tubules lined by two rows of epithelial cells may be found within the tumour nodules. A characteristic feature is the presence of eosinophilic PAS positive globules throughout the entire neoplasm, sometimes surrounded by neoplastic cells in pseudorosette fashion. These globules are composed of basement membrane material. Sometimes the stroma shows striking oedema.

Spiradenoma in children may show a different histopathologic pattern. The neoplastic cells appear more immature, making the distinction between clear and dark neoplastic epithelial cells difficult, and the neoplasm may be misinterpreted as a mesenchymal neoplasm {1206}.

Spiradenoma and cylindroma show significant morphological overlap. In some patients with multiple lesions, some tumours show features of spiradenoma, and others features of cylindroma. This supports the notion that spiradenoma and cylindroma are closely related, probably representing two morphologic expressions of the same basic neoplastic process {846,2280}.

Immunoprofile

The tumour cells express cytokeratins, and the tubular structures are CEA positive {1801,2465}. Inflammatory cells scattered within the neoplastic aggregations have been identified as abundant T lymphocytes and Langerhans cells.

Histogenesis

The histochemical and immunohistochemical studies have not clarified the histogenesis of spiradenoma. The frequent association of spiradenoma and cylindroma, a likely apocrine neoplasm, and the sporadic association of spiradenoma with neoplasms with follicular differentiation such as trichoepithelioma {2500}, support an apocrine line of differentiation for spiradenoma on the basis of the common embryologic origin for the three elements of the folliculo-sebaceous-apocrine unit. This is furthermore supported by some examples of spiradenoma that show decapitation secretion in the cells lining the luminal border of the tubular structures. Therefore, the qualifying term of "eccrine" that almost invariably is applied to spiradenoma is inaccurate.

Prognosis and predictive factors

Spiradenoma is a benign neoplasm. Because of the sharp demarcation of the tumour from the surrounding stroma, excision is easily accomplished. Several examples of carcinomas arising in long-standing spiradenomas have been described. In those instances, enlargement of a nodule that had been stable for many years seems to be the sign of malignant transformation {89,240,539, 699,884,2602}. It appears to be accompanied by increased expression of p53 protein {239}.

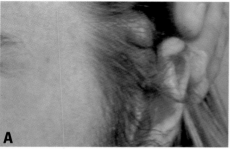 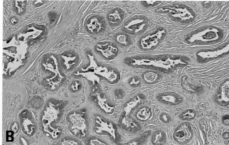 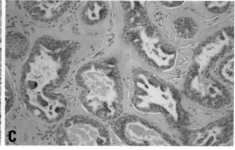

Fig. 3.31 Tubular adenoma. **A** A skin-coloured smooth surfaced nodule on the left parietal scalp. **B** Multiple irregularly shaped tubular glandular structures within a partly sclerosed stroma. **C** Banal appearing tubular glandular elements lined by a double layer of epithelial cells within a sclerosed stroma. The peripheral layer is cuboidal in appearance and the luminal layer demonstrates decapitation secretion. The lumina are filled with cellular debris and granular eosinophilic material.

Cylindroma

Definition
Cylindroma is a relatively undifferentiated benign adnexal neoplasm with a mosaic microscopical pattern. Cylindroma commonly occurs as a hybrid with spiradenoma, an event that has been referred to as cylindrospiradenoma or spiradenocylindroma {301,846,1543,1600}.

ICD-O code   8200/0

Synonyms
Cylindrospiradenoma {301}, spiradenocylindroma {1600}

Epidemiology
Cylindromas may be solitary or multiple, arising on a sporadic basis or as part of Brooke-Spiegler syndrome. There is no sex predilection.

Etiology
The etiology is unknown. A link to chromosome 9 seems likely for multiple spiradenomas and cylindromas in the context of the Brooke-Spiegler syndrome, as the gene has been mapped to 9p21 {951,1538}.

Localization
The vast majority of cylindromas occur on the scalp or face, especially in the vicinity of the ear. Uncommonly, cylindromas develop on the trunk or proximal extremity.

Clinical features
Cylindromas are typically smooth, dome-shaped hairless red-brown papules and nodules. Extensive scalp involvement can create clinical morphology resembling a headpiece ("turban tumour").

Cylindroma can rarely be found as a secondary neoplasm within naevus sebaceous.

Histopathology
Cylindroma is a mostly dermal and sometimes subcutaneous neoplasm with a multinodular, circumscribed pattern at scanning magnification. Individual nodules are composed of mosaic nests of undifferentiated basaloid cells with small darkly-staining nuclei and scant cytoplasm; individual nests fit tightly and neatly within larger nodules in a pattern that has been likened to that of a jigsaw puzzle. The nests of cylindroma are commonly surrounded by a rim of densely eosinophilic PAS-positive basement membrane material, and the nests are also punctuated by small round "droplets" with similar staining qualities. Hybrid lesions with areas of cylindroma and spiradenoma in juxtaposition are not uncommon {301,846,1543,1600}.

Immunoprofile and histogenesis
Refer to the previous chapter on spiradenoma.

Prognosis and predictive factors
Simple excision is usually curative. Malignant transformation is extremely uncommon.

Tubular and tubular papillary adenoma

Definition
Tubular apocrine adenoma is a benign dermal adnexal neoplasm demonstrating apocrine differentiation that typically occurs in a broad age group of women on the scalp region.

ICD-O code
Tubular adenoma   8211/0
Tubular papillary adenoma
                         8263/0

Synonyms
Apocrine adenoma, tubular adenoma, tubulopapillary hidradenoma, papillary tubular adenoma

Epidemiology
Tubular apocrine adenomas occur sporadically with a female predilection {1361}. A broad age group may be affected {1361}. Some neoplasms may occur in association with a syringocystadenoma papilliferum {76,489,1111, 2364} and can also arise within an organoid naevus {1111,1361,2394}.

Localization
Tubular apocrine adenomas commonly occur on the scalp and less often at other sites including the leg, trunk, axillary and anogenital areas {1361}.

Clinical features
Tubular apocrine adenomas present as asymptomatic solitary nodules that are skin-coloured to pink-red in appearance with either a smooth or irregular appearance {1361}. Most tumours range in overall dimension between 1 to 2 cm but rarely may be as large as 7 cm {1361}.

Histopathology
Tubular apocrine adenomas are well-circumscribed dermal neoplasms that may extend into the subcutis. They have an overall lobular architecture and are typically encased by a fibrous stroma. The lobules consist of multiple irregularly shaped tubular structures that have a double to several layered epithelial lining.

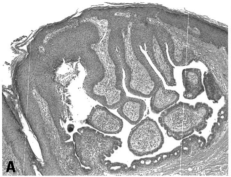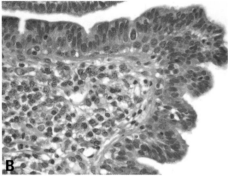

Fig. 3.32 Syringocystadenoma papilliferum. **A** Keratinizing squamous epithelium at the surface merges with columnar epithelium in the deeper portions of the tumour. **B** Papillary projections are lined by pseudostratified columnar epithelium, and plasma cells are typically noted in the stroma.

The peripheral epithelial layer consists of cuboidal to flattened cells (myoepithelial) and the luminal layer of columnar cells that demonstrate decapitation secretion. In some tubules papillary cellular extensions that are devoid of stroma project into the lumina. Additionally, cellular debris and eosinophilic granular material are identified within some lumina {1361}. The neoplasm lacks cytologic atypia and mitotic activity. Overlying epidermal hyperplasia may be present. In those neoplasms that occur in conjunction with syringocystadenoma papilliferum {76, 489,2364}, the tubular adenoma component is typically present underlying the syringocystadenoma component. The differential diagnosis includes apocrine adenocarcinoma and papillary eccrine adenoma. In contrast to apocrine adenocarcinoma tubular apocrine adenomas lack cytologic atypia, are well circumscribed and possess a peripheral myoepithelial layer {1751}. Tubular apocrine adenomas resemble papillary eccrine adenomas in many respects and previously these were believed to be related neoplasms {489}. However on the basis of morphologic criteria (papillary eccrine adenomas lack decapitation secretion) and enzyme histochemistry and ultrastructural analysis demonstrating differences in differentiation (apocrine versus eccrine) they are now believed to represent distinct neoplasms. In some instances both eccrine and apocrine differentiation may be observed making a distinction between these neoplasms impossible {771}. The terms tubulopapillary hidradenoma {705} and papillary tubular adenoma {2335} have been suggested for cases with apocrine and eccrine differentiation.

Histogenesis
Enzyme histochemistry {1361} and ultrastructural analysis {1361,2394} have demonstrated tubular apocrine adenomas to be of apocrine differentiation.

Prognosis
Tubular apocrine adenomas are benign slow-growing neoplasms. Simple excision is curative.

Syringocystadenoma papilliferum

Definition
Syringocystadenoma papilliferum is a benign adnexal neoplasm that occurs in association with an organoid naevus such as naevus sebaceous in at least one-third of cases.

ICD-O code
8406/0

Synonyms
Syringoadenoma

Epidemiology
Syringocystadenoma papilliferum occurs with equal frequency in both sexes. It is a tumour of childhood or adolescence, with many examples noted at birth. These lesions tend to increase in size at puberty, and sometimes multiply in number as well as becoming more papillomatous over time.

Clinical features
The majority of syringocystadenomas affect the head and neck area, typically as one or more warty papules, sometimes in a linear array, or as a solitary grey or red plaque. Scalp and neck are favoured sites; those on the scalp are typically alopecic. Syringocystadenomas may develop during puberty in a pre-existing naevus sebaceous, and at least one-third are associated with an underlying organoid naevus.

Histopathology
Histologically, endophytic invaginations of epithelium extend from the epithelial surface into the dermis. Typically squamous epithelium is present at the surface of the invaginations, and is contiguous with a double layer of cuboidal and columnar epithelium in the deeper portions of the lesion. Within the dermis, broad villous projections protrude into cystic spaces. Columnar epithelium is present toward the lumen of the spaces, and simple cuboidal epithelium can be seen at the periphery. Decapitation secretion of luminal cells is a frequent finding. Plasma cells are consistently numerous within the stroma, and are a highly reproducible finding in the stroma of syringocystadenomas.

The differential diagnosis includes hidradenoma papilliferum, which differs clinically by location in the perineal region, and histologically by dermal nodules showing a more complex papillary growth pattern, and absence of plasma cells in the stroma. The epithelial lining of the two lesions shows histologic overlap, however.

Precursor lesions
Approximately one-third of cases arise in organoid naevi.

Histogenesis
Syringocystadenomas show differentiation that is predominantly apocrine in pattern, but eccrine origin has been suggested in some cases, as exemplified by immunohistochemical labelling with eccrine marker IKH-4 {1109}. An intriguing finding is the presence of IgA and secretory component within the epithelial cells in syringocystadenomas, and IgA and well as IgG within the plasma cells {2420}. This observation suggests that plasma cells are attracted to tumour epithelium via a mechanism similar to that used by glands of the normal secretory immune system.

Somatic genetics
Allelic deletions of the patched gene 9q22 and loss of heterozygosity at 9p21

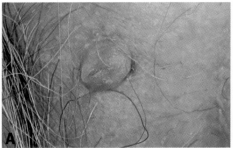
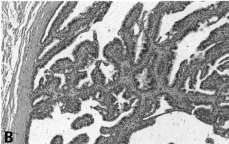
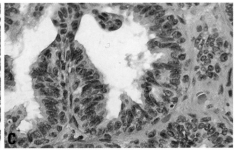

Fig. 3.33 Hidradenoma papilliferum. **A** Hidradenoma papilliferum of the vulva. A polypoid exophytic lesion involving the left labius majus of an elderly woman. **B** The neoplasm shows a prominent papillary pattern. **C** Columnar cells shows evidence of decapitation secretion in their luminal border.

(p16) have been reported in syringocystadenoma papilliferum {281}.

Prognosis and predictive factors
Syringocystadenomas are benign and simple excision is curative.

Hidradenoma papilliferum

Definition
Hidradenoma papilliferum is a benign cystic and papillary neoplasm that almost always develops in the vulval and perianal regions of middle-aged women.

ICD-O code   8405/0

Epidemiology
Most cases appear in women, although there are also reports in males {588, 1441,1697,2421}. The neoplasm is rare in Black patients. The age of presentation ranges from 20-90 years {2428, 2435}.

Localization
The skin of the vulva and perianal regions are the most frequently involved areas {588,1106,1441,1565,1568,1697, 2324,2421}, although rare examples of extra-genital or ectopic hidradenoma papilliferum have been reported on postauricular skin {247}, eyelids {1106, 1697,2056,2421}, external auditory canal {1718}, face {1106,1697} scalp {845}, axilla {1106,2421}, upper limb {2421}, back {727,1106} and thigh {2421}.

Clinical features
The lesion appears as a slow-growing cystic dermal nodule, usually asymptomatic, although it sometimes ulcerates and bleeds. The neoplasm is a unilateral skin-coloured nodule, papule or polypoid exophytic lesion, most commonly located on the labius majus.

Histopathology
At scanning magnification, hidradenoma papilliferum consists of a cystic neoplasm composed of elongated tubules and large papillary structures with a frond-like pattern. The papillae are composed of a central axis of connective tissue lined by two layers of epithelial cells. The basal layer is composed of pale-staining cuboidal myoepithelial cells and the luminal layer is made up by columnar cells with decapitation secretion. The cystic cavity and the lumina of the tubular structures contain apocrine secretions in the form of eosinophilic homogeneous material.
The epithelial cells at the periphery are flattened, and decapitation secretion is less evident, as a consequence of the pressure exerted by the cyst contents. The stroma surrounding the cystic cavity is composed of compressed fibrous tissue that is separated from the normal adjacent dermis by clefts. These clefts are responsible for the tendency of the neoplasm to shell out easily after incision of the epidermis.
In contrast with syringocystadenoma papilliferum, hidradenoma papilliferum is not connected with follicular infundibula and there are not plasma cells in the axis of connective tissue of the papillations. Sometimes, neutrophils are scattered within the connective tissue framework.

Immunoprofile
Immunohistochemical studies demonstrated that epithelial cells lining the papillations express low-molecular weight cytokeratins. The luminal border of the cells lining tubular structures is also decorated by carcinoembryonic antigen, epithelial membrane antigen and gross cystic disease fluid protein-15. Immunostains for S-100 protein and high-molecular-weight keratins are nega-

tive {2257}. Neoplastic epithelial cells lining tubules and papillations also express strong immunoreactivity for androgen and oestrogen receptors {1739}.

Histogenesis
Both the histopathologic and ultrastructural characteristics of hidradenoma papilliferum support an apocrine line of differentiation, although some authors have postulated the possibility of origin from Wolffian ducts or accessory mammary glands {576,1633}.

Prognosis and predictive features
Hidradenoma papilliferum is a benign neoplasm cured by simple excision. Malignant transformation is a very uncommon event {588,1730,2274,2460}. A case of adenosquamous carcinoma of the vulva developing from a pre-existing hidradenoma papilliferum has also been reported {142}.

Mixed tumour (chondroid syringoma)

Definition
Cutaneous mixed tumours are benign adnexal tumours of skin composed of epithelial and stromal elements with a wide spectrum of patterns. These tumours are histologically analogous to mixed tumours of the salivary gland, but lack the tendency for local recurrence seen in the latter lesions.

ICD-O code   8940/0

Synonyms
Chondroid syringoma, mixed tumour of skin.

Epidemiology
Mixed tumours most often occur as solitary slowly growing nodules on the head

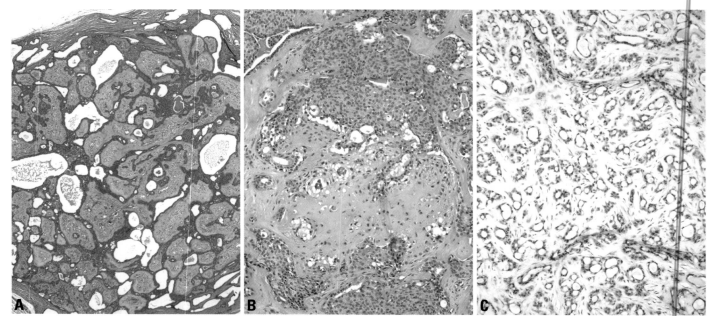

Fig. 3.34 Mixed tumour (chondroid syringoma). **A** Well-circumscribed mixed tumour with branching tubules and myxochondroid stroma. **B** Mixed tumour with epithelial tubules embedded in a myxoid and hyaline stroma. **C** Predominantely ductal epithelial pattern of mixed tumour.

and neck of adults, although other sites may be affected. There is a male predilection. Most lesions are between 1-3 cm in diameter, although examples as large as 6 cm have been reported {1182}.

Clinical features
Cutaneous mixed tumours present as asymptomatic dermal nodules, with no specific distinguishing clinical characteristics.

Histopathology
At low power, cutaneous mixed tumours are well-circumscribed lesions located in the dermis and/or subcutis. A biphasic growth pattern can be readily detected, with epithelial elements embedded within a myxoid, chondroid, or fibrous stroma. The epithelium often shows a pattern of branching tubules, sometimes with decapitation secretion suggesting apocrine differentiation. Solid cords and islands of epithelium as well as single cells may also be present. In some cases, the epithelial elements are composed of small non-branching tubules that may contain eosinophilic cuticles. Follicular differentiation occurs in some mixed tumours, in the form of follicular germinative cells, shadow cells, or sebocytes. Mixed tumours may exhibit clear cell change within the epithelial cells. In an estimated 40% of cases, mixed

tumours contain hyaline cells characterized by an ovoid shape, dense ground-glass or hyaline-like cytoplasm, and an eccentric nucleus {85}. The cells resemble plasma cells, and have been called plasmacytoid cells. In some cases, hyaline cells are the predominant cell type, leading to the term hyaline-cell rich chondroid syringoma {735}. The presence of hyaline cells appears to be of no prognostic significance, although such cells may present a diagnostic challenge to the unsuspecting pathologist {735}.

Immunoprofile
Immunohistochemical studies reveal staining of the inner layer of epithelial cells with cytokeratin, CEA, and EMA, and staining of the outer cellular layer with S100 and vimentin {2559}.
The stroma of mixed tumours usually comprises at least half of the lesion, and may show variable patterns of differentiation, including myxoid, fibroblastic, fibrocartilagenous, chondroid, and even osteoid components. Combinations of matrix components are the rule. Despite the name chondroid syringoma, chondroid areas may be absent in the stroma. The stroma stains strongly for alcian blue with hyaluronidase resistance.

Differential diagnosis
In mixed tumours where stroma predominates, the differential diagnosis includes

entities such as myxoma. In other lesions with abundant epithelial elements, the differential diagnosis includes benign adnexal tumours such as hidradenoma and syringoma, depending on the pattern of epithelial growth.

Histogenesis
It is generally accepted that there are both apocrine and eccrine variants of mixed tumours. Ultrastructural studies confirm that myoepithelial cells surround the epithelial cells, and appear to produce the stromal components of the lesions {2423}. The stroma of mixed tumours contains matrix components such as types II and IV collagen, tenascin, fibronectin, and laminin {773}. Ultrastructural and immunohistochemical studies of hyaline cells in mixed tumours suggest these cells derive from both the epithelial and stromal components of the lesions, possibly representing a regressive process {85}.

Prognosis
Cutaneous mixed tumours are benign lesions cured by simple excision.

Malignant tumours with follicular differentiation

S. Kaddu
L. Requena

Pilomatrical carcinoma

Definition
Pilomatrical carcinoma is the malignant counterpart of pilomatricoma.

ICD-O code   8110/3

Synonyms
Pilomatrix carcinoma, matrical carcinoma, invasive pilomatrixoma, malignant pilomatrixoma, matrix carcinoma.

Epidemiology
Pilomatrical carcinoma is an extremely rare tumour. Most cases present in adults with a broad age range {28,804,954, 2064}. The mean age at the time of diagnosis is about 48 years. The male to female ratio is 2:1.

Etiology
The majority of pilomatrical carcinomas develop de novo, although malignant transformation from a pre-existing pilomatricoma has been reported {2064}. It is conceivable that proliferating pilomatricoma, a variant of pilomatricoma that

occurs mainly in middle aged and elderly individuals, may represent an intermediate precursor lesion.

Localization
Pilomatrical carcinomas mostly occur in the head and neck, upper extremities and buttocks. Rare tumours have been reported in the axilla and inguinal regions.

Clinical features
The clinical appearance of pilomatrical carcinoma is generally not distinctive. Patients show solitary, occasionally ulcerated or fungating nodules ranging in size from 1-10 cm in diameter. Skin nodules are often of long duration ranging from several months to years before diagnosis, although occasional cases of recent onset and a history of rapid growth have been reported.

Histopathology
The tumour is a large, asymmetrical, poorly circumscribed dermal or dermal-subcutaneous mass composed of several, irregularly shaped and variously sized

aggregations of basaloid cells (matrical and supramatrical cells) {28,804,954, 2064}. Foci of cornified material containing shadow cells are characteristically observed within the basaloid cell aggregations. Some neoplasms show a variable desmoplastic stroma surrounding the basaloid cell aggregations. Focal connections of basaloid cell aggregations to the overlying epidermis and/or ulceration are often noted. Basaloid cells exhibit hyperchromatic nuclei, with one or more prominent nucleoli and ill-defined cytoplasmic margins as well as variable numbers of occasionally atypical mitotic figures (up to 10 mitoses per high-power field). Foci of geographical necrosis, calcification and ossification are observed. Mitotic activity is not a reliable indicator of malignancy, because mitoses are common in pilomatricoma. Other parameters, such as an infiltrative growth pattern, as well as angiolymphatic, perineural, and bone invasion, are more reliable features {804,2064}.

Immunoprofile
Immunohistological studies have previ-

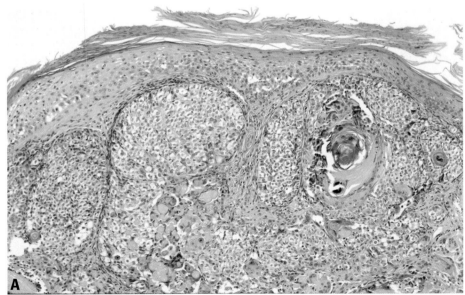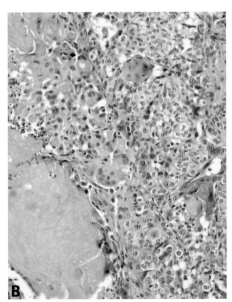

Fig. 3.35 Pilomatrical carcinoma. **A** The neoplastic cells are present in apposition to the epidermis. **B** A large mass of shadow (ghost) cells is present. The clear cells have more nuclear pleomorphism than in the pilomatricoma.

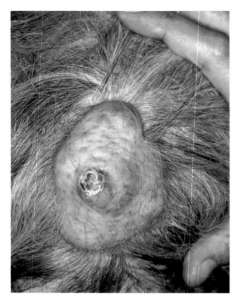

Fig. 3.36 Proliferating tricholemmal tumour. A large tumour on the scalp of an elderly woman.

ously revealed keratin staining in both basaloid and shadow cells {556}.

Prognosis and predictive factors

Treatment of choice is by surgical excision with adequate margins. Mohs micrographic surgery technique may be useful in treating some patients. Pilomatrical carcinoma is a mainly locally aggressive tumour which often recurs if not completely removed but very rarely shows distant metastases. Metastatic spread is evidenced by involvement of regional lymph nodes, lungs and/or bone.

Proliferating tricholemmal tumour

Definition

Proliferating tricholemmal tumour is a solid-cystic neoplasm that shows tricholemmal differentiation similar to that of the isthmus of the hair follicle.

ICD-O code   8103/1

Synonyms and historical annotation

Epidermoid carcinoma in sebaceous cyst {252,416} subepidermal acanthoma {1458}, proliferating epidermoid cyst {1152}, invasive hair matrix tumour of the scalp {1910}, trichochlamydocarcinoma {1053}, giant hair matrix tumour {583}, proliferating tricholemmal cyst {321}, proliferating pilar cyst {68,92}, proliferating follicular cystic neoplasm {23}, proliferating tricholemmal cystic squamous cell carcinoma {1631}, proliferating isthmic cystic carcinoma. These different names reflect the distinct histogenetic and biologic interpretations for this neoplasm among different authors.

Epidemiology

The neoplasm is more frequent in women than in men and most patients are elderly {2069}.

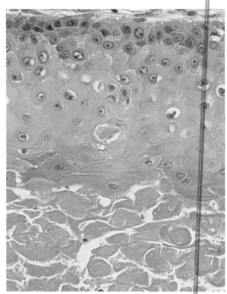

Fig. 3.37 Proliferating tricholemmal tumour. The lobules of the neoplastic epithelium show tricholemmal keratinization, characterized by peripheral palisading of small basaloid cells and large keratinocytes with ample eosinophilic cytoplasm that develop abrupt keratinization without previous granular layer, resulting in compact orthokeratotic eosinophilic keratin. This type of keratinization is similar to that of the outer sheath at the level of the isthmus of the hair follicle.

Localization

More than 90% of the lesions are situated on the scalp. Other described locations, in decreasing order of frequency, include face, trunk, back and forehead {2069}.

Clinical features

The tumour is a solitary, multilobular, large, exophytic mass, which may develop within a naevus sebaceous {866, 1874}. Multiple lesions are very rare. The size ranges from 2-10 cm in diameter, although lesions up to 25 cm in diameter have been described {407}. Alopecia and ulceration can be found.

Macroscopy

The lesions often show a multilobular appearance. The cystic structures often contain compact keratin and calcified material.

Histopathology

Proliferating tricholemmal tumour occurs on a morphologic continuum. On one end of the spectrum, it consists of a well-circumscribed solid and cystic neoplasm which involves the dermis and sometimes extends to the subcutaneous tis-

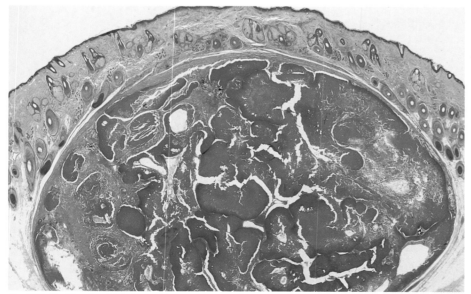

Fig. 3.38 Proliferating tricholemmal tumour. At scanning power the neoplasm appears as a well-circumscribed cystic neoplasm involving deeper dermis and subcutaneous tissue of the scalp.

play features of transepidermal elimination of shadow cells (perforating pilomatricoma) or a keratoacanthoma-like pattern. Old pilomatricoma lesions reveal no epithelial components but show irregularly shaped, partially confluent, focally calcified or metaplastically ossified shadow cell areas embedded in a desmoplastic stroma, with little or no inflammatory infiltrate. Extramedullary haematopoiesis has been observed in some regressing and old pilomatricoma lesions.

A subset of pilomatricomas, also termed "proliferating pilomatricoma", is characterized by the presence of relatively large, solid or solid-cystic basaloid cell areas with small foci of shadow cells {1170}. This variant presents mainly in middle aged and elderly individuals. "Matricoma" represents another unusual pilomatricoma variant characterized by discrete, small, solid aggregations of basaloid cells with several connections to pre-existing infundibula at different points {28}.

Molecular and cytogenetics
Derivation of pilomatricomas from the hair matrix has been underlined by recent biochemical studies demonstrating prominent staining of tumour cells with antibodies directed against LEF-1, a marker for hair matrix cells. Mutations in the gene CTNNB1 have been detected in up to 75% of pilomatricomas studied implicating beta-catenin/LEF misregulation as a possible cause of hair matrix cell tumourigenesis {438}. In another study, all 10 pilomatricomas examined were found to display strong bcl-2 immunostaining, a proto-oncogene well known to help in suppressing apoptosis in benign and malignant tumours {712}. This finding supports a role for faulty suppression of apoptosis in the pathogenesis of pilomatricomas.

Prognosis and predictive factors
Treatment is recommended mainly to avoid a foreign body reaction and inflammation with eventual scarring. Surgical excision is usually curative, but occasional recurrences may be observed. Spontaneous regression has been reported in a few cases. Malignant transformation has only been suspected in a single case of pilomatrical carcinoma {2064}.

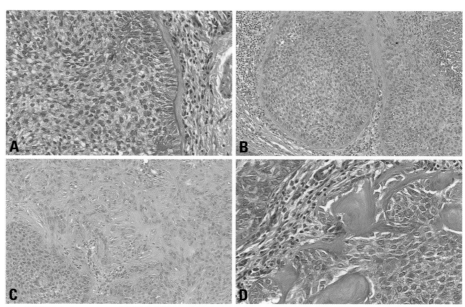

Fig. 3.43 Tricholemmoma. **A** Thick PAS-positive basement membrane. **B** Focal necrosis within bulbous follicular hyperplasia. Thickened basement membrane. **C** Desmoplastic stroma with entrapped bizarre epithelial strands ("pseudoinvasive interface"). **D** PAS-positive desmoplastic stroma and basement membrane.

Tricholemmoma

Definition
Tricholemmoma (TL) is a benign folliculo-infundibular proliferation occurring frequently but not exclusively on the face of adults. Multiple tricholemmomas may be associated with Cowden disease.

ICD-O code
Tricholemmoma   8102/0
Multiple tricholemmomas 8102/0

Synonyms
Trichilemmoma

Epidemiology
TL is a relatively common cutaneous proliferation that occurs mostly in adults and affects both sexes equally {323}. Multiple TLs, often in conjunction with acral keratoses, palmar pits, and oral fibromas, are a cutaneous marker of Cowden disease (multiple hamartoma and neoplasia syndrome) {322,325,681,2025,2247, 2249-2251}.

Localization
TL arises on the head and neck, almost exclusively on the face, favouring the centrofacial area. Rarely, TL may occur in naevus sebaceous {410,1979}.

Clinical features
Patients usually present with a solitary asymptomatic exophytic centrofacial lesion which is either wart-like with verrucous and keratotic features or dome shaped with a smooth surface. Individual lesions are small, varying in diameter between 3 and 8 mm {28}. Multiple facial TLs are almost invariably associated with Cowden disease {2247,2249-2251}.

Histopathology
Most cases of TL present as a sharply circumscribed superficial exo-endophytic proliferation with a papillated surface. There is marked parakeratosis, hyperkeratosis, and wedge-shaped hypergranulosis of the infundibula, in conjunction with a collarette of embracing adnexal epithelium {28,323}. TL does not involve the interfollicular epidermis. The dominating histological pattern of TL is that of a bulbous infundibular hyperplasia with tricholemmal differentiation, akin to the outer root sheath of the hair follicle {28}. There are one or more bulbous lobules, always in continuity with the epidermis. These lobules consist of numerous pale and clear isomorphic epithelia, most of which are PAS positive. At the periphery, pale columnar cells are arranged in a palisade, bordered by a prominent PAS-

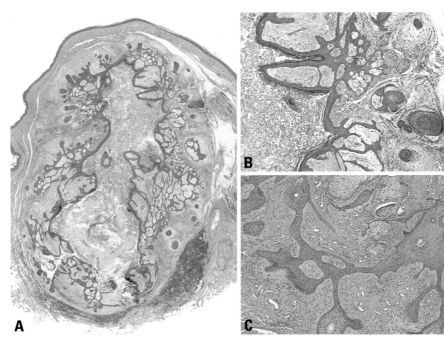

Fig. 3.44 Trichofolliculoma. **A** Note reticulate pattern of vellus follicles in devolution. **B** Detail. Reticulate epithelial strands, sebaceous lobules and few vellus follicles. **C** Note sebaceous lobules and dense fibrotic stroma. Vellus follicles in different stages of devolution.

and type IV collagen-positive basement membrane. Central foci of epidermal / infundibular keratinization, occasional small and inconspicuous squamous eddies, and keratinous microcysts in larger lesions are occasional findings {28}. There are no mitoses.

Desmoplastic tricholemmoma is a variant of TL characterized by a highly desmoplastic stroma with broad zones of sclerosis and distinctive artifactual clefts. Instead of "pushing" smooth lobular contours there may be a pseudoinvasive interface akin to pseudocarcinomatous epithelial hyperplasia, simulating carcinomatous growth {1079,2333}.

Differential diagnosis

Warts, basal cell carcinomas, squamous cell carcinomas, trichoblastomas, seborrhoeic keratoses, and keratosis follicularis inversa may contain areas of tricholemmal differentiation {31,1931}. The tumour of the follicular infundibulum exhibits a plate-like pattern with interconnecting horizontally-oriented epithelial strands. Inverted follicular keratosis consists of basaloid and squamous epithelia, associated with large numbers of squamous eddies (i.e. concentric layers of squamous cells in a whorled pattern, sometimes keratinized).

Histogenesis

According to strict topographical anatomical criteria, TL arises from the follicular infundibulum and differentiates toward the outer [tricholemmal] root sheath {28}. Its superficial folliculo-infundibular location militates against the classification of TL as a neoplasm of the lower portion of the hair follicle (i.e. the [outer] tricholemmal sheath).

However, it is still a matter of debate whether TL is of hamartomatous/neoplastic {318,991,1906,1931} or of viral origin {15,28,31}. The detection of HPV DNA in tricholemmomas by PCR {2688} favours the latter view of TL as a resolving verruca vulgaris with tricholemmal differentiation {15,28, 31}.

Prognosis and predictive factors

TL is an entirely benign cutaneous neoplasm. Multiple TLs are a hallmark of Cowden disease and should prompt a search for internal malignancy.

Trichofolliculoma

Definition

Trichofolliculoma (TF) is a follicularly differentiated hamartoma generally appearing during adult life.

ICD-O code   8101/0

Epidemiology

TF represents a rare hamartoma mostly occurring during adulthood (with a wide range of ages between 11 and 77 years {28}) without sex predilection {887}.

Localization

TF favours the head and neck region, foremost the face. Most lesions are situated around the nose {887}.

Clinical features

TF presents as a solitary asymptomatic dome-shaped lesion with a smooth surface and a widely dilated central ostium from which a small tuft of delicate white hairs emerges. Lesions are small, ranging between 0.5 and 1.0 cm in diameter {28}.

Histopathology

The main histological features of TF are reflected by its "Caput Medusae" pattern {28}: embedded in a highly fibrocytic stroma, large numbers of vellus follicles with upper and lower segments like those of normal follicles radiate from the perimeter of a dilated infundibulum.

TF is a symmetrical, well-circumscribed, vertically oriented lesion composed of three components: infundibulo-cystic, follicular, and stromal {28}. The centre of the lesion is occupied by one or more widely dilated infundibulo-cystic structures that are continuous with the epidermis and open to the surface of the skin through an ostium. The cystic lumina may be filled with innumerable corneocytes and vellus hairs. From the epithelial walls of the infundibular cystic spaces smaller infundibula radiate, to which are attached vellus follicles in various numbers. These vellus follicles are not associated with muscles of hair erection or with sebaceous ducts, albeit sebaceous cells arranged as solitary units or in lobules may occur within the lining epithelium of the central infundibulo-cystic structure.

The morphology of the individual vellus follicles may vary from normal to strikingly aberrant {28}. Normal vellus follicles may exhibit all stages of the follicular cycle {2106}. The whole lesion is embedded in a cellular connective tissue sheath, which is separated from the adjacent normal dermis by prominent shrinkage clefts. The highly fibrocytic stroma which surrounds the individual vellus follicle resembles perifollicular sheath {28}. The existence of considerable numbers of Merkel cells in all trichofolliculomas underlines their classification as hamartomas with follicular differentiation {967}.

Variants

TF is a complex lesion with protean features {28}. Some of these are caused by the evolutionary and devolutionary alteration of the vellus hair follicles in their regular biological cycles {2106}. In this context, folliculo-sebaceous cystic hamartoma {1275,2187} may be interpreted as a TF at its very late stage with nearly complete regression of the transient follicular epithelium, but with concurrent growth and maturation of sebaceous elements {2105}. Sebaceous trichofolliculoma {1846} exhibits distinct sebaceous lobules at its outer circumference, but lacks vellus follicles that radiate from the epithelial lining of the dilated infundibulum. The latter criterion militates against the classification of sebaceous trichofolliculoma as a true TF {28}. Hair follicle naevus is regarded as a TF that was histologically sampled at its periphery {28}. There is a striking predominance of mature vellus follicles and the central infundibular lumen may be quite inconspicuous.

Prognosis and predictive factors

TF represents an entirely benign cutaneous hamartoma with no reports of tumour progression or aggressive clinical course.

Pilar sheath acanthoma

Definition

Pilar sheath acanthoma is a follicular neoplasm differentiated toward the permanent part of the hair follicle, to wit, the infundibulum and the isthmus. [The infundibulum is an extension of epidermis to meet the isthmus, but both function as part of the follicular sheath].

Synonyms
Infundibuloisthmicoma

Clinical features

Pilar sheath acanthomas affect adults of either sex, and are identified usually on the face. They are small, solitary papules up to 5 mm in diameter, with a central 1-

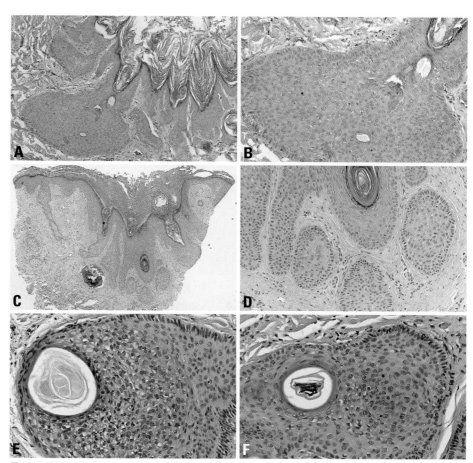

Fig. 3.45 Pilar sheath acanthoma. **A** The characteristic infundibular and isthmic differentiation is stereotyped. Note the lack of a hair filament or inner root sheath. **B** The lobule contains red-pink corneocytes, characteristic of the isthmus. **C** This pilar sheath acanthoma does not have the obvious widened ostium, but it does contain the lobules of isthmic epithelium. **D** The lobules have a nearly syncytial pattern. **E** This lobule has clear-cell changes and syncytial, pink cell changes. Note the lack of inner sheath or hair filament. **F** The small, partly cornified cyst seen here contains no hair filament. Parts of the transient portion of the follicle are rarely seen in pilar sheath acanthoma.

2 mm punctum, lacking hair filaments, and will express corneocytes if squeezed. There are no known associated syndromes and no known genetic abnormalities within the neoplasms {29, 232,473,1570,2212,2402}.

Histopathology

The classical example consists of a patulous infundibulum that connects with lobules of epithelium differentiated toward both the infundibulum and the isthmus. This differentiation results in blue-gray (infundibular) and pink (isthmic) corneocytes that fill the follicular canal. There can be a minor component of stem or bulb (or both) differentiation in some examples. Consequently there is, as a rule, no evidence of hair filaments in these neoplasms.

Differential diagnosis

Pilar sheath acanthoma should be differentiated from dilated pore (Winer), trichofolliculoma, and fibrofolliculoma/trichodiscoma. Dilated pore is an infundibular cyst that has proliferated minimally, but lacks isthmic differentiation.

Trichofolliculoma is a hamartoma and contains fully formed vellus hair follicles that radiate around a centrally positioned cyst. Fibrofolliculoma/trichodiscoma is also a hamartoma found characteristically in the Birt-Hogg-Dubé syndrome and that contains thin strands of infundibular epithelium connected so that fenestrations of delicate fibrous stroma are found within. Additionally, considerable stroma, lacking epithelium, is often identified (trichodiscoma).

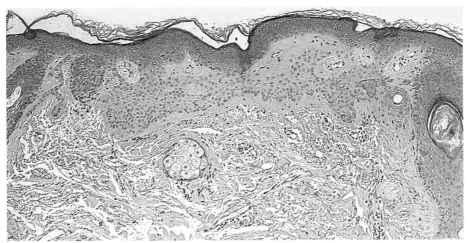

Fig. 3.46 Histopathology of a typical tumour of the follicular infundibulum, with horizontal proliferation of pale keratinocytes in the papillary dermis. Note the connection with the overlying epidermis.

Prognosis and predictive factors
The neoplasm is benign; no treatment is necessary.

Tumour of the follicular infundibulum

Definition
Tumour of the follicular infundibulum (TFI) is a benign epithelial neoplasm of follicular origin.

Synonym
Infundibular tumour.

Epidemiology
TFI is an uncommon tumour occurring in adults, mainly after the age of 50. In two studies, TFI accounted for less than 10 per 100,000 skin samples. They can be observed on the face of patients with Cowden syndrome or on the surface of naevus sebaceous.

Localization and clinical features
Solitary TFI is mainly localized on the face and presents as a small flesh-coloured nodule, resembling basal cell carcinoma. Multiple or eruptive TFI present as hundreds of symmetrically distributed hypopigmented geometric macules localized on the face, neck, trunk, or on the periocular area. Sun exposure increases the contrast between normal skin and the tumours.

Histopathology
TFI is a plate-like horizontal proliferation of pale keratinocytes, which is localized in the papillary dermis and shows multiple connections with the overlying epidermis or with the infundibulum. The cells are paler and larger than normal keratinocytes and their cytoplasm stains with PAS. The tumour is sharply circumscribed and limited by a dense network of elastic fibres easily demonstrated by orcein staining. Desmoplastic and sebaceous variants have been described {557,1485}.

Histogenesis
TFI derives from the normal follicular infundibulum. The occurrence of multiple TFI suggests a possible genetic basis, which remains to be established.

Prognosis and predictive factors
The prognosis is good, except in rare patients with multiple TFI who may develop basal cell carcinomas.

Fibrofolliculoma / trichodiscoma

Definition
Fibrofolliculoma and trichodiscoma are different developmental stages in the life of one single benign appendageal hamartomatous tumour, which differentiates towards the mantle of the hair follicle {27}. Fibrofolliculoma represents the early and trichodiscoma the late stage in the development of this lesion {27}.

ICD-O code   8391/0

Synonyms
Trichodiscoma first was erroneously thought to arise from or to differentiate toward the hair disk (Haarscheibe) and therefore bears this name {1836}. Fibrofolliculoma was often used for perifollicular fibroma in the past. Neurofollicular hamartoma and trichodiscoma are the same {2048}. "Mantleoma" was used as the overall term for both fibrofolliculoma and trichodiscoma {27}.

Epidemiology
Fibrofolliculomas/trichodiscomas are rare appendageal tumours, occurring equally in males and females, usually not before the third decade of life.

Etiology
The etiology of the solitary lesions is unknown. The Birt-Hogg-Dubé (BHD) gene was mapped to 17p11.2 {1256}.

Localization
The preferred sites of location are the face, neck and chest.

Clinical features
Fibrofolliculomas and trichodiscomas cannot be distinguished clinically {248}.

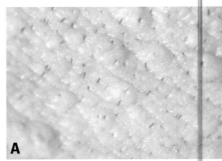
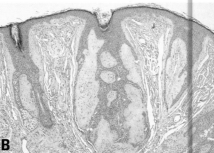

Fig. 3.46A Fibrofolliculoma / trichodiscoma. **A** Multiple fibrofolliculomas and trichodiscomas in a patient with BHD. **B** Fibrofolliculoma. Three adjacent dilated follicular infundibula with bizarre mantle-like proliferations are embedded in a prominent specialized stroma, well demarcated from the surrounding dermis.

plify the nomenclature of the different benign sebaceous adnexal tumours and to summarize them under one name {2003}.

Genetics

Little is known about the genetics of sebaceous adenoma. Most of the tumours occur as solitary lesions but a few examples of SA are part of the spectrum of different sebaceous tumours in MTS. By immunohistochemistry it is possible to look for a loss of MSH-2, MLH-1 repair proteins. Tumours related to a mismatch repair gene defect show a microsatellite instability in a high percentage {1334}.

Prognosis and predictive factors

Sebaceous adenomas are benign tumours. If the patient has Muir-Torre syndrome, the prognosis depends on the associated internal malignancies.

Sebaceoma

Definition

Sebaceoma is a benign, adnexal neoplasm with sebaceous differentiation. It is characterized by multiple, smooth-bordered lobules and cystic spaces composed primarily of immature sebaceous cells admixed with randomly scattered mature sebocytes.

ICD-O code   8410/0

Synonyms

Sebaceous epithelioma, basal cell epithelioma with sebaceous differentiation, and sebomatricoma.

Epidemiology

Sebaceomas are rare sebaceous neoplasms that may be associated with the Muir-Torre syndrome {1624,2114}. They typically arise in late adulthood with the mean age of diagnosis being at approximately 70 years of age, but may be seen in early adulthood {2378}. The tumours have a predilection for females.

Localization

Sebaceomas occur mainly on the face and scalp, with rare cases reported on the trunk {226,636,1710,1749,1922, 2258,2378}.

Clinical features

Clinically, sebaceomas present as yellow to orange solitary papules on the head and neck {636,2258,2378}. Those lesions associated with the Muir-Torre syndrome may be multiple {347,1624, 2114}. They are slow-growing neoplasms and do not recur after excision {636, 2258,2378}.

Histopathology

Architecturally sebaceoma is composed of multiple well-circumscribed lobules of various size centred on the dermis. The lobules often contain ducts and cystic areas containing holocrine secretion and only rarely do they connect with the overlying epidermis. A brightly eosinophilic cuticular material lines both the ducts and cysts, similar to what is seen in the normal sebaceous ducts.

Cytologically the neoplasm is comprised predominantly of small, uniform basaloid cells with bland nuclear features admixed with haphazardly distributed mature-appearing sebaceous cells. The mature sebaceous cells have abundant vacuolated cytoplasm and ovoid nuclei, which often have a scalloped nuclear membrane. Rare typical mitoses may be seen, however, atypical mitosis and necrosis are not features of sebaceoma. The surrounding stroma is dense, eosinophilic connective tissue. There is no cleft seen between the neoplasm and the stroma, as is the case with basal cell carcinoma.

A wide variety of patterns have been described for sebaceoma, sometimes even within the same neoplasm. These include reticulated, cribriform and glandular {634,1710}. There have been reports of a variant with eccrine differentiation, a pigmented variant and a sebaceoma that arose in a seborrhoeic keratosis {226,1749,1922}. Those lesions that arise in Muir-Torre syndrome may have a keratoacanthoma-like architecture {347}.

Immunoprofile

Immunohistochemistry demonstrates positivity with high-molecular weight keratin. EMA stains most mature sebocytes, and thus will only show positivity of the mature vacuolated sebaceous cells scattered amongst the tumour, while the basaloid cell compartment will be negative {1710}. Several reports have demonstrated loss of heterozygosity as well as

microsatellite instability in a marker gene located near hMSH2 in patients with sebaceoma and Muir-Torre syndrome {1332,1536}. By immunohistochemistry it is possible to look for a loss of MSH-2, MLH-1 repair proteins {1334}.

Prognosis and predictive factors

Sebaceoma is a benign neoplasm that does not recur after treatment or metastasize. It may be a marker of Muir-Torre syndrome, in which case the patient has a high risk of internal malignancies.

Cystic sebaceous tumour

Definition

Cystic sebaceous tumour is a large distinctive tumour with is almost always associated with Muir-Torre syndrome (MTS) {1999}.

ICD-O code   8410/0

Epidemiology

Cystic sebaceous tumours occur nearly exclusively in MTS, which is a phenotypical variant of the hereditary non polyposis colon cancer syndrome (HNPCC). MTS is inherited in an autosomal-dominant fashion and is caused by genetic alterations within the DNA mismatch repair system. Patients often have a family history of malignancies and most are affected with a variety of internal malignancies such as colon cancer, urothelial cancer, endometrial cancer and others. MTS patients develop a broad spectrum of different sebaceous skin tumours, which may be difficult to classify {347, 1624}, and keratoacanthomas. Among the sebaceous tumours, CSTs are unique because they serve as diagnostic markers for the syndrome. MTS has a male preponderance and is clinically diagnosed mostly in adults older than 40 years.

Localization

The upper trunk is the most common location.

Clinical features

CSTs are usually solitary, but rarely can be multiple. They resemble hair follicle cysts and present as dermal nodules. In patients diagnosed with internal malignancies CST is often excised in order to rule out a metastatic skin lesion.

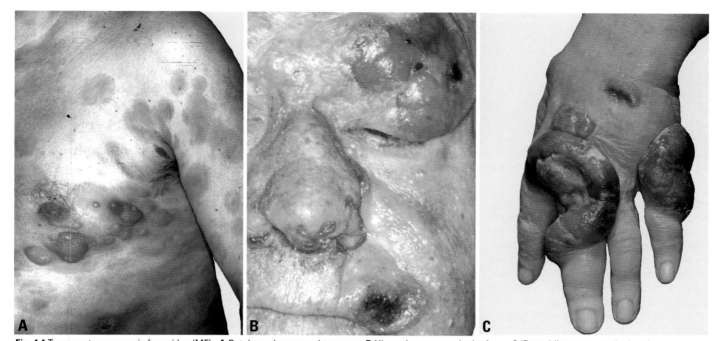

Fig. 4.4 Tumour-stage mycosis fungoides (MF). **A** Patches, plaques and tumours. **B** Ulcerating tumours in the face. **C** 'Fungoid' tumours on the hands.

the presence of more than 25% blast cells may be observed.

Immunoprofile
The immunophenotypical prototype of MF is CD2+, CD3+, CD4+, CD5+, CD45RO+, CD8, TCR-beta+, CD30-. During progression of the disease loss of CD7, 2 and 5 can occur. Helpful in the diagnosis is the loss of CD7, CD2, CD5, or CD4 in the epidermotropic cerebriform cells. During progression of the disease especially when transformation is present CD4 positive epidermotropic cells can have a cytotoxic phenotype (TIA-1, Granzyme B). In the transformed stage the blast cells can express CD30. Besides the CD4 prototype, a small number of MF cases have a CD8 positive cytotoxic phenotype (TIA-1 and gran-

zyme B). These cases have the same clinical behaviour as the CD4 positive cases.

Prelymphomatous precursor lesions
The term "parapsoriasis" is confusing and requires explanation. It encompasses a number of different pathologic states clinically manifested by chronic recalcitrant erythematous scaling lesions {311,312,1375}.
Two groups of parapsoriasis can be differentiated {337}. The benign form 'parapsoriasis en plaques' (Brocq disease), never evolve into malignant lymphoma. The large plaque forms (LPP) with poikiloderma (prereticulotic poikiloderma, parapsoriasis en grandes plaques poikilodermiques, poikiloderma vasculare atrophicans, parapsoriasis lichenoides,

parakeratosis variegata) or without poikiloderma (parapsoriasis en plaques, premalignant type, parapsoriasis en grandes plaques simples), may after several decades evolve into mycosis fungoides or CTCL in up to 10-50% of cases. Few large (more than 5 cm in diameter) patches show pityriasiform scaling with (poikilodermatous variant) or without telangiectasia and netlike pigmentation. There is no palpable infiltration.
Histologically lesions in large plaque parapsoriasis (LPP) are different from MF or other CTCL. Under patchy parakeratosis there is slight atrophy of the epidermis, due to loss of rete ridges. The subepidermal zone is free of lymphocytes, which accumulate in a band-like arrangement in the upper dermis, spar-

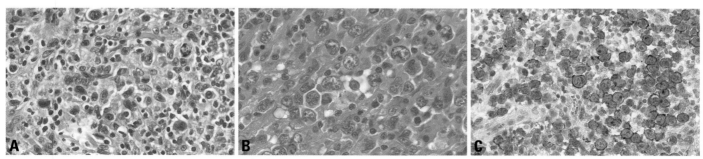

Fig. 4.5 Histopathology of transformed mycosis fungoides(MF). **A** Large-cell pleomorphic transformation. **B** Large cell anaplastic transformation. **C** Immunohistochemistry reveals CD30 positive tumour-cells.

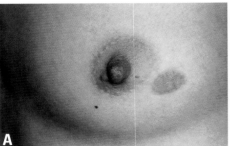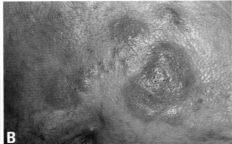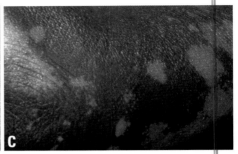

Fig. 4.6 A Plaque in mono-lesional mycosis fungoides (MF). **B** Symptomatic mucinosis follicularis in MF. **C** Hypo-pigmented lesions in MF.

ing the papillary region. There is no significant epidermotropism as usually seen in early stages of mycosis fungoides. The poikilodermatous variant of the diseases in addition shows dilated blood vessels in the upper dermis. T-cell receptor gamma gene rearrangement, which is clonal in about half of the patients with LPP, is without any prognostic significance {2186}. There is no significant difference between the observed and expected survivals in patients with LPP.

Histogenesis

Mature skin homing T cells that express the cutaneous lymphocyte antigen (CLA) enabel them to specifically home into the skin. Functionally, the neoplastic cells in MF express TH2 phenotype, which accounts for many systemic changes associated with MF due to the production of a TH2-specific cytokine pattern (IL-4, IL-5, IL-10) leading to fever, oedema, eosinophilia, increase of IgE or IgA, and impaired delayed type reactivity {656,2445}.

Somatic genetics

There have been a few reports on familial occurence of MF or CTCL {2160} and on a possible association of HLA-DR5 with MF {2004}. HLA class II susceptibility alleles, i.e. HLA-DRB1*11, HLA-DQB1*03 and HLA-DRB1*1104 are more prevalent among patients with MF and are likely to be important in the pathogenesis of MF {1039,1118}. T-cell receptor beta and gamma chain genes are clonally rearranged. In advanced cases with extracutaneous involvement, the same clone is usually detected in the skin and in the extracutaneous lesions. In transformed cases the same clone is present in the pre-existing lesions and the high-grade lymphoma {207}.

In advanced stage, the rate of chromosomal aberrations, especially of chromosomes 1, 6 and 11, increase with the activity of the disease and has prognostic significance in patients with MF. Aberrations of chromosomes 8 and 17 are especially associated with active or progressive disease.

Chromosomal abnormality possibly results in increased genetic instability as a basic prerequisite for the development of CTCL. In G-banding studies, numerical aberrations of chromosomes 6, 13, 15, and 17, marker chromosomes, and structural aberrations of chromosomes 3, 9, and 13 were increased in MF {1209}. In contrast to nodal lymphomas, the large cell transformation in cutaneous T-cell lymphoma (CTCL) is not associated with t(2;5)(p23;q35) chromosomal translocation {613,1420}.

Increased expression of C-myc, p62, TP53 and proliferation markers (PCNA) has been found in advanced stages of MF as compared to early stages of MF suggesting a relationship between levels of these proteins and aggressiveness of CTCL {1192}.

Prognosis and predictive factors

The majority of MF patients show an indolent clinical course over years or decades. The prognosis of the disease is defined by its stage. Patients with early

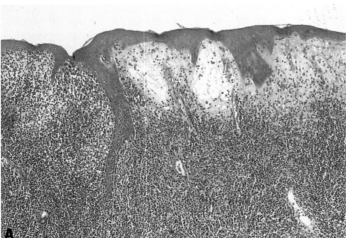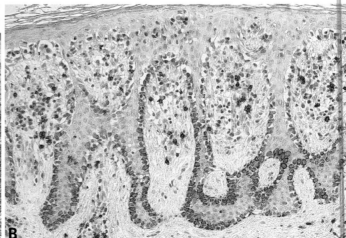

Fig. 4.7 Mycosis fungoides (MF). **A** Bullous variant of MF. **B** Immunohistochemistry shows CD8 positive tumour-cells lining up in the basal layer.

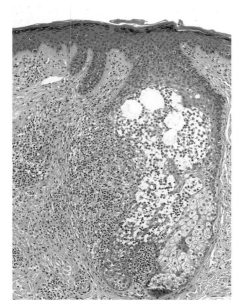

Fig. 4.8 Mucinous follicular variant of MF.

stages, i.e. with patches or thin plaques, without involvement of lymph nodes, peripheral blood or other extracutaneous compartment have an excellent prognosis with survival similar to that of an age, sex, and race-matched population {2575}.

Advanced stage and age above 60 years of age indicate a poor prognosis. When extracutaneous involvement or transformation into high-grade lymphoma occurs, expected survival is usually less than one year {2367,2412}.

Variants

Apart from the classical form of MF, there are several variants of this disease with unusual or atypical clinical and/or histopathological features. These comprise follicular, bullous, dyshidrotic, granulomatous, hypopigmented, poikilodermic, hyperpigmented, pigmented purpu-

ra-like, unilesional, palmoplantar, hyperkeratotic/verrucous, vegetating/papillomatous, ichthyosiform, pustular and other forms {1234}.

Pagetoid reticulosis, syringotropic MF, folliculotropic (pilotropic) and granulomatous MF also are variants and deserve special emphasis.

Pagetoid reticulosis

Pagetoid reticulosis, in its localized form also referred to as Woringer-Kolopp disease (WKD) {302,2550} clinically presents as a solitary, slowly growing psoriasiform crusty or hyperkeratotic patch or plaque, typically on a distal limb.

The histological hallmark is the sponge-like disaggregation of the epidermis by small to medium-sized lymphoid cells (pagetoid) which immunophenotypically correspond to those found in MF in most of the cases {336}. However, the neoplastic cells in WKD often demonstrate a higher proliferation rate (>30%) in comparison to lymphocytes in patch or plaque stage MF (<10%), and in some cases infiltrates in WKD may contain high numbers of CD30+ cells {937}. CD8+ {792} variants have also been reported. There exists a disseminated form featuring the same distinct pagetoid pattern of the infiltrate {1252}, which is now regarded as a separate disease, primary cutaneous aggressive epidermotropic CD8+ cytotoxic T-cell lymphoma.

Syringotropic MF

Syringotropic MF represents a rare variant of MF {2586} showing a solitary well circumscribed red-brown plaque with hair loss in the affected area. Histology reveals predominant involvement of

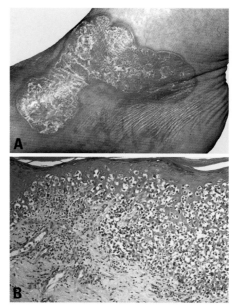

Fig. 4.9 Pagetoid reticulosis. **A** Solitary psoriasiform lesion on the foot. **B** Pagetoid reticulosis showing sponge-like disaggregation of the epidermis by invading haloed lymphoid cells.

irregularly proliferating eccrine sweat glands by small cerebriform lymphocytes {343,2586}.

Folliculotropic MF

Follicular MF, also referred to as pilotropic MF {776} is a rare variant, histopathologically characterized by infiltrates of atypical T lymphocytes around and within the epithelium of the hair follicles with sparing of interfollicular skin. The follicles may show cystic dilatation and/or cornified plugging. There may or may not be mucinosis. When present, mucinous degeneration of the follicular epithelium varies from focal spots of mucin deposition to complete destruction of follicles with mucin lakes. The folliculotropism is

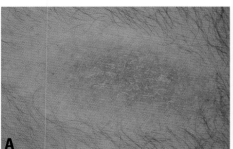
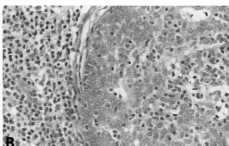
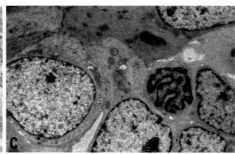

Fig. 4.10 Syringotropic cutaneous T-cell lymphoma (CTCL). **A** Cutaneous patch with hair-loss. **B** Infiltration of a sweat gland. **C** EM showing the convoluted nucleus of a neoplastic cell between acinar cells.

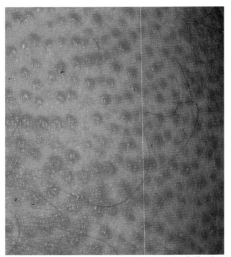

Fig. 4.11 Pilotropic lymphoid infiltrate in follicular mycosis fungoides (MF).

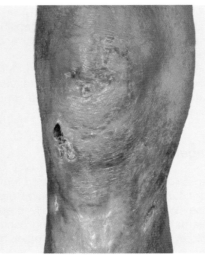

Fig. 4.12 Granulomatous MF. Granulomatous plaques with ulceration on the leg.

possibly due to an increased expression of skin-selective homing receptors and adhesion molecules in the follicular epithelium {1805}. A recent study has demonstrated that follicular MF shows a more aggressive behaviour and a worse prognosis than classical MF {829,2411}.

Granulomatous MF

Granulomatous MF is characterized by the histological presence of a granulomatous reaction {584}, sometimes featuring a sarcoidal or granuloma annulare-like pattern. Multinucleated giant cells may be present {1387}.
The prognostic and clinical significance of a granulomatous reaction in MF remains uncertain {454}.

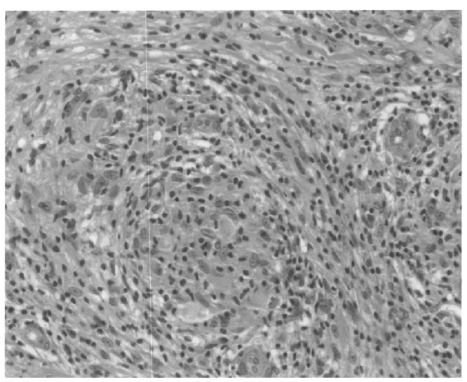

Fig. 4.13 Granulomatous mycosis fungoides (MF) with sarcoidal infiltrate pattern.

Sézary syndrome

R. Russell-Jones
M. Bernengo
G. Burg
L. Laroche

S. Michaelis
E. Ralfkiaer
E. Vonderheid
S. Whittaker

Definition

Sézary syndrome (SS) is a rare variant of cutaneous T-cell lymphoma (CTCL), characterized by erythroderma, blood involvement and a poor prognosis. Neoplastic lymphocytes are typically mature T-helper cells with cerebriform nuclei. Criteria for the diagnosis of SS include the demonstration of a peripheral blood T-cell clone by molecular or cytogenetic methods; an expanded CD4+ population resulting in a CD4:CD8 ratio > 10, and immunophenotypic abnormalities such as absent expression of T-cell antigens (CD2, CD3. CD4 and/or CD5). Sézary syndrome (SS) is part of a broader disease spectrum, erythrodermic CTCL. The presence of a clonal T-cell population in the peripheral blood distinguishes SS from reactive disorders that exhibit erythroderma and circulating cells with cerebriform nuclei (pseudo-SS) {777}.

ICD-O code

9701 / 3

Epidemiology

Sézary syndrome accounts for less than 5% of all cutaneous T-cell lymphomas {2523}. It occurs almost exclusively in adults, characteristically presents over the age of 60 and has a male predominance {2523}.

Etiology

SS is of unknown etiology. However, a syndrome clinically indistinguishable from SS is occasionally seen in HTLV-1 associated lymphoma/leukaemia.

Clinical features

SS comprises a clinical triad of pruritus, erythroderma and lymphadenopathy. The pruritus is commonly intractable and sufficiently severe to prevent the patient sleeping or pursuing a normal life. Additional clinical features include alopecia, ectropion, nail dystrophy, palmoplantar keratoderma and leonine facies. Bacterial skin infection is common in Sézary patients and may lead to a marked deterioration in their cutaneous disease. An increased prevalence of secondary malignancies, both cutaneous and systemic, has been reported in SS and attributed to the immunoparesis associated with loss of normal circulating CD4 cells {2075}.

Tumour spread and staging

Haematological involvement was defined in the TNM classification of MF as more than 5% atypical circulating lymphocytes (B1), but was not included as part of the Bunn-Lamberg staging system {1356}. Sézary patients are all T4/B1 (erythroderma with blood involvement) but staging will vary from stage III if there is no lymph node involvement to IVB if there is bone marrow involvement. In practice, most cases of SS are staged as IVA. In 1988, the definition of B1 was increased from 5 to 20%, by the NCI, but was still not included as part of the staging system {2071}.

The problem is that erythrodermic CTCL represents a spectrum and that any attempt to distinguish SS from cases that show a lesser degree of haematological involvement is necessarily arbitrary. An alternative approach is to develop a staging system that incorporates both lymph node status and haematological stage. A haematological staging system

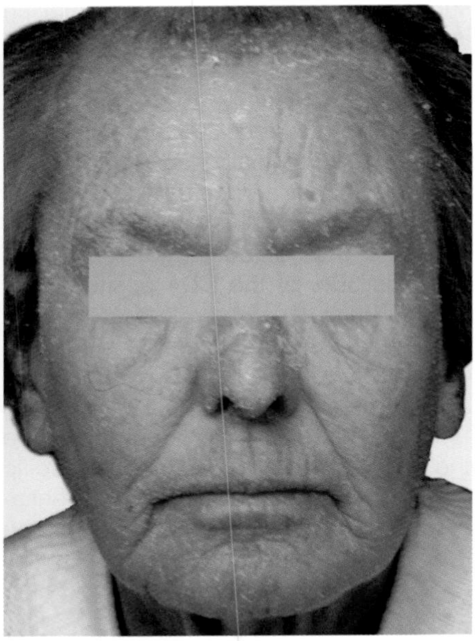

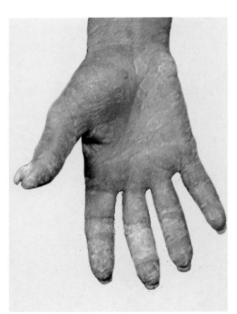

Fig. 4.14 Erythroderma and scaling of the face in Sézary syndrome.

Fig. 4.15 Palmar hyperkeratosis and onychodystrophy in Sézary syndrome.

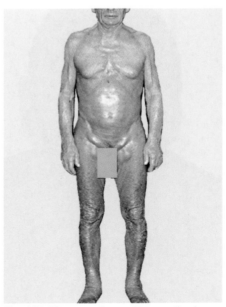

Fig. 4.16 Sézary syndrome. Note erythroderma, oedema of the skin, and swelling of lymph nodes.

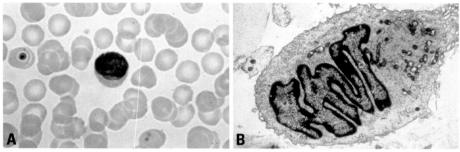

Fig. 4.17 Morphology of Sézary cells. **A** Blood film and **B** Ultrastructure showing a typical convoluted nucleus.

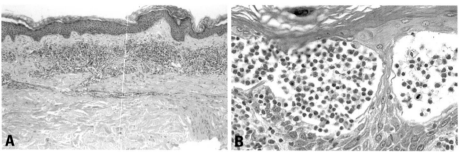

Fig. 4.18 Sézary syndrome. **A** Band-like infiltrate in the epidermis without epidermotropism. **B** Intraepidermal Pautrier microabscesses.

comprising five categories (H0-H4) was proposed by Russell-Jones and Whittaker {1998}, and subsequent data showed an increase in disease-specific death rates for each category with the most significant change occurring at H2, defined by 5% Sézary cells with a T cell clone demonstrated by PCR, or a T cell clone demonstrated by Southern blot analysis only {2077}. The need for a haematological staging system has also been recognised by the International Society for Cutaneous Lymphoma ISCL {2444}. Currently this is being tested in a larger, multi-centre study under the auspices of the ISCL.

Histopathology

Despite minor differences {1099}, the range of histological changes in SS are not dissimilar to those seen in patients with mycosis fungoides {2135}. Epidermotropism is a variable feature, and the size of Sézary cells varies in the skin as it does in blood. Only 2/3 of the skin biopsies and 73% of patients had diagnostic changes in the skin biopsies.

Other causes of erythroderma need to be differentiated from SS, particularly drug induced erythroderma and chronic actinic reticuloid, both of which may show a high proportion of activated lymphocytes with cerebriform nuclei {2135}. In cases with a non-specific histology, the differential diagnosis would include other causes of erythroderma such as eczema or psoriasis.

Immunoprofile

A typical Sézary cell is a mature helper T cell with a memory phenotype. A classic immunoprofile is CD2, CD3, CD4, CD5, CD45RO positive and CD8 negative {1368,2526}. The majority of Sézary cells are also CLA positive {1827} and CD7 negative, and this latter feature has been proposed as a method of distinguishing Sézary cells from normal lymphocytes {957}. However, further studies have shown that the neoplastic cell population is present in both the CD7 positive and CD7 negative subset in the same patient {657}. More recently, Bernengo et al. have demonstrated that CD4 positive Sézary cells typically loose the CD26 marker and that a diagnosis of SS or MF with haematological involvement can be made if the CD26 negative subset exceeds 30% of the CD4 positive cells {215}.

Complete loss of T cell antigens such as CD2, CD3, CD4, or CD5 is present in approximately 2/3 of patients with SS {957}. An alternative approach would be the identification of a tumour-specific antigen {669}. Recently two differentiation antigens P140 and SCS have been reported in circulating Sézary cells and P140 was also found in skin-infiltrating cells of patients with SS {1715}.

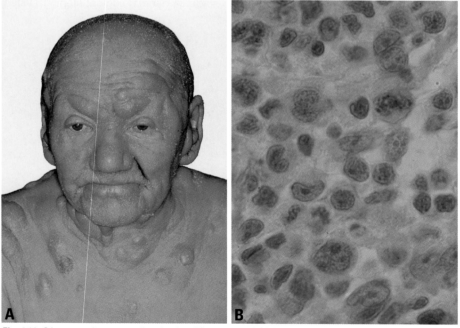

Fig. 4.19 Sézary syndrome transforming into blast-stage. **A** Multiple nodules and tumours. **B** Large atypical cells in blastic transformation of Sézary syndrome.

Histogenesis

The postulated cell of origin is a mature peripheral T cell which has skin-homing properties and exhibits a helper-cell phenotype.

Somatic genetics

Recurrent chromosomal translocations have not been detected in Sézary syndrome, but complex clonal numerical and structural chromosomal abnormalities are common and associated with a poor prognosis {1505,2343}. M-FISH techniques have shown a high rate of unbalanced translocations and associated deletions often involving chromosomes 1p, 10q, 14 and 15 {1505}. CGH studies have identified a consistent pattern of chromosomal gains/deletions (1p, 10q, 13q, 19, 17p losses and 4/4q, 17q and 18 gains) which, with the exception of 17q gains in Sézary syndrome, are identical to mycosis fungoides suggesting a similar pathogenesis {1210,1504}.

Allelic losses on 1p, 9p, 10q and 17p have been confirmed by LOH studies and a high rate of microsatellite instability (MSI) has also been detected {2079, 2080}. These findings suggest that dysregulated genes at these chromosomal loci are involved in the pathogenesis {1554,2078}. There is a high rate of genomic instability as indicated by the presence of chromosomal instability {1505}. Constitutive activation of Stat 3 and chromosomal amplification of JUNB, a member of the AP-1 transcription factor complex, have been identified in Sézary syndrome {1089,1506}. A recent cDNA array study in Sézary syndrome has confirmed the presence of JUNB overexpression and has also revealed overexpression of other genes associated with a TH2 phenotype such as Gata-3 and RhoB {1211}. These array findings appear to allow the identification of a poor prognostic group {1211}.

Prognosis and predictive factors

Sézary syndrome has a poor prognosis with a median survival of 2 to 4 years depending on the exact definition used {777,1271,2044,2523}. Absolute Sézary cell count and lymph node involvement are independent prognostic factors. In addition, large cell transformation and the development of skin tumours on a background of erythroderma are poor prognostic signs.

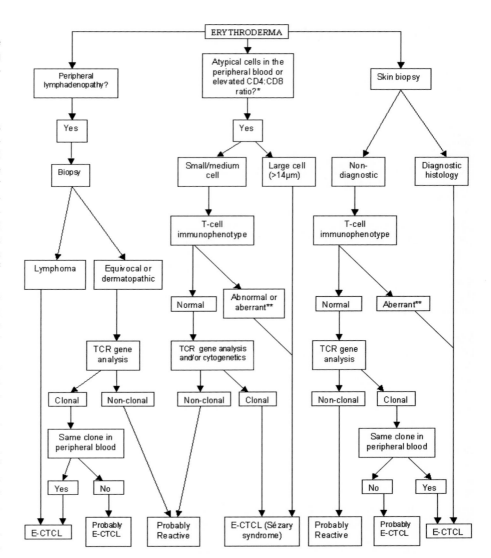

Fig. 4.20 Diagnostic pathways for the differential diagnosis of erythroderma. Algorithm for the evaluation and diagnosis of erythroderma due to cutaneous T-cell lymphoma (E-CTCL) vs. 'reactive' causes of erythroderma. TCR, T-cell receptor. *A CD4/CD8 ratio > 10 or an absolute Sézary cell count of 1x 10^9 L^{-1} have been proposed as diagnostic criteria for Sézary syndrome (SS), but this algorithm requires additional immunophenotypic or genotypic data. Even so, a Sézary cell count > 1x 10^9 L^{-1} or a CD4/CD8 ratio > 10 increases the probability of neoplasia, and separates SS from E-CTCL with a lesser degree of blood involvement. **Abnormal T-cell immunophenotype = an increased population of CD4+ cells that are CD26 (> 30%) or p140+. CD7 is less reliable. Aberrant T-cell immunophenotype = loss of pan T-cell markers such as CD2, CD3 or CD5, and/or double-negative T cells (CD4 and CD8). In skin, the loss of CD7 from epidermal lymphocytes is CTCL specific.
From: R. Russell-Jones {1997}.

Granulomatous slack skin

W. Kempf
D.V. Kazakov
S. Michaelis
G. Burg
P. LeBoit

Definition
Granulomatous slack skin (GSS) is clinically characterized by the development of bulky skin lesions in the major skin folds and histologically by a granulomatous infiltrate composed of small lymphocytes and scattered multinucleated giant cells containing nuclei arranged in a wreath-like fashion.

Synonyms
Progressive atrophying chronic granulomatous dermohypodermitis

Epidemiology
GSS is a rare form of primary cutaneous T-cell lymphoma. GSS usually appears in the third or fourth decade, but can also affect children {373}. GSS occurs almost exclusively in Whites. The male to female ratio is 2:1 to 3:1 {490}.

Clinical features
GSS begins with slightly infiltrated, poikilodermatous sharply demarcated patches and plaques. Predilection sites are the intertriginous areas, especially the axillary and inguinal folds. After years, pathognomonic bulky pendulous skin folds develop as a result of progressive destruction of elastic fibres. The lesions then resemble cutis laxa. Occasionally ulceration occurs. Regional lymphadenopathy may be present. In contrast to granulomatous MF, GSS is in almost all cases confined to intertriginous areas, and runs a more benign course than classic MF {1387}.

Histopathology
Early lesions of GSS display a bandlike infiltrate of small lymphocytes without significant nuclear atypia {1379}. More advanced lesions show a dense lymphocytic infiltrate throughout the entire dermis. Nuclear atypia of lymphocytes is less pronounced than in granulomatous MF. The diagnostic hallmark is numerous multinucleated histiocytic giant cells, which are scattered throughout the background of the dense lymphocytic infiltrate. These giant cells contain 20-30 nuclei located at the periphery of the cytoplasm. Elastophagocytosis and emperipolesis (phagocytosis of lymphoid cells by giant cells) are present. Elastic stains demonstrate the loss of elastic fibres at the sites of the infiltrates in all dermal layers. On occasion, involvement of large vessels occurs. Ultrastructurally, the lymphocytes show hyperchromatic cerebriform nuclei similar to those seen in mycosis fungoides and Sézary syndrome {490}. Specific infiltration of regional lymph nodes or internal organs exhibiting similar features as in the skin has been observed in rare cases.

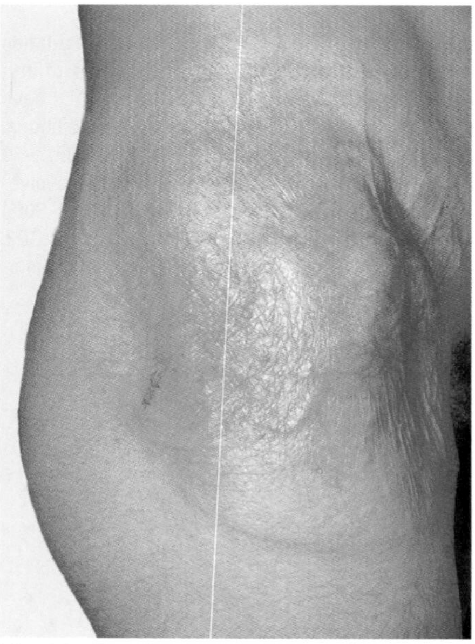

Immunoprofile
The lymphoid tumour cells display a T helper phenotype with expression of CD3, CD4 and CD45RO. There may be loss of other T-cell markers like CD5 or CD7. In rare cases, the tumour cells express CD30.

Genetics
Clonal rearrangement of TCR genes can be found in most cases and is a useful diagnostic tool in early stages of the disease {1382}. Trisomy 8 has been reported in two cases {136,2442}.

Histogenesis
The tumour cells represent skin-homing T-helper cells.

Prognosis and predictive factors
The disease has a long natural history with a slowly progressive course over decades. Occasionally involvement of regional lymph nodes is found, but does not seem to affect survival. Although life expectancy is not reduced by GSS *per se*, other cutaneous and nodal lymphomas such as mycosis fungoides, Hodgkin lymphoma and peripheral T-cell lymphomas occur in approximately 20 – 50% of the patients, often years or even decades after the manifestation of GSS {202,490,1729,2413}.

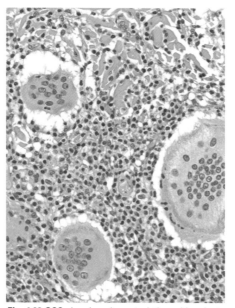

Fig. 4.21 Granulomatous slack skin (GSS). Large slightly infiltrated plaque in the groin.

Fig. 4.22 GSS showing characteristic multinucleated giant cells with emperipolesis of lymphocytes.

CD30+ T-cell lymphoproliferative disorders

W. Kempf
R. Willemze
E.S. Jaffe
G. Burg
M.E. Kadin

CD30-positive T-cell lymphoproliferative disorders (LPD) of the skin (CD30+LPD) represent a distinctive group of primary cutaneous T-cell lymphoma. The spectrum of CD30+ LPD includes lymphomatoid papulosis (LyP), primary cutaneous anaplastic lymphoma (C-ALCL) and borderline cases which differ in their clinical and histological presentations {191, 1174,1225,1795,2520}.

A feature common to all is the expression of CD30, a cytokine receptor belonging to the tumour necrosis factor receptor superfamily.

The term 'borderline lesions' has been applied to lesions that show clinical presentation of one entity (e.g. C-ALCL) but histological features of another one (e.g. LyP). This discrepancy may result in difficulties to assign such lesions to a distinct entity. Clinical presentation plays a crucial role in such discordant cases.

Lymphomatoid papulosis (LyP)

Definition
LyP is a chronic recurrent lymphoproliferative skin disease with self-regressing papulo-nodular skin lesions and atypical lymphoid cells in a polymorphous inflammatory background {1466}.

ICD-O code   9718/1

Epidemiology
LyP is a rare disease with an estimated prevalence of 0.1 to 0.2 cases per 100 000 and a male to female ratio of 1.5:1 {2456}. Mostly people in the third and fifth decades are affected, but children can also be involved.

Localization
Although no definite predilection site has been identified, LyP lesions more often arise on the trunk, especially the buttocks, and extremities.

Etiology
The cause of the disease is unknown. Endogenous retroviral elements have been identified in LyP lesions {1242}. Interaction of CD30 and CD30L as well as TGF-beta and its receptor play an important role in growth regulation, including regression of tumoural lesions {1177,1648}.

Clinical features
LyP is characterized by grouped or disseminated asymptomatic papules and/or nodules, which regress spontaneously after a few weeks, sometimes leaving behind varioliform scars {1174}. Often new lesions develop concurrently in the same or another body region. Larger nodules up to 2 cm can develop and persist for months {2524}. Clinicopathologic variants of LyP include regional follicular and pustular forms {2076}.

Histopathology
The histological features of LyP are variable and depend on the stage of the lesions and disease. Three histologic subtypes (types A, B and C) have been delineated {2524} which represent a spectrum with overlapping features {2148}. In fully developed LyP lesions, there is a wedge-shaped diffuse dermal infiltrate which contains medium-sized to large pleomorphic or anaplastic lymphoid cells with irregular nuclei, sparse chromatin and mitotic activity. Some of the large atypical lymphoid cells resemble Reed-Sternberg cells. Ulceration may be present. In type A lesions, scat-

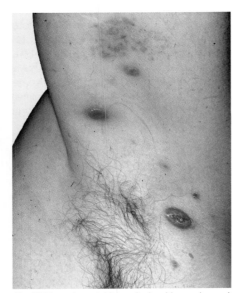

Fig. 4.23 Lymphomatoid papulosis with papules and ulcerating nodules.

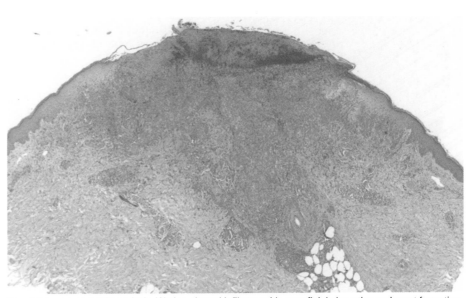

Fig. 4.24 Lymphomatoid papulosis. Wedge-shaped infiltrate with superficial ulceration and crust formation.

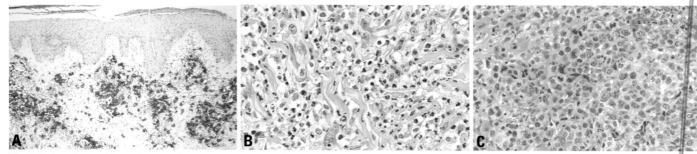

Fig. 4.25 Lymphomatoid papulosis. **A** Grouped and scattered CD30+ lymphocytes of various sizes. **B** Mixed infiltrate consisting of large atypical lymphocytes, eosinophils and neutrophils (LyP, type A). **C** 1325. Cohesive sheets of large atypical lymphocytes with only few neutrophils (LyP, type C).

tered tumour cells are intermingled with numerous inflammatory cells such as neutrophils, eosinophils and histiocytes. Type C lesions show cohesive sheets of large atypical lymphoid cells with only a few intermingled reactive inflammatory cells. The rare type B is characterized by an epidermotropic infiltrate of small atypical lymphoid cells with cerebriform nuclei and histologically resembles mycosis fungoides. Various histologic types may be present in individual patients at the same time.

Due to an overlap of histologic features between LyP and primary as well as secondary cutaneous ALCL, final diagnosis depends on correlation of clinical presentation and histologic findings.

Immunohistochemistry
A hallmark of the large atypical lymphoid cells is their positivity for CD30 {1173, 1227}. The large atypical lymphoid cells

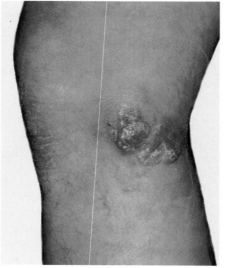

Fig. 4.26 Primary cutaneous anaplastic CD30+ large-cell lymphoma. Solitary large ulcerated nodule on the leg.

in LyP are of T-cell origin with a CD3+, CD4+, CD8-. In 10% of the cases tumour cells express CD56+ {193}. Usually CD2 and CD5 are expressed, whereas often CD7 and sometimes CD3 are absent. In addition, expression of activation markers such as HLA-DR and CD25 (interleukin 2-receptor) is found. Cytotoxic molecules such as TIA-1 and granzyme B are expressed in 70% of the cases {1342}. CD56 is generally negative {968}. CD15, a marker for Reed-Sternberg cells in Hodgkin lymphoma, is usually not expressed in LyP. In contrast to the tumour cells expressing CD30 as in LyP type A and type C, the small atypical lymphocytes present in LyP type B are usually negative for CD30.

Genetics
Clonal rearrangement of T cell receptor genes can be found in at least 40% of LyP lesions. Cytogenetic studies have demonstrated chromosomal deletions and rearrangements of chromosomes 1, 7, 9 and 10 {1813}. The t(2;5)(p23;q35) translocation is not detected in LyP {613}.

Histogenesis
LyP represents a proliferation of activated skin-homing T-cells with a unique cytotoxic phenotype (TIA-1+).

Prognosis and predictive factors
LyP exhibits a favorable prognosis with 5-year-survival rates of 100% {191,1795}. So far, there are no data indicating that any kind of therapeutic intervention in LyP alters the natural history of the disease or prevents progression to other malignant lymphomas {650}. Other cutaneous and nodal lymphomas such as mycosis fungoides, Hodgkin lymphoma and systemic or cutaneous CD30+ large T-cell lymphoma (LTCL) develop in 5-

20% of patients with LyP {191,1174}. Long-term follow-up is therefore recommended. These lymphomas are usually referred to as LyP-associated malignant lymphomas. They can develop prior to, concurrent with, or after the manifestation of LyP {1175} and result in a fatal outcome in 2% of patients {191}. No risk factors have been identified which definitely indicate likely progression to associated lymphomas in LyP patients. So far, only fascin expression is found at a significantly higher rate in LyP cases associated with systemic lymphomas {1243}.

Primary cutaneous anaplastic large-cell lymphoma

Definition
Primary cutaneous anaplastic lymphoma (C-ALCL) is a neoplasm composed of large atypical lymphocytes of either pleomorphic, anaplastic or immunoblastic cytomorphology and expression of the CD30 antigen by the majority, i.e. more than 75% of tumour cells. Primary cutaneous and primary nodal CD30+ ALCL are distinct clinical entities that can have similar morphologic features and some overlap in immunophenotype, but differ in age of onset, genetic features, etiology and prognosis {600,2259,2493}.

ICD-O-code   9718/3

Synonyms
Regressing atypical histiocytosis, EORTC: Primary cutaneous large cell T cell lymphoma CD30+

Epidemiology
C-ALCL is the second most common form of cutaneous T-cell lymphoma with an incidence of 0.1-0.2 patients per 100,000. This form of lymphoma affects

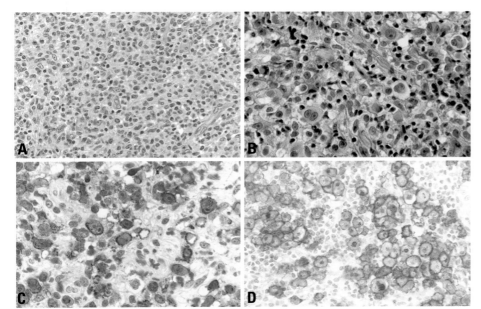

Fig. 4.27 CD30+ primary cutaneous anaplastic large-cell lymphoma. **A** Large cells in a background of histiocytes, plasma cells and small lymphocytes. **B** Large atypical cells in CD30+ anaplastic large-cell lymphoma. **C** Scattered tumour cells expressing CD30. **D** Expression of CD30 by almost all tumour cells.

mainly people in their sixth decade with a male to female ratio of 2-3:1 {191,1226}, but it can also occur in childhood. C-ALCL is a common form of cutaneous T-cell lymphoma in HIV-infected individuals {1248}.

Localization
The extremities, head and buttocks are predilection sites {196,1228}.

Clinical features
ALCL usually presents as an asymptomatic, solitary firm nodule which rapidly grows and often ulcerates {1174}. Approximately 20% of the patients have multifocal disease, i.e. two or more lesions at multiple anatomic sites {191}. Involvement of regional lymph nodes can occur. Other extra-cutaneous spread is rare. If there is no therapeutic intervention, spontaneous regression occurs in 10-40% of the tumour lesions {191,1226}.

Histopathology
There is a dense nodular infiltrate extending through all levels of the dermis into the subcutis. Epidermotropism may be found. The infiltrate consists of cohesive sheets of large, cells with irregularly shaped nuclei and one or multiple nucleoli and an abundant, clear or eosinophilic cytoplasm. Mitoses are frequent. Clusters of small reactive lymphocytes are found within and around the tumour. Eosinophils, plasma cells, and accessory dendritic cells usually are not prominent in C-ALCL. Variants of C-ALCL include neutrophil-rich or pyogenic CD30+ ALCL presenting histologically with small aggregations or scattered CD30+ medium to large pleomorphic lymphoid cells within an extensive infiltrate of neutrophils {341,1549}.

Immunohistochemistry
C-ALCL displays an activated T-cell phenotype with expression of T-cell associated antigens CD2, CD3, CD4 and CD45RO, activation markers such as CD25 (IL-2R), CD30, CD71 and HLA-DR, and frequent expression of cytotoxic molecules such as TIA-1, granzyme B and perforin {290,1342}. CD30 must be expressed by at least 75% of the large pleomorphic or anaplastic lymphoid cells. Variable loss of T cell antigens (CD2, CD3, CD5 and CD7) can be found

{1228}. In contrast to systemic (nodal) ALCL, C-ALCL does not express EMA, but may express the cutaneous lymphocyte antigen (CLA, HECA-452) and homeobox gene HOXC5 {243}. C-ALCL is consistently negative for the anaplastic lymphoma related tyrosine kinase (ALK).

Genetics
Clonal rearrangement of T cell receptor genes is detected by Southern blot and PCR in most cases (over 90%) of C-ALCL {1467}. The translocation t(2;5) (p23;q35) resulting in expression of NPM-ALK protein (p80), which is a characteristic feature of systemic anaplastic large cell lymphomas, is rarely if ever found in C-ALCL {228,613}. Systemic ALCL may present with cutaneous disease, and the identification of ALK-expression is helpful in this distinction.

Histogenesis
Activated skin-homing T-cell.

Prognosis and predictive factors
C-ALCL has a favourable prognosis with 5 year-survival rates of 90% {191,1795}. Up to 40% of C-ALCL show spontaneous regression {198}. Regional lymph nodes may be involved, but the survival rate is similar to patients with skin lesions only {191}. Other extracutaneous spread occurs in 10% of the patients, especially in those with multiple grouped or multifocal tumour lesions with a fatal outcome in only a minority of the patients {191}.
Spontaneous regression and age less than 60 years are associated with a better prognosis, while extracutaneous disease and higher age tend to have a worse outcome. Cytomorphology (anaplastic or pleomorphic and immunoblastic) seems not to be a prognostic factor {191,1795}.

Subcutaneous panniculitis-like T-cell lymphoma

E.S. Jaffe
G. Burg

Definition

Subcutaneous panniculitis-like T-cell lymphoma (SPTCL) is a T-cell lymphoma with preferential infiltration of subcutaneous tissue by atypical lymphoid cells of varying size, often with marked tumour necrosis and karyorrhexis.

ICD-O code   9708/3

Historical annotation

In the historical literature, most cases of SPTCL were probably diagnosed as histiocytic cytophagic panniculitis {562, 1527}.

Epidemiology

Subcutaneous panniculitis-like T-cell lymphoma is a rare form of lymphoma, representing less than 1% of all non-Hodgkin lymphomas. It occurs in males and females equally, and has a broad age range. Cases have been reported in children under the age of two years. Most cases occur in adults {1060,1341,2026, 2480}.

Etiology

Unknown. In most patients the disease presents sporadically.

Localization

Patients present with multiple subcutaneous nodules, usually in the absence of other sites of disease. The most common sites of localization are the extremities and trunk.

Clinical features

Clinical symptoms are primarily related to the subcutaneous nodules. The nodules range in size from 0.5 cm to several cm in diameter. Larger nodules may become necrotic, but ulceration of cutaneous lesions is rare. Systemic symptoms, most commonly fever, are variable but usually present. Some patients may present with a haemophagocytic syndrome with pancytopenias, fever, and hepatosplenomegaly {338,863,2480}. Lymphadenopathy is usually absent.

Histopathology

The infiltrate extends diffusely through the subcutaneous tissue, usually without sparing of septae. The overlying dermis and epidermis are typically uninvolved. The neoplastic cells range in size from small cells with round nuclei and inconspicuous nucleoli to larger transformed cells with hyperchromatic nuclei. The lymphoid cells have a moderate amount of pale-staining cytoplasm. A helpful diagnostic feature is the rimming of the neoplastic cells surrounding individual fat cells {1341}. Admixed reactive histiocytes are frequently present, particularly in areas of fat infiltration and destruction. The histiocytes are frequently vacuolated, due to ingested lipid material. Vascular invasion may be seen in some cases, and necrosis and karyorrhexis are common. However, the infiltrates usually are confined to the subcutaneous tissue, with sparing of the dermis. This feature is helpful in the differential diagnosis from other lymphomas involving skin and subcutaneous tissue. The necrosis is primarily apoptotic in nature, possibly related to the release of cytotoxic molecules {1341,2133}. Cutaneous γδ T-cell lymphomas can have a panniculitis-like component, but commonly show both dermal and epidermal involvement in addition to subcutaneous disease {1060, 1341,2026,2366}. Plasma cells and reactive lymphoid follicles are generally absent, in contrast to lupus profundus panniculitis, and other forms of lobular panniculitis.

In some cases of SPTCL the infiltrates in initial phases may appear deceptively benign, and the differential diagnosis with benign panniculitis may be difficult {338,863}.

Immunoprofile

SPTCL is derived from αβ cells, T-cells with a cytotoxic profile. The cells are usu-

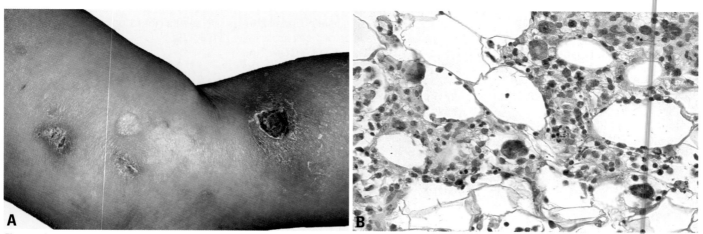

Fig. 4.28 Subcutaneous panniculitis-like T-cell lymphoma (SPLTCL). **A** Erythematous plaques and nodules on the leg with ulceration. **B** Diffuse infiltration of subcutaneous tissue simulating lobular panniculitis. Large atypical cells rimming around fat lobules.

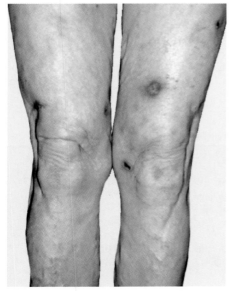

Fig. 4.29 Subcutaneous panniculitis-like T-cell lymphoma (SPLTCL). Subcutaneous erythematous plaques and nodules on the legs.

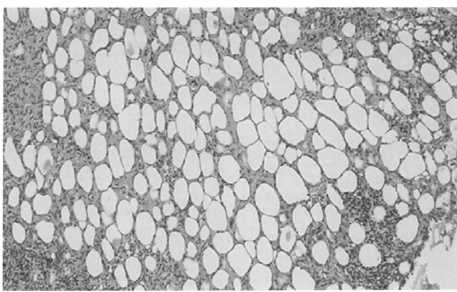

Fig. 4.30 Subcutaneous panniculitis-like T-cell lymphoma (SPLTCL) Lobular panniculitis-like infiltrate of neoplastic lymphoid cells.

ally CD8-positive, with expression of cytotoxic molecules including granzyme B, perforin, and T-cell intracellular antigen (TIA-1) {1341,2026}. However, in contrast to other cytotoxic TCLs related to the innate immune system (enteropathy-type T-cell lymphoma, extranodal NK/T-cell lymphoma), the cells are negative for granzyme M (metase) {694, 1122,1325,2564}. The neoplastic cells are capable of producing a number of cytokines and chemokines, a feature that is related to development of systemic symptoms and the haemophagocytic syndrome {338,2340}. Cutaneous γδ T-cell lymphomas {119,338,1341,2026} are distinguished from SPTCL, even if a panniculitis-like component is present.

Histogenesis
Mature cytotoxic T-cell of the adaptive immune system.

Precursor lesions
Oligoclonal T-cell populations may be found in some cases of lobular panniculitis, suggesting the potential for clonal evolution in rare cases {1484}. However, progression from cytophagic panniculitis without monoclonality to SPTCL rarely if ever occurs {1527}.

Somatic genetics
The neoplastic cells show rearrangement of T-cell receptor genes, and are negative for Epstein-Barr sequences.

Prognosis and predictive factors
Dissemination to lymph nodes and other organs is uncommon and usually occurs late in the clinical course. The natural history is often aggressive {694,863,917, 1300,2026}. A haemophagocytic syndrome is a frequent complication in αβ cases and usually precipitates a fulminant downhill clinical course. However, if therapy for the underlying lymphoma is instituted and is successful, the haemophagocytic syndrome may remit.

Primary cutaneous peripheral T-cell lymphoma, unspecified

E. Ralfkiaer
R. Willemze
C.J.L.M. Meijer
R. Dummer
E.S. Jaffe

S.H. Swerdlow
E. Berti
W Kempf
G. Burg
L. Cerroni
J.R. Toro

Definition

A heterogeneous group of cutaneous T-cell lymphomas that do not fit into one of the well-defined subtypes of T-cell lymphoma/leukaemia. Three provisional entities have been separated: Cutaneous γδ T-cell lymphoma, primary cutaneous aggressive epidermotropic CD8+ cytotoxic T-cell lymphoma and primary cutaneous small-medium CD4+ T-cell lymphoma.

ICD-O code   9709/3

Synonyms and historical annotation

The category of the peripheral T-cell lymphomas, unspecified (PTL) was introduced in the REAL classification {960} and was maintained in the WHO classification {1369}. It encompasses per definition all T-cell neoplasms that do not fit into any of the better defined subtypes of T-cell lymphoma/leukaemia. As such it constitutes a heterogeneous group of diseases. These conditions are most frequently systemic {1121}. Primary cutaneous PTL are rare and constitute less than 10% of all cutaneous T-cell lymphomas (CTCL) in large series {195}. They correspond to the CD30-negative CTCL in the EORTC classification and show an aggressive behaviour in most cases {195,2523}. Therefore, distinction between "primary" and "secondary" cutaneous involvement seems less important for this category.

Although it is still controversial how these tumours can be grouped into separate diseases, recent investigations have suggested that some disorders within this broad group of neoplasms can now be separated out as provisional entities. For the remaining diseases that do not fit into either of these provisional entities (Table 4.1), the designation PTL, unspecified, is maintained.

Cutaneous γδ T-cell lymphoma

Definition

Cutaneous γδ T-cell lymphoma (CGD-TCL) is a lymphoma composed of a clonal proliferation of mature, activated gd T-cells expressing a cytotoxic phenotype. This group includes cases of subcutaneous panniculitis-like T-cell lymphoma (SPTCL) with a gamma/delta phenotype. In the WHO classification 2001, these were grouped together with SPTCL of αβ origin {1121}, but they show distinctive features and seem to be more closely related to other CGD-TCL {192,1060, 1533,2026,2366}. A similar and possibly related condition may present primarily in

mucosal sites {98}. Whether cutaneous and mucosal γδ TCLs are all part of a single disease, i.e. muco-cutaneous γδ TCL, is not yet clear {1122,2539}.

Epidemiology

CGD-TCLs are rare, with approximately 50 cases reported {1533,1665,2366}. In one series they represented <5% of cutaneous T-cell lymphomas {1879}. Most cases occur in adults. There is no reported sex predilection.

Table 4.1
Characteristic features of three provisional cutaneous T-cell lymphomas.

	Skin lesion	Pattern of infiltration	Cytology	Phenotype	EBV	Behaviour
γδ-TCL	Patches, plaques, tumours, disseminated	E, D, S	Medium-large, pleomorphic	TCRd1+, CD3+, CD4-, CD8-, CyAg+, CD56 +/-	-	A
AECD8+	Eruptive nodules, hyperkeratotic patches/ plaques, disseminated	E	Medium-large pleomorphic	bF1+, CD3+, CD4-, CD8+, CyAg+	-	A
PTL, CD4+	Solitary nodules, tumours	D, S	Small-medium pleomorphic	bF1+, CD3+, CD4+, CD8-	-	I

Abbreviations: γδ-TCL= gamma delta-T-cell lymphoma; AECD8+= aggressive, epidermotropic, CD8+ cytotoxic T-cell lymphoma; E=epidermal; D=dermal; S=subcutaneous; CyAg= cytotoxic antigens (TIA-1, granzyme B, perforin); EBV= Epstein-Barr Virus; A =aggressive; I=indolent.

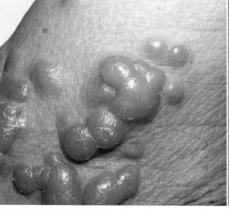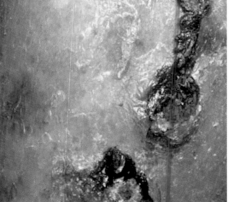

Fig. 4.31 Cutaneous γδ T-cell lymphoma presenting with skin tumours.

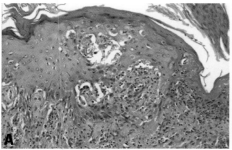 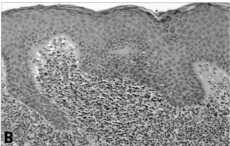 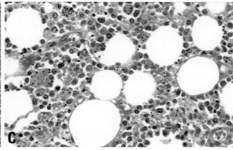

Fig. 4.32 Cutaneous γδ T-cell lymphoma. **A** The infiltrates may be epidermotropic, **B** dermal **C** subcutaneous or combined.

Etiology

The distribution of disease reflects the localization of normal γδ T cells, which are believed to play a role in host mucosal and epithelial immune responses {268}. Impaired immune function associated with chronic antigen stimulation may predispose to the development of mucosal and CGD-TCLs {98,2539}. Epstein-Barr virus (EBV) is generally negative in CGD-TCLs, but may be positive in primary γδ TCL in mucosal sites {98,1191,2366,2539}.

Clinical features

The clinical presentation is variable. The disease may be predominantly epidermotropic and present with patches/plaques, or it may be predominantly deep dermal/subcutaneous with necrotic tumours or nodules, resembling subcutaneous panniculitis-like T-cell lymphoma (SPTCL) of αβ type {192,221,1060,1533, 1665,1879,2026,2366}. The lesions are often mainly present on the extremities {2366}, but other sites may be affected as well {1533,2365}. Patients with CGD-TCL usually lack involvement of lymph nodes, spleen, and bone marrow, but the disease may disseminate to extranodal/mucosal sites. A haemophagocytic syndrome may occur in patients with panniculitis-like tumours {119,2365}.

Histopathology

The neoplastic cells are generally medium to large in size with coarsely clumped chromatin {2366}. Large blastic cells with vesicular nuclei and prominent nucleoli are infrequent. Apoptosis and necrosis are common, often with angioinvasion {1533}. Three major histologic patterns of involvement are present: epidermotropic, dermal, and subcutaneous. However, usually more than one histologic pattern is present in the same patient in different biopsy specimens or within a single biopsy specimen {2366}. Epidermal infiltration may occur as mild epidermotropism to marked pagetoid reticulosis-like infiltrates {221,1665,1879}. Subcutaneous nodules may be panniculitis-like or more solid in appearance and may show rimming of fat cells, similar to SPTCL of αβ origin {1533}. Dermal and epidermal involvement often coexists with subcutaneous disease, in contrast to SPTCL of αβ origin, which is mainly or exclusively subcutaneous in distribution {192,1060, 2026}.

Immunoprofile

The cells are CD3+, CD2+, CD7 +/-, but usually negative for CD5 {2539}. Most CGD-TCLs lack both CD4 and CD8, but some are CD8+ {2366}. The cells are positive for TCR-δ, but lack βF1 of the αβ T-cell receptor. The absence of βF1 may be used to infer a γδ origin under appropriate circumstances {1151,2026,2365}. The cells are positive for TIA-1 and the cytotoxic proteins granzyme B, granzyme M, and perforin {1325,1341, 1533}. CD56 is frequently expressed {1533}.

Histogenesis

Functionally mature and activated cytotoxic γδ T-cells of the innate immune system.

Somatic genetics

The cells show clonal rearrangement of the TCR gamma gene. TCR beta may be rearranged or deleted, but is not expressed. Cases with predominant subcutaneous involvement express Vδ2, but this has not been studied in other CGD-TCL {1860,2026}. EBV is generally negative in primary CGD-TCL {98,119}.

Prognosis and predictive factors

Patients have aggressive disease resistant to multiagent chemotherapy and/or radiation {1665,2366}. In a recent series of 33 patients, 22 (66%) died within 5 years of diagnosis, and in the same study TCRδ1 expression was an independent predictor of survival {2366}. Among 33 patients with CGD-TCL, there was a trend for decreased survival for patients who had subcutaneous fat involvement in comparison with patients who had epidermotropic or dermal disease only. Age, sex, and lymphadenopathy did not have any discernible prognostic impact {2366}.

Primary cutaneous aggressive epidermotropic CD8+ cytotoxic T-cell lymphoma

Definition

A cutaneous T-cell lymphoma characterized by epidermotropic infiltrates of CD8-positive, cytotoxic T-cells of αβ origin. The behaviour is aggressive in most cases {223}.

Epidemiology

This disease occurs mainly in adults and is rare with approximately 30 cases published worldwide {36,192,223,1533, 2062}.

Clinical features

The clinical presentation is characterized by sudden eruptions of localized or disseminated papules, nodules and tumours, often with central ulceration and necrosis. Superficial, hyperkeratotic patches and plaques may also be present {36,223}. The disease may resemble epidermotropic variants of other cutaneous T-cell lymphomas and is similar, if not identical to cases described as generalized pagetoid reticulosis of the Ketron-Goodman type {1252,1533}. Classical MF, which may express CD8 in rare cases {1456,1880, 2062,2510}, usually does not show overt destruction and necrosis and has a more protracted behaviour with progression over years from patches to plaques and tumours. The disease may disseminate to other visceral sites (lung, testis, central nervous system, oral mucosa), but lymph nodes are often spared {223}.

Histopathology
The histological and cytological appearance is very variable ranging from a lichenoid pattern with marked, pagetoid epidermotropism and subepidermal edema to deeper, more nodular infiltrates. The epidermis may be acanthotic or atrophic, often with necrosis, ulceration and blister formation {36,223}. Invasion and destruction of adnexal skin structures are commonly seen {1533}. Angiocentricity and angioinvasion may be present {1533}. Tumour cells are small-medium or medium-large with pleomorphic or blastic nuclei {223}.

Immunoprofile
The tumour cell have a βF1+, CD3+, CD8+, Granzyme B+, perforin+, TIA-1+, CD2-, CD4-, CD5-, CD7-/+ phenotype {36,223,2062}. EBV is generally negative {192,1533}.

Histogenesis
Skin homing, CD8-positive, cytotoxic T-cells of αβ type.

Somatic genetics
The neoplastic T-cells show clonal TCR gene rearrangements. Specific genetic abnormalities have not been described.

Prognosis
These lymphomas have an aggressive clinical course with a median survival of 32 months {36,223,1533,2062}.

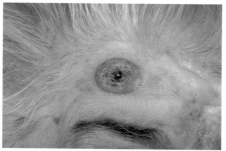

Fig. 4.33 Primary cutaneous aggressive epidermotropic CD8+ cytotoxic T-cell lymphoma presenting with an ulcerated skin tumour.

Primary cutaneous small-medium CD4+ T-cell lymphoma

Definition
A cutaneous T-cell lymphoma characterized by a predominance of small to medium-sized CD4-positive pleomorphic T-cells with clinical features different from MF. Most cases have a favourable clinical course {195,878}.

Epidemiology
A rare disease, accounting for 5-10% of cutaneous lymphomas in large series {195,878}.

Clinical features
Characteristically, these lymphomas present with a solitary plaque or tumour, generally on the face, the neck or the upper trunk {195}. Less commonly, they present with one or several papules, nodules or tumours, but always without patches typical of mycosis fungoides {195,783,2267}.

Histopathology
These lymphomas show dense, diffuse or nodular infiltrates within the dermis with tendency to infiltrate the subcutis.

Epidermotropism may be present focally. There is a predominance of small/medium-sized pleomorphic T cells {195,783, 2267}. A small proportion (<30%) of large pleomorphic cells may be present {195}. A considerable admixture with small reactive lymphocytes and histiocytes may sometimes be observed {2074}.

Immunoprofile
By definition these lymphomas have a CD3+, CD4+, CD8-, CD30- phenotype sometimes with loss of pan T-cell markers {195,783}. Cytotoxic proteins are generally not expressed {195}.

Histogenesis
Skin homing, CD4-positive T-cell.

Somatic genetics
The TCR genes are clonally rearranged {783,878}. Demonstration of clonality is a useful criterion for distinction from pseudo-T-cell lymphomas, which may also present with a solitary plaque or nodule. No consistent cytogenetic abnormalities have yet been identified.

Prognosis and predictive factors
These lymphomas have a rather favourable prognosis with an estimated 5-year survival of 60-80% {195,783, 878,2267}. Cases presenting with solitary or localized skin lesions seem to have an especially favourable prognosis {195,878}.

Primary cutaneous PTL, unspecified

Definition
The designation PTL, unspecified is maintained for cutaneous T-cell lym-

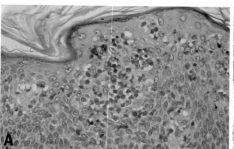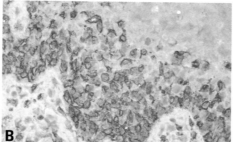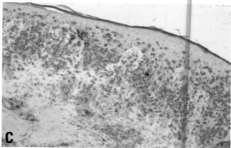

Fig. 4.34 Primary cutaneous aggressive epidermotropic CD8+ cytotoxic T-cell lymphoma. **A** The neoplastic infiltrate is markedly epidermotropic and pleomorphic and is **B** positive for CD3 and **C** for CD8.

phomas that originate from mature, transformed T-lymphocytes and that do not fit into any of the better defined subtypes of mature cutaneous T-cell neoplasms. Hence, other categories of T-cell lymphoma must be excluded. These include the three provisional entities described above. Furthermore, given the wide variety of histologic appearances of tumour stage mycosis fungoides (MF), a diagnosis of MF should always be ruled out by complete clinical examination and an accurate clinical history.

Epidemiology
These tumours account for 5 to 10% of all primary cutaneous T cell or NK cell lymphomas {195}. All ages may be affected, but the disease is most common in adults.

Clinical features
Most lymphomas in this category present with rapidly growing tumours or nodules that may be multiple or (more rarely) solitary or localized {195,197,878,2523}. No sites of predilection have been recorded.

Histopathology
Skin infiltrates are most often diffuse, but nodular or band-like patterns can be seen. Epidermotropism is mild or absent in most cases. The tumour cells are medium to large, usually with markedly pleomorphic nuclei. Rare cases may show a predominance of cells that are more immunoblastic in appearance {197,2523}. Small reactive lymphocytes, eosinophils and plasma cells may be present {195}, but the inflammatory background is usually not as pronounced as it can be in nodal malignancies.

Immunoprofile
The tumour cells express T-cell associated antigens (CD2, CD3, CD5), but usually lack CD7; most cases are CD4+, but rare tumours may be CD8+ or positive (or negative) for both CD4 and CD8 {195}. Cytotoxic antigens (TIA-1+, granzyme B) are usually not expressed {195}. Occasional tumour cells may be CD30-positive.

Histogenesis
Skin homing T-cells.

Precursor lesion
There are no known precursor lesions. As

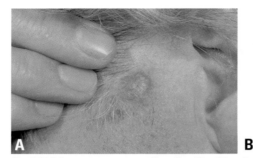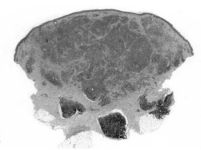

Fig. 4.35 Primary cutaneous small-medium T-cell lymphoma. **A** Small-medium CD4+ T-cell lymphoma with a solitary skin nodule on the face. **B** Nodular infiltrates of lymphocytes involving the entire dermis and superficial part of subcutaneous tissues.

mentioned, cases of transformed MF may closely resemble peripheral T cell lymphoma unspecified and can only be distinguished on clinical grounds.

Somatic genetics
The TCR genes are clonally rearranged. No consistent cytogenetic abnormalities have yet been identified.

Prognosis and predictive factors
The prognosis is poor with 5-year survival rates of less than 20% {195,878}. Cases with immunoblastic morphology may have an even more aggressive behaviour {197,2523}. Cases with solitary/localized lesions seem to behave just as aggressively as those with multiple lesions {195}.

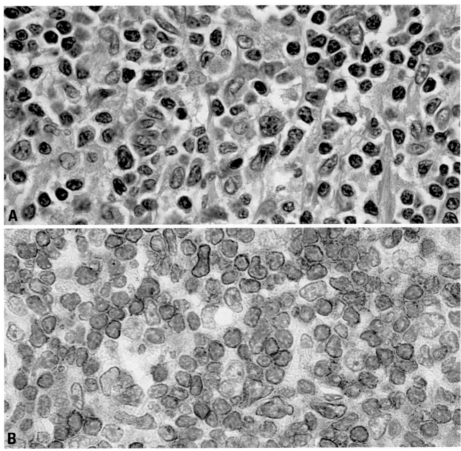

Fig. 4.36 Cutaneous small-medium pleomorphic T-cell lymphoma. **A** Small-medium lymphocytes with pleomorphic nuclei predominating. **B** Staining for CD3 confirms the T-cell lineage of the lymphocytes.

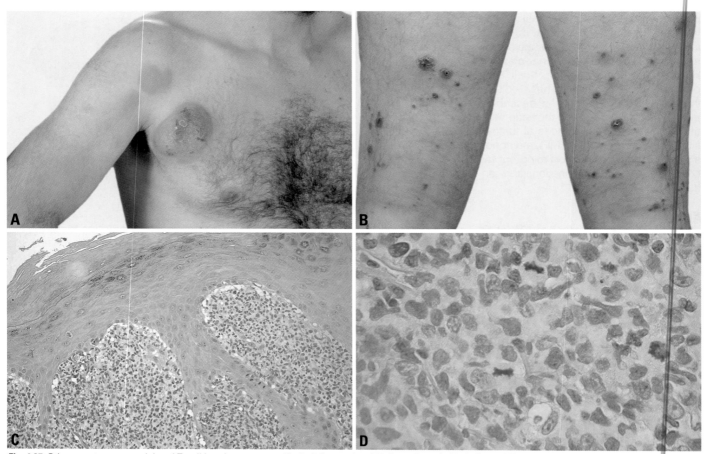

Fig. 4.37 Primary cutaneous peripheral T-cell lymphoma, unspecified. **A** Grouped and **B** disseminated skin lesions. **C** The dermal neoplastic infiltrate is dense and **D** consists of large, pleomorphic cells with irregular nuclei and numerous mitoses.

Cutaneous adult T-cell leukaemia / lymphoma

Y. Tokura
E.S. Jaffe
C. A. Sander

Definition
Adult T cell leukaemia / lymphoma (ATLL) is a malignancy of mature CD4+ T cells caused by the human T-cell leukaemia virus type I (HTLV-1).

ICD-O code   9827/3

Synonyms
Adult T-cell leukaemia (ATL)

Epidemiology
ATLL is endemic in some regions of the world, especially in southwest Japan, the Caribbean islands, South America, and parts of Central Africa {1848,2392}.

Etiology
ATLL develops in 1% to 5% of individuals infected with HTLV-1 after more than 2 decades of viral persistence. In most patients viral exposure occurs early in life, and incidence figures are related to the place of birth, not residence.
HTLV-1 proviral DNA is monoclonally integrated in the malignant T cell. HTLV-1 encodes the transcriptional activator Tax, which can transform T cells by increasing the expression of a unique set of cellular genes involved in T cell proliferation {1589}.

Localization
Based on organ involvement and severity, ATLL is divided into four clinical categories: acute, chronic, lymphoma, and smoldering types {2171}. Cutaneous involvement is seen in up to 50% of patients. Lymph nodes, liver and spleen are frequently involved.

Clinical features
Patients with ATLL exhibit various cutaneous manifestations. The most frequent manifestation is nodules/tumours (33.9%), followed by red papules (22.6%), erythematous plaques (19.4%) and macules (6.5%) {2142}. Nodules/ tumours usually occur as solitary or several lesions on limited sites, whereas multiple papules tend to be distributed over large areas of the body. Subcutaneous tumours (4.8%), erythroderma (3.5%), and purpura (1.6%) are less frequent, and alopecia, folliculitis, erythema multiforme, and prurigo are rarely seen.
In addition to the four clinical types, the cutaneous type of ATLL has been proposed to indicate skin-limited lesions without lymph node involvement or leukaemic involvement {1144}. ATLL limited to the skin may be considered part of the smouldering type. Two patterns of skin involvement are seen, i.e., tumoural and erythematopapular. The tumoural subtype has been reported to have a worse prognosis than the erythematopapular one.

Histopathology
Individual skin lesions of ATLL exhibit varying degrees of tumour cell infiltration from the epidermis to subcutaneous tissue. Epidermotropism of the malignant T-cells is present in the majority of cases,

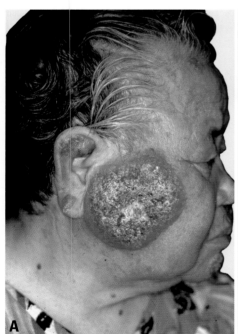
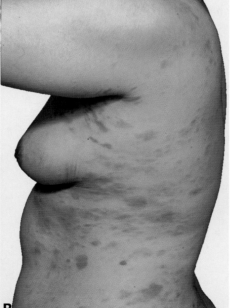
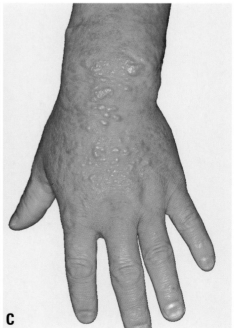

Fig. 4.38 Adult T-cell leukaemia/lymphoma (ATLL) **A** A large tumour on the right cheek. **B** Multiple erythematous plaques on the trunk. **C** Multiple papules on the hand and forearm.

and even Pautrier microabscesses, indistinguishable from those of mycosis fungoides and Sézary syndrome, are often seen. The cells have medium- to large-sized pleomorphic nuclei, and occasionally show mitoses. Nuclear irregularity may be marked, with polylobated flower cells often seen in the blood and tissues. Eosinophils may be intermingled with lymphocytes. In some cases, the tumour cells infiltrate mainly in the subcutaneous tissue {2142,2171}.

Immunohistochemistry
In general, the malignant T cells are positive for CD3, CD4, CD25, and CD45RO but negative for CD7. CD8, CD19, and CD20 {2171}. CD30 expression may be seen in larger transformed cells.

Prognosis and predictive factors
The prognosis of ATLL patients with skin lesions is dependent on clinical and histological factors, and relates to the four main clinical subtypes. It has been suggested that cases of the smoldering type of ATLL have a poorer prognosis if there are deep dermal cutaneous infiltrates, as compared to cases in which skin manifestations are absent, or only present as superficial infiltration {2142}.

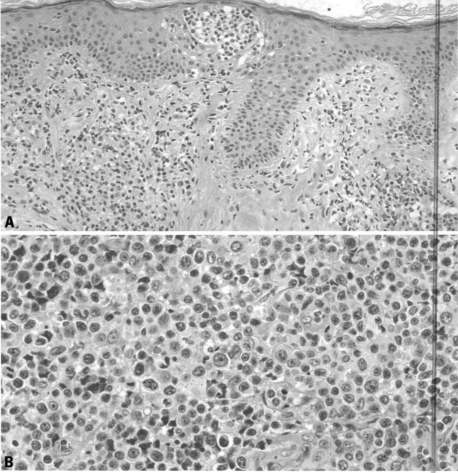

Fig. 4.39 Adult T-cell leukaemia/lymphoma (ATLL). **A** Erythematous macule, showing infiltration of atypical lymphocytes in the upper dermis with Pautrier microabscess. **B** Tumour, massive infiltration of pleomorphic lymphocytes in the dermis.

Extranodal NK/T-cell lymphoma, nasal-type

S. Kohler
K. Iwatsuki
E.S. Jaffe
J.K.C. Chan

Definition
Extranodal NK/T-cell lymphoma, nasal-type, is an EBV+, nearly always extranodal lymphoma of small, medium or large cells usually with an NK-cell, or more rarely cytotoxic T-cell phenotype. The skin is the second most common site of involvement after the nasal cavity/nasopharynx, and skin involvement may be a primary or secondary manifestation of the disease.

ICD-O code: 9719/3

Synonyms
REAL: angiocentric T-cell lymphoma; EORTC used to include in CTCL, large cell, CD30- and CTCL, pleomorphic, small/medium-sized

Epidemiology
Extranodal NK/T-cell lymphoma is a rare disease occurring in adults, with a male predominance. This lymphoma is more prevalent in Asia, Central America and South America.

Etiology
It is universally associated with EBV, and genetic factors play a role in susceptibility to the disease {443,1689}.

Localization
The majority of patients present with skin lesions affecting more than one anatomic region, most commonly the trunk and extremities {443,1660}.

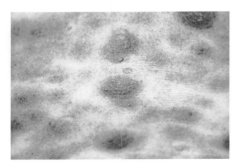

Fig. 4.40 Extranodal NK/T-cell lymphoma, nasal-type. Clinical appearance with violaceous tumour nodules.

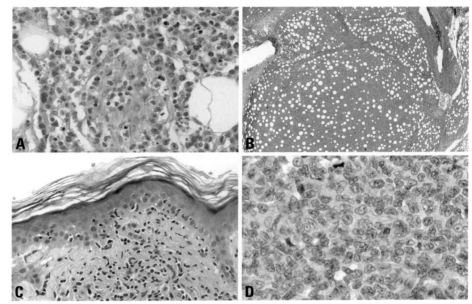

Fig. 4.41 Extranodal NK/T-cell lymphoma, nasal-type. **A** Angiocentricity and angiodestruction. **B** Involvement of the subcutis. **C** Focal epidermotropism, present in approx. 30% of cases. **D** Cytologic detail showing medium-sized cells with irregular nuclear foldings.

Clinical features
Cutaneous involvement consists of tumour nodules and plaques. Systemic symptoms such as fever, malaise and weight loss are common. Some cases are accompanied by a haemophagocytic syndrome. The disease is closely related to aggressive NK-cell leukaemia, which also may have cutaneous manifestations, and is also EBV-associated.

Histopathology
A dense dermal infiltrate is often centred on the skin appendages and blood vessels resulting in a column-like low power appearance {1689}. Prominent angiocentricity and angiodestruction are often accompanied by extensive necrosis {443,1689}. Extension into the subcutis is common. Approximately 30% of cases show at least focal epidermotropism {1689}. The mitotic rate is high and apoptotic bodies are numerous. NK/T-cell lymphoma has a broad cytologic spectrum ranging from small to large cells, with most cases consisting of medium-sized cells. The cells often exhibit irregular nuclear foldings, moderately dense chromatin, and pale cytoplasm.

Immunoprofile
The most common immunophenotype is: CD2+, CD56+, surface CD3-, cytoplasmic CD3ε+, CD43+ and cytotoxic granules + (TIA-1, granzyme B, perforin) {1325}. Occasional cases are CD56-, but then require EBV positivity or presence of cytotoxic granules for diagnosis; otherwise they should be classified as peripheral T-cell lymphoma, unspecified. LMP-1 is inconsistently expressed, with EBER in situ hybridization preferred for diagnosis.

Genetics
The T-cell receptor is usually in germline configuration.

Prognosis and predictive factors
Extranodal NK/T-cell lymphoma presenting in the skin is a highly aggressive tumour with a median survival of less than 15 months {443,1660}. The most

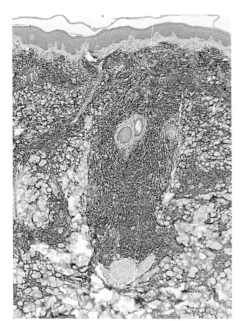

Fig. 4.42 Nasal type NK/T-cell lymphoma (EBV+), immunostained for CD56. Almost all cells are CD56 positive.

important factor predicting poor outcome is the presence of extracutaneous involvement at presentation {1660}. Preliminary data indicate that co-expression of CD56 and CD30 may be associated with a better prognosis {1660,1690}.

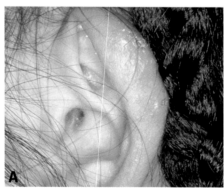

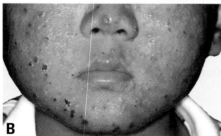

Fig. 4.43 Hydroa vacciniforme-like cutaneous T-cell lymphoma. **A** Infiltrate on the sun-exposed ear-lobe. **B** Papules, vesicles and crusted erosions on face of young boy.

Hydroa vacciniforme-like cutaneous T-cell lymphoma

Definition
Hydroa-vacciniforme-like cutaneous T-cell lymphoma is a rare EBV-associated lymphoma of cytotoxic T-cell or NK-cell origin that affects children, characterized by a vesiculopapular skin eruption that clinically resembles hydroa vacciniforme.

Synonym
Angiocentric cutaneous T-cell lymphoma of childhood

Epidemiology
Hydroa vacciniforme-like CTCL affects children and teenagers, with almost all reported cases being from Latin America (such as Peru, Bolivia, Mexico) {166, 1479,1991} and Asia (such as Korea and Japan). Boys and girls are affected in an equal ratio {471,765}.

Etiology
The strong association with EBV suggests a pathogenetic role of the virus and genetic predisposition, as in extranodal NK/T-cell lymphoma. The anatomic distribution of the skin lesions suggests sun exposure as a risk factor although tests for minimal erythema doses are usually within normal limits.

Localization
The lesions occur predominantly in sun-exposed areas, particularly the face and limbs.

Clinical features
Patients present with facial and hand oedema and a papulovesicular eruption that affects sun-exposed and to a lesser extent sun-protected areas. Individual lesions start with oedema and erythema and then progress to vesicles, necrosis, ulceration, crusts, and heal as varicelliform scars. Fever, wasting, hepatosplenomegaly, lymphadenopathy and hypersensitivity to insect bites are common. Some cases are accompanied by a haemophagocytic syndrome. The disease may progress to lymph node and visceral involvement.

Histopathology
The infiltrate consists of medium-sized atypical lymphoid cells set in an inflammatory background. The depth of the infiltrate seems related to the age of the lesion {166}. A fully developed lesion shows a dense dermal infiltrate with epidermotropism and extension into the fat in a lobular fashion. Ulceration is common. The infiltrate is often angiotropic/angioinvasive and in addition may display a periadnexal and perineural growth pattern.

Immunoprofile
The tumour cells are cytotoxic T-cells, that have often lost expression of some pan T-cell markers. The most common phenotype is: CD2+, CD3+, CD8+, CD43+, CD45RO+, TIA-1+, Granzyme B+; CD4-, CD5-, CD7-. CD56 is variably positive, but CD57 is negative. CD30 reactivity can be seen in a subset of cells (<30%).

Somatic genetics
The T-cell receptor gene is clonally rearranged {166,1479}, although in cases of NK-cell derivation, T-cell receptor genes are germline.

Prognosis
The prognosis is poor, with a 2-year survival rate of 36% {166}.

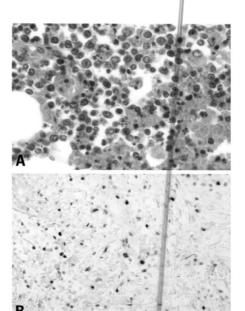

Fig. 4.44 A Subcutaneous infiltrate of tumour cells with prominent cytophagocytosis. **B** In situ hybridization showing EBER+ tumour cells.

Cutaneous involvement in primary extracutaneous T-cell lymphoma

W. Kempf
E. Ralfkiaer
D.V. Kazakov
E.S. Jaffe

Systemic peripheral T-cell lymphoma (PTL), unspecified, involves the skin in approximately 20-30% of the cases {836, 1453}. Skin lesions may be present at diagnosis or can develop during disease progression. Lesions are most often tumours or nodules that may be solitary or multiple. No sites of predilection have been recorded. The histological and phenotypic features are identical to the systemic disease. The prognosis is very poor {104,690,836,1453}.

Systemic anaplastic large cell lymphoma (ALCL)

Primary systemic anaplastic large cell lymphoma affects lymph nodes and extranodal sites, including in 20% of the cases the skin. The skin lesions may be present at diagnosis or can develop at relapse or during disease progression. The skin lesions are usually tumours or nodules that can be solitary or multiple. No sites of predilection have been recorded. The histological, phenotypic and genotypic features are identical in lymph nodes and the skin. The tumour cells are most often large with abundant cytoplasm and characteristic so-called hallmark cells with eccentric, horseshoe- or kidney-shaped nuclei often with an eosinophilic region near the nucleus. The principal morphological variants are the small cell variant and the histiocyte rich variant {809}. It is important to distinguish these lesions from primary cutaneous ALCL. The histological appearance of systemic cases is usually more monomorphic with infrequent tumour giant cells. The tumour cells in systemic ALCL express a cytotoxic phenotype and are positive for CD30 and EMA. CD3 is negative in more than 75% of cases {191, 1121}. CD5 and CD7 are often negative. CD2, CD4 and CD43 are more useful and are expressed in a significant proportion of cases. ALK expression and t(2;5) or variant translocations involving ALK and fusion partners other than NPM are present in the majority of cases {706, 809}. The natural history is aggressive but long term complete remissions can be obtained in most patients with ALK-positive disease {191}.

Angioimmunoblastic T-cell lymphoma (AITL)

ICD-O code   9705/3

Skin lesions in angioimmunoblastic T-cell lymphoma (AITL) occur in half of the cases, usually as a generalized maculopapular eruption simulating viral exanthem or drug eruption, or as urticaria, purpura, erythemato-squamous plaques, prurigo-like lesions, erythroderma, erosions and necrotic lesions. The disease occurs mostly in middle-aged or elderly people without gender preponderance {787}. Other findings are fever, weight loss, night sweats, lymphadenopathy, hepato- and splenomegaly, anaemia, an elevated sedimentation rate, leukocytosis, neutropaenia or thrombocytopaenia, as well as polyclonal hypergammaglobulinemia. AITL exhibits an aggressive course with a median survival ranging from 11 to 30 months and a fatal outcome

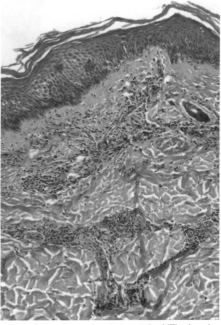

Fig. 4.45 Cutaneous involvement in AITL. A polymorphous perivascular infiltrate is present in the superficial dermis

in 50 to 70% of patients.
Histologically, the skin lesions are characterized by nonspecific subtle superficial perivascular infiltrates composed of eosinophils and lymphocytes without atypia accompanied by hyperplasia of capillaries. Admixed plasma cells and histiocytes can be found {2087}. Clonal T cell receptor rearrangement has been reported in some cases {1522}. However, it is not clear whether the cutaneous manifestations are generally due to tumour cell involvement or a secondary phenomenon related to cytokine production.

Cutaneous marginal zone B-cell lymphoma

W. Kempf
E. Ralfkiaer
L. Duncan

G. Burg
R. Willemze
S.H. Swerdlow
E.S. Jaffe

Definition

Primary cutaneous marginal zone B-cell lymphoma (MZL) is an indolent lymphoma composed of small B cells including marginal zone (centrocyte-like) or monocytoid cells, lymphoplasmacytoid cells and plasma cells. It is considered part of the broad group of extranodal marginal zone B-cell lymphomas commonly involving mucosal sites (mucosa associated lymphoid tissue, MALT). Primary cutaneous immunocytoma, primary cutaneous plasmacytoma and cutaneous follicular lymphoid hyperplasia with monotypic plasma cells are considered variants of MZL.

ICD-O code   9699/3

Synonyms

EORTC (1997): Primary cutaneous immunocytoma / marginal zone B-cell lymphoma

Epidemiology

MZL most commonly affects adults aged over 40 years. There is no clear gender preponderance {132,2141}.

Etiology

In Europe, Borrelia burgdorferi DNA has been identified in some cases of MZL suggesting that it may play an etiological role. {433}. However, no association of Borrelia with CBCL has been found in the United States and Asia {2547}.

Localization

MZL is predominantly localized on the upper extremitites, and less often head and trunk.

Clinical features

In most cases, cutaneous MZL presents with red to violaceous plaques or nodules with an erythematous border {2141}. Ulceration and visceral dissemination are

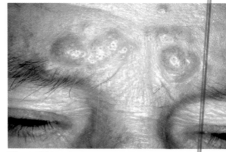

Fig. 4.48 Marginal-zone lymphoma. Firm nodules on the forehead.

uncommon. MZL with secondary spread to the skin is often multifocal {1418}.

Histopathology

The infiltrate is characterized by residual reactive lymphoid follicles surrounded by pale staining cuffs of tumour cells. Reactive germinal centres with distinct mantle zones are commonly found in early lesions but may become colonized by tumour cells as the disease progresses. The interfollicular infiltrate is composed of small to medium-sized, centrocyte-like or monocytoid cells with slightly irregular nuclei, moderately dispersed chromatin, inconspicuous nucleoli and a rim of pale cytoplasm {2234,2362}. Variable numbers of lymphoplasmacytoid cells and plasma cells are typically present at the periphery of the infiltrates or in the subepidermal area. Intranuclear PAS positive pseudoinclusions (Dutcher bodies), are commonly found, particularly in plasma cell rich forms of MZL. Diffuse infiltrates almost completely consisting of monocytoid cells, lymphoepithelial lesions with infiltration of sweat glands and the presence of very immature plasma cells should raise suspicion of secondary cutaneous involvement.

Immunoprofile

The neoplastic cells express CD19+, CD20+, CD22+, CD79a+, but are negative for CD5-, CD10-, bcl-6, CD23-. CD43 may be positive {132}. In contrast to FL, the tumour cells are bcl-2+, but negative for bcl-6 and CD10 {603,1418}. Reactive

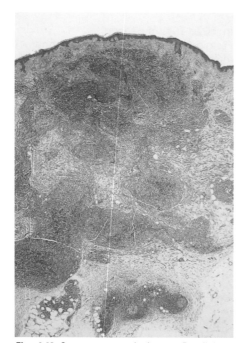

Fig. 4.46 Cutaneous marginal zone B-cell lymphoma. Infiltrate extends through dermis to subcutaneous tissue.

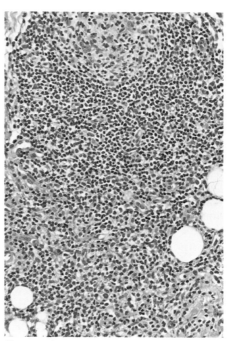

Fig. 4.47 Cutaneous marginal zone B-cell lymphoma. Neoplastic cells surround a residual germinal centre.

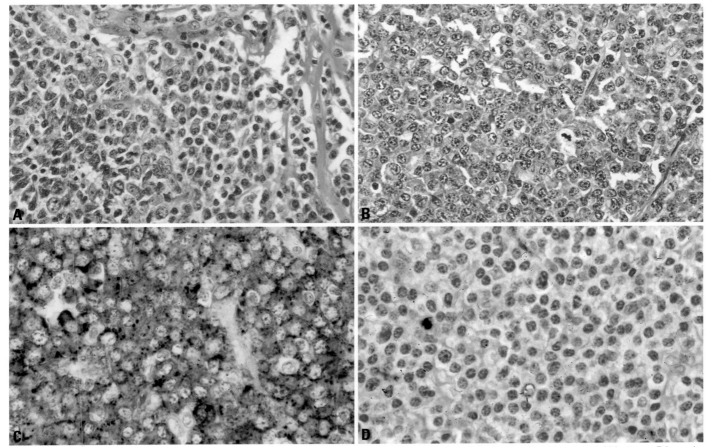

Fig. 4.49 Plasmacytoid cells in cutaneous marginal zone B-cell lymphoma. **A** Monoclonal plasma cells are admixed with cells with monocytoid features. **B** In a subsequent biopsy from the same patient, all of the cells have a plasmacytic morphology and express monoclonal Ig light chains. **C** Kappa. **D** Lambda.

germinal centres are bcl-6+ and bcl-2-. Anti-CD21 staining often reveals regular and irregular networks of follicular dendritic cells (FDC) in reactive follicles, but not associated with tumour cells. The lymphoplasmacytoid cells and the plasma cells show monotypic expression of immunoglobulin light chains. There are numerous admixed reactive T-cells.

Precursor lesion
Cutaneous lymphoid hyperplasia due to Borrelia infection may mimic MZL and has been postulated to represent a precursor lesion in some circumstances.

Histogenesis
Post germinal centre B-lymphocyte with plasmacytic differentiation and gene expression pattern {2273}.

Somatic genetics
IgH genes are clonally rearranged. The most common translocation in gastric MZL, the t(11;18) involving the API2/MLT genes, has not been demonstrated in primary cutaneous MZL {1418,2141,2279}. However, the t(14;18)(q32;q21) involving IGH and MALT1 was reported in approximately one third of cases in a small series. Fas gene mutations are present in

a minority of cases, similar to MZL of other extranodal sites. Abnormalities of BCL10 are absent {906}.

Prognosis
MZL shows a protracted clinical course with a tendency for recurrences. However, the prognosis is favourable with 5-year-survival rates between 90 and 100%. Transformation into diffuse large B cell lymphoma occurs infrequently {2141}.

Cutaneous follicle centre lymphoma

N. Pimpinelli
E. Berti
G. Burg
L. Duncan
N. L. Harris
E.S. Jaffe

H. Kerl
M. Kurrer
W. Kempf
C.J.L.M. Meijer
M. Santucci
S.H. Swerdlow
R. Willemze

Definition

Primary cutaneous follicle centre lymphoma (PCFCL) is defined as a tumour of neoplastic follicle centre cells (FCC), usually a mixture of small and large cleaved cells (centrocytes) and, to a lesser extent, large noncleaved cells (centroblasts) with prominent nucleoli. The growth pattern varies from follicular to follicular and diffuse to diffuse.

ICD-O Code   9690/3

Synonyms

Kiel: centroblastic-centrocytic (follicular, follicular and diffuse), centroblastic.
Working formulation: follicular, follicular and diffuse (predominantly small cleaved, mixed small cleaved and large cell, predominantly large cell).
WHO: follicular lymphoma, diffuse follicle centre lymphoma, diffuse large B-cell lymphoma.
EORTC (1997): follicular centre cell lymphoma.
Reticulohistiocytoma of the dorsum (Crosti disease): {220}.

Epidemiology

Primary cutaneous B cell lymphoma (CBCL) in Europe account for up to 25% of cutaneous lymphomas, manifesting predominantly in middle-aged adults, with no gender predominance {2523}, and having an incidence rate of 0.1-0.2 per 100,000 persons per year {1831}. Among primary CBCL, marginal zone B cell lymphoma and FCL are by far the most common subtypes {744,1281, 2576}.

Etiology

The etiology of primary cutaneous FCL is unknown.

Localization

Most patients have local or regional disease. Trunk and head and neck regions are by far the most frequent localizations {429,744,2061,2523}. Presentation with multifocal skin lesions is observed in a small minority of patients.

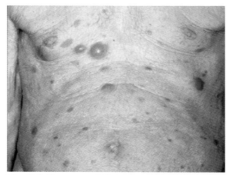
Fig. 4.50 Cutaneous follicle centre lymphoma. Firm nodules on the trunk.

Clinical features

The clinical presentation consists of firm erythematous to violaceous plaques, nodules or tumours of variable size. Larger nodules may be surrounded by small papules and slightly infiltrated, sometimes figurate plaques. The skin surface is smooth. Lesions may be present for months to many years {220, 2061,2523}.

Histopathology

The infiltrates show a spectrum of growth patterns, with a morphologic continuum from follicular to follicular and diffuse to diffuse. The lesions are by definition composed of a mixture of centrocytes (which may be small and/or large) and centroblasts in varying proportion. Small centrocytes and a predominantly follicular growth pattern are more frequently found in small, early lesions. A predominance of large neoplastic cells, particularly large centrocytes or multilobated cells and less frequently centroblasts (not in confluent sheets), are generally found in more advanced lesions (large nodules or tumours) {2523}. When morphologically identifiable, follicles are often ill-defined and show a monotonous population of FCC, lack starry sky histiocytes, and generally have an attenuated or absent mantle zone, different from cutaneous follicular hyperplasias {425, 429,603,864,1397}. The infiltrates are found primarily in the dermis, with extension into subcutaneous tissue seen in larger nodules. The overlying epidermis is generally unaffected.

Immunoprofile

The cells express B-cell markers including CD19, CD20, and CD22, and may show (more often in cryostat sections)

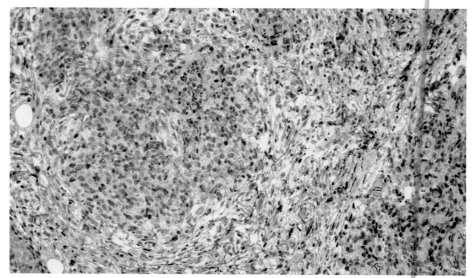
Fig. 4.51 Primary cutaneous follicle centre lymphoma. Neoplastic bcl6+ cells surround and infiltrate a reactive follicle with bcl6+ germinal center.

monotypic staining for surface immu-
noglobulins (sIg). However, absence of
detectable sIg staining is common in
tumours showing a diffuse population of
large FCC. In PCFCL, neoplastic cells
consistently express Bcl-6 protein, while
CD10 is variably expressed (often positive in follicular cases and more fequently
negative in lesions with diffuse pattern of
growth) {425,429,823,1042,1832, 2061}.
Bcl-2 protein is usually not expressed but
may be faintly positive, less than reactive
T-cells {38, 209, 425, 603, 774, 1042,1
622}. The follicles are associated with follicular dendritic cells, positive for CD21,
CD23, and CD35. Residual, scattered
FDC may be sometimes found in diffuse
large cell infiltrates. Neopastic cells are
constantly CD5- and CD43-negative.
Admixed T-cells may be abundant and
sometimes predominant, particularly in
small, early lesions.

Histogenesis
Mature germinal centre derived B-lymphocyte {2273,2523}.

Somatic genetics
Clonally rearranged immunoglobulin
genes are present. Bcl-2 gene
rearrangement and t(14;18) chromosomal translocation are absent in most
cases {209,430,467,1622,1820,2523}.
Inactivation of p15 and p16 tumour suppressor genes by promotor hypermethy-
lation has been reported in about 10%
and 30% of PCFCL, respectively {468}.
Chromosomal imbalances have been
identified by comparative genomic hybridization (CGH) analysis in a minority of
PCFCL, but a consistent pattern has not
emerged {942,1503}.

Prognosis and predictive factors
Primary cutaneous FCL have an excellent prognosis (>95% 5-year survival).
Local recurrences, most often near the
initial site of cutaneous presentation, may
develop but will not influence clinical outcome. Cytologic grade or growth pattern
(follicular or diffuse) do not appear to
have an impact on prognosis in patients
with primary cutaneous disease. Locally

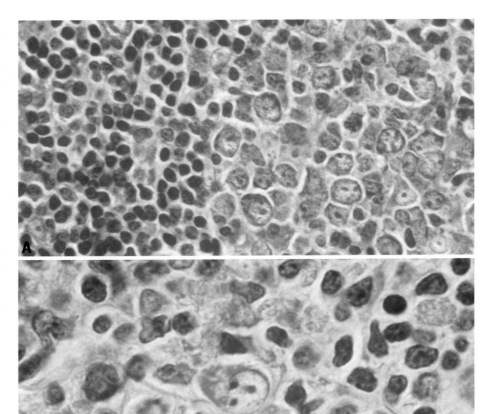

Fig. 4.52 Cutaneous follicle centre lymphoma, follicular growth pattern. **A** Small and large follicle centre
cells. **B** Detail of large follicle centre cells

directed forms of therapy, most commonly radiation or surgical excision (small,
isolated lesions), are generally effective {194, 429, 1283, 1824, 1825, 1938,
2060, 2061, 2202, 2523}.

Secondary cutaneous follicular lymphoma (FL)

Patients more often present with multiple
lesions in non-contiguous skin sites
{429,2060}. Unlike PCFCL, neoplastic
cells strongly express CD10 and Bcl2,
and show t(14:18) translocation in most
cases. These secondary cutaneous
forms are managed like a systemic lymphoma. Whether cutaneous involvement
by FCL has an impact on prognosis is
presently unknown.

Cutaneous diffuse large B-cell lymphoma

G. Burg
E.S. Jaffe
R. Willemze
C. Dommann-Scherrer
S.H. Swerdlow

W. Kempf
M Kurrer
H Kutzner
J. Wechsler
N.L. Harris

Definition
Primary cutaneous diffuse large B-cell lymphomas (DLBCLs) are neoplastic proliferations showing a completely diffuse growth pattern consisting of large transformed B-cells without significant admixture of centrocytes.

The most common variant, DLBCL, leg-type, usually occurs on the leg and less frequently at other sites. Other variants are referred to as DLBCL, other and comprise T-cell/histiocyte-rich LBCL, plasmablastic lymphoma and lesions that do not fulfill the criteria for a DLBCL, leg type.

ICD-O code   9680/3

Diffuse large B-cell lymphoma (DLBCL), leg-type

Epidemiology
Approximately 5-10% of cutaneous B-cell lymphomas are classified as DLBCL, leg type. The median age is around 70 years, and the tumours are more common in females than males {2432}. DLBCL of the skin is rare in children {1005}.

Clinical features
DLBCL, leg type occurs primarily in elderly females who present with rapidly developing multiple tumours, most commonly on the leg but sometimes at other localizations. Therefore analogous to the "nasal-type" designation for a distinct extranodal variant of NK/T-cell lymphomas, the term "DLBCL, leg-type" is chosen for all cutaneous diffuse large B-cell lymphomas with the designated cytological and immunophenotypic features. Clinically multiple disseminated or aggregated dome shaped red tumours with a firm consistency and a shiny surface without scaling are seen. Ulceration may occur in advanced stages.

Histopathology
The tumour cells diffusely infiltrate the dermis with a destructive growth pattern, often obliterating adnexal structures. The infiltrate may extend into subcutaneous tissue. The epidermis is often spared, with a Grenz zone. The infiltrate is composed of medium to large sized B cells, which are usually monomorphic in appearance. Cells may resemble immunoblasts, and less commonly centroblasts. There is usually a minimal inflammatory component and little stromal reaction.

Immunohistochemistry
The tumour cells are positive for CD20 and CD79a, negative for CD10 and CD138, have variable BCL-6 expression and are usually strongly positive for BCL-2 protein and MUM-1/IRF-4 {1797}. These features have been shown in nodal DLBCL to correlate with an activated B-cell gene expression profile, which is usually predictive of a more aggressive clinical course {1041, 1977}.

Histogenesis
Transformed peripheral B cell of probable post germinal centre origin {816}.

Somatic genetics
The immunoglobulin genes are clonally rearranged. The BCL-2/JH translocation is absent {814,905,2472}. Recent studies using gene expression profiling have identified increased expression of genes associated with cellular proliferation. The gene expression profile of the leg-type of tumour resembles that of activated B-cell type of nodal or systemic DLBCL {1041}. Significant differences have not been identified among tumours of the leg-type arising in different sites {814,1797}.

The primary cutaneous large B-cell lymphoma of the leg-type can be seen in a variety of anatomic locations and is not restricted to the leg {1797}.

Prognosis and predictive factors
In multivariate analysis, BCL-2 expression, multiple skin lesions, and age remained independent prognostic factors. The 5-year disease-specific survival rates in BCL-2–positive and BCL-2–negative patients were 41% and 89%, respectively (P < .0001) {1732A,1797, 1819A}. Thus, these studies support the identification of DLBCL leg type, as a clinically and biologically distinctive group.

Diffuse large B-cell lymphoma, other

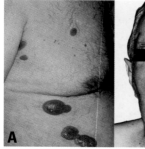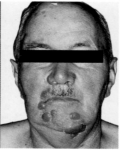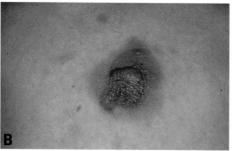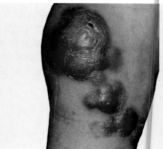

Fig. 4.53 Diffuse large B-cell lymphoma. **A** Dome-shaped nodules and tumours without ulceration on the trunk and in the face. **B** Soft tumour surrounded by an erythematous infiltrate on the back. **C** Aggregation of non-ulcerated nodules and tumours confined to a limited area of the lower leg.

Definition

The term DLBCL, other, refers to diffuse lymphomas composed of large transformed B-cells that lack the typical features of DLBCL, leg-type, and do not conform to the definition of primary cutaneous follicle centre lymphoma. These tumours may be comprised of a monomorphic population of centroblast-like cells, but with a mixed inflammatory background.

BCL-2 protein may be negative, whereas BCL-6 will usually be expressed. The presence of multiple lesions is a poor prognostic indicator; such cases must be distinguished from secondary involvement by DLBCL.

There are some primary cutaneous follicle centre lymphomas in which the majority of tumour cells are centroblasts. Previously these lesions have been categorized as DLBCL by most observers {864,877,879,1263}. These lymphomas invariably contain a population of centrocytes as well as some reactive cells. A focal follicular growth pattern may be seen. Despite the predominance of centroblasts, clinical studies have suggested that these lymphomas have an benign clinical course, and may usually be treated in a conservative manner. Based on the clinical behaviour and the spectrum of cytological composition, these tumours are classified under the single heading of cutaneous follicle centre lymphoma.

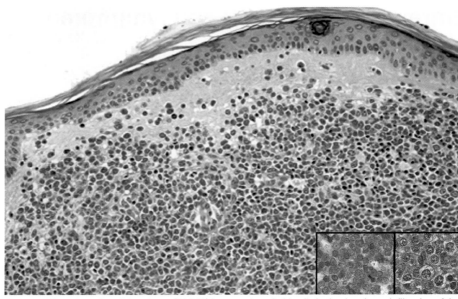

Fig. 4.54 Diffuse large B-cell lymphoma (DLBCL) leg type. Lymphoid cells in the dermis; no infiltration of the epidermis. Left insert: lymphoid cells with strong immunoreactivity for BCL-2. Right insert: large, densely packed lymphoid cells.

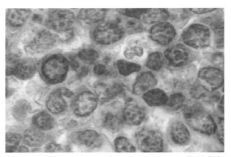

Fig. 4.55 Diffuse large B-cell lymphoma (DLBCL), leg type. BCL-2 staining of atypical lymphoid cells.

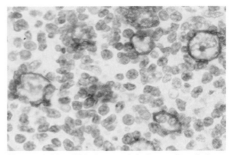

Fig. 4.56 T-cell/histiocyte-rich large B-cell lymphoma. CD20 staining highlights the few neoplastic B-cells intermingled in a dense infiltrate of reactive T-cells.

T-cell / histiocyte-rich large B-cell lymphoma

T-cell / histiocyte-rich large B-cell lymphoma is an unusual morphological variant of "diffuse" LBCL {1886} that rarely occurs primarily in the skin {645,1423}. It is characterized by a small number of large neoplastic B-cells (<10%), scattered within an abundant background of small reactive T-lymphocytes with or without histiocytes. Some T-cell/histiocyte-rich large B-cell lymphomas may represent progression from a more indolent B-cell lymphoma {645,2042}.

Plasmablastic lymphoma

Plasmablastic lymphomas rarely may present as a primary cutaneous lymphoma. The tumour cells can be positive for Epstein-Barr virus (EBV), and have a phenotype that reflects terminal stages of B-cell differentiation (CD20-, MUM-1+, CD138+, EMA+). Plasmablastic lymphomas are usually a heterogenous group of disease entities {524} and can be encountered in settings of immunodeficiency, HIV-associated, or iatrogenic {617,985}.

Secondary skin involvement by diffuse large B-cell lymphoma

Secondary skin involvement most commonly shows localisation of the disease on the trunk and the extremities {1263}. The prognosis is worse than in primary DLBCL, which can be controlled by local treatment modalities, particularly if one is dealing with a single lesion.

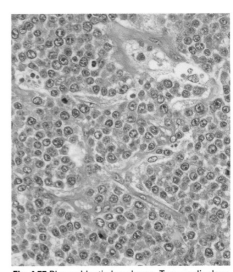

Fig. 4.57 Plasmablastic lymphoma. Tumour displays a spectrum of immunoblasts, plasmablasts, and plasma cells between collagen bundles.

Intravascular large B-cell lymphoma

H. Kutzner
E.S. Jaffe

Definition
Intravascular large B-cell lymphoma (IL) is a rare disease with multiorgan involvement, which also affects the skin. This extranodal subtype of diffuse large B-cell lymphoma (DLBCL) is characterized by the presence of large lymphoid cells within the lumina of small to medium-sized blood vessels, particularly capillaries and postcapillary venules. Skin is a common site of presentation, but most patients have systemic disease at time of diagnosis {696,2523}.

ICD-O code   9680/3

Synonyms
Intravascular lymphomatosis; intravascular lymphoma; angioendotheliomatosis proliferans systematisata; malignant angioendotheliomatosis; angiotropic large cell lymphoma (Lukes-Collins), diffuse large B-cell lymphoma (REAL) intravascular large B-cell lymphoma (WHO).

Epidemiology
IL is rare and can occur at any age, but most patients are in their 6th – 9th decade of life. Male to female ratio is 0.8 (range 0.7 – 5.0) {2566}.

Localization
Dermatological manifestations are present in up to one third of patients. Sites of predilection are the lower extremities, but lesions may involve all parts of the integument. A wide range of organ involvement has been described: central nervous system, skin, adrenal glands, thyroid, gastrointestinal system, kidneys, lungs, genitourinary tract, and eye {275}. At autopsy, involvement of the majority of organs is seen despite the absence of prior clinical manifestations or mass lesions {1257}.

Clinical features
The clinical manifestations are predominantly neurologic (85%) {214} and dermatologic {633} and are attributed to vascular occlusion. There is a notable absence of lymphadenopathy, splenomegaly or circulating lymphoma cells in the majority of cases {631,684, 837, 1257,2387}.
There is a plethora of different skin lesions including tender, indurated nodules, livedo-like reticulate erythema, linear erythematous streaks, and painful indurated telangiectasias. Lesions may imitate phlebitis, panniculitis, or vasculitis {1809}.

Histopathology
The angiotropic lymphoid infiltrate often spares the dermis, requiring deep biopsies including parts of the subcutaneous fat. The large neoplastic lymphoid cells are usually confined to the lumina of capillaries and postcapillary venules {1809, 2513}, albeit extravascular involvement may occur {1257}. Tumour cells are large with vesicular nuclei, prominent nucleoli, and frequent mitoses. Fibrin thrombi in the upper and deep dermal plexus, with partial occlusion of the vascular lumina, and few entrapped hyperchromatic lymphocytes are typical of IL presenting with reticulate and livedoid erythema.

Immunoprofile
Tumour cells usually express B-cell associated antigens and may coexpress CD10 or CD5. {406,697,953,1193,1253, 2566}. Although most IL present with overexpression of theBCL-2 protein {1257} they lack BCL-2 gene rearrangement {1193,2566}. These cases have to be distinguished from other intravascular lymphomas of different lineages {112, 113,633,697,736,1355,2138,2143}.
The precise mechanisms of lymphoid-endothelial interaction leading to vascular occlusion and thrombotic events are

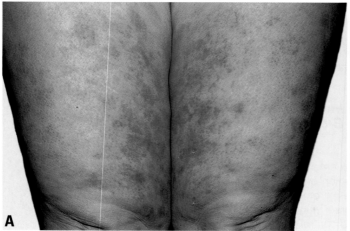

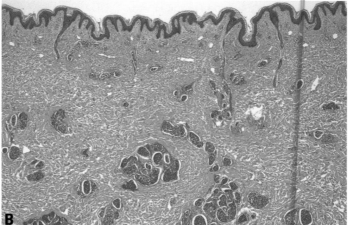

Fig. 4.58 Intravascular large B-cell lymphoma. **A** Involvement of the cutis with livedoid palpable erythema. **B** Dilated dermal vessels filled with densely packed neoplastic lymphoid cells.

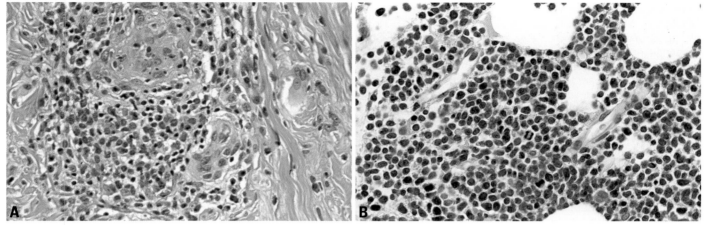

Fig. 4.64 Mantle cell lymphoma. **A** Perivascular infiltrate of small atypical lymphoid cells. **B** Densly packed small atypical lymphoid cells showing polygonal or indented nuclei and homogeneous chromatin staining.

{654,1422}. Gene profiling has suggested the presence of a small subset of cases that lack cyclin D1 abnormalities {1978}. Other primary and mostly secondary abnormalities are also described {376,1045,2303}.

Prognosis and predictive factors
MCL has a median survival of 3-5 years with those having "non-nodal" disease doing better {376,1756,2301,2303}. Adverse prognostic indicators include a high proliferative fraction, probably blastoid morphology, secondary genotypic abnormalities and blood involvement (at least in patients with nodal disease). Whether skin involvement in particular is an independent prognostic indicator is uncertain.

Burkitt lymphoma

Definition
Burkitt lymphoma is a mature B-cell neoplasm composed of relatively uniform medium sized transformed B-cells with a C-MYC translocation {630}.

ICD-O code   9687/3

Epidemiology
BL occurs in children in equatorial Africa (endemic), primarily in children and young adults elsewhere (sporadic) and in immunodeficient patients. There is a male predominance.

Etiology
Endemic BL and a minority of sporadic BL are Epstein-Barr virus positive.

Clinical features
BL usually presents as an extranodal mass often in the abdomen or, in endemic cases, in jaw or other facial bones. Other patients have a leukaemic presentation. Cutaneous involvement in BL appears to be extremely rare and at least usually is associated with disease at other sites {123,141,349,700}. It has rarely been described as occurring with ulceration from direct invasion from underlying bony lesions {349}, as distinct cutaneous lesions at relapse {123} and in 12% of autopsied cases of American BL (2 cases) {141}.

Histopathology
Histologic sections show a diffuse proliferation of medium sized transformed lymphocytes with relatively round nuclei with several nucleoli and a narrow rim of very amphophilic/basophilic cytoplasm. There are many apoptotic bodies and tingible body macrophages creating a starry sky appearance. Skin involvement demonstrates a diffuse but sometimes patchy dermal and subcutaneous infiltrate with a Grenz zone {123,700}.

Immunohistochemistry
Immunophenotypic studies demonstrate CD5-, CD10+,BCL-2-, CD20+ mature B-cells with surface immunoglobulin expression.

Histogenesis
Germinal centre/post germinal centre B-cell

Somatic genetics
All cases have clonal immunoglobulin

gene rearrangements and a C-MYC translocation, most often with a t(8;14)(q24;q32) {1483}. Many, if not all, cases also have C-MYC mutations {230, 1483}.

Prognosis and predictive factors
BL is an aggressive but curable neoplasm with a 5-year overall survival of 44% {3}.

Chronic lymphocytic leukaemia / small lymphocytic lymphoma

Definition
Chronic lymphocytic leukaemia/small lymphocytic lymphoma (CLL/SLL) is a mature B-cell neoplasm composed of small, usually CD5+, CD23+, cyclin D1- B-cells with relatively round nuclei having clumped chromatin {1662}. Especially in lymph nodes, there is often an associated minor population of prolymphocytes and paraimmunoblasts that form proliferation centres.

ICD-O code
Chronic lymphocytic leukaemia
                    9823/3
Small lymphocytic lymphoma
                    9670/3

Epidemiology
CLL is the most common type of leukaemia in the West and SLL are reported to account for 6.7% of non-Hodgkin lymphomas {3,1064}.

Clinical features

CLL/SLL is seen most commonly in middle aged and older adults with a male predominance. It usually presents with blood and marrow involvement, frequent adenopathy and sometimes hepatosplenomegaly. Skin involvement is reported in 2% of patients without a marked predilection for any region of the body and occurs in patients who also have blood involvement {273,1167}. The face and scalp are frequent sites of involvement. It may be present either at the time of diagnosis or, much more frequently, develops subsequently {431}. Lesions may be single or multiple erythematous macules, papules, violaceous plaques, nodules or tumours either occurring in a limited or less frequently more generalized area {431,1167}. Atypical presentations include chronic paronychia, papulovesicular eruption and finger clubbing. Skin involvement may occur at sites of previous viral (eg, herpes zoster, herpes simplex) or Borrelia burgdorferi infection {427} and at sites of epithelial neoplasms {2215}. Spontaneous regression of CLL infiltrates at least at sites of prior herpetic infection may occur {2449}. In contrast to the absence of virus in at least most of the lesions in viral scars, B. burgdorferi DNA is found in at least some cutaneous CLL lesions {427}.

Histopathology

Histologic sections demonstrate a diffuse proliferation of small relatively round lymphocytes with condensed chromatin with lymph node biopsies typically demonstrating paler (pseudofollicular) proliferation centres where the cells have more abundant pale cytoplasm, more dispersed chromatin and sometimes prominent central nucleoli. The latter cells represent paraimmunoblasts and some of the former cells prolymphocytes.

Cutaneous lesions show a patchy perivascular, nodular, more diffuse or rarely band-like dermal infiltrate of small, usually but not always round, lymphocytes with occasional single lymphocytes in the epidermis and frequent extension into the subcutaneous tissue {431}. Patients with more than one biopsy can demonstrate more than one growth pattern. There may be overlying epidermal changes infrequently including ulceration. Proliferation centres are seen only in a minority of cases although there may be scattered larger cells in other cases {427}. A minority of cases have admixed eosinophils, neutrophils, and/or histiocytes. A granulomatous reaction may be present especially in some of the lesions arising in scars following prior viral infection {432}. Cutaneous CLL associated with granuloma annulare-like changes has also been reported {797}.

Immunoprofile

Immunophenotypic studies demonstrate a characteristic CD5+, CD43+, CD10-, CD23+, FMC7-, cyclin D1-, weakly CD20+ monoclonal B-cell population with weak surface immunoglobulin expression {1662}. In the cutaneous lesions, the admixed T-cells present are mostly of CD4+ type {431}.

Histogenesis

Mature B-cell most likely of memory type (including cases with either mutated or unmutated immunoglobulin heavy chain genes) {586,1288,1976}.

Somatic genetics

All cases have clonal immunoglobulin gene rearrangement although oligoclonal bands suggesting admixed reactive B-cells may also be present in the cutaneous lesions {431}. In some cases the immunoglobulin genes show somatic hypermutation and in others they do not {586,943,1288,1976}. There are no chromosomal abnormalities specific for CLL/SLL; however, the most commonly described abnormalities include 13q and 11q deletions, trisomy 12 and 17q deletion {643}.

Genetic susceptibility

There is an inherited susceptibility to CLL; however, the critical genes remain to be determined {1064}.

Prognosis and predictive factors

CLL/SLL is one of the indolent lymphoid neoplasms. Clinically advanced stage, 17q deletions, unmutated immunoglobulin genes, CD38 and ZAP-70 expression include some of the more important adverse prognostic indicators {553,643, 943,1662,1760,2518}. Most do not believe that skin involvement portends an adverse outcome; however, it has been reported that cases with >5% medium and large-sized B-cells, admixed reactive cells and epidermal changes did worse than those without these features and there are reports in the literature suggesting a poor outcome following any cutaneous involvement {427,432,1167}. Transformation to a large cell lymphoma (Richter syndrome), Hodgkin lymphoma or prolymphocytic leukaemia is also associated with an aggressive course {826}. Richter syndrome can present as cutaneous lesions {427,2578}.

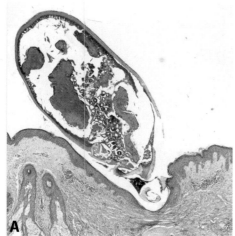 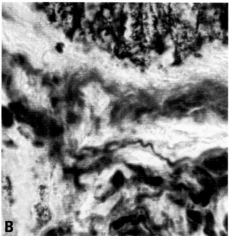

Fig. 4.73 A Head of Ixodes ricinus fixed to the skin. **B** Borrelia burgdorferi in the dermis, silver stain.

Histologically there is a scant sleeve-like perivascular lymphocytic infiltrate in the mid or deep dermis.

Lymphomatoid contact dermatitis has been reported as a reaction to various allergens (i.e. nickel, Peru balsam) or drugs (diphenylhydantoin) inducing mycosis fungoides-like features {1975}. Genotyping has shown clonal rearrangement in some cases. Such cases may be closely related to "clonal dermatitis" some of which develop into overt CTCL {2545,2546}. Histologically, eczematous features with epidermotropism of lymphocytes and accumulations of CD1a-positive Langerhans cells may be found. Actinic reticuloid is a chronic photoallergic infiltrative dermatitis of light exposed areas associated bearing a clinical and histological resemblance to malignant lymphoma, especially to Sézary syndrome. Histologically there is a dense infiltrate of lymphocytes mixed with many polyclonal plasma cells, eosinophils and macrophages.

There is a considerable overlap between T- and B-PSL in persistent nodular arthropod-bite reaction, nodular scabies and inflammatory molluscum contagiosum which show a dense polymorphous infiltrate consisting of a mixture of T-cells, B-cells, macrophages and predominantly eosinophilic granulocytes.

Lymphomatoid papulosis even though showing biologic features of pseudolymphoma is considered to belong to the group of lymphomas since despite spontaneous regression of single lesions, the

disease is not curable and may show transitions to other lymphomas.

PSL with predominant B-cell infiltrates

Lymphadenosis benigna cutis (LABC) {124} – the prototype of this group of B-PSL – is synonymous with lymphocytoma cutis. In Europe it is most commonly caused by infection with Borrelia burgdorferi after a tick bite (Ixodes ricinus). However, other microbiological (medicinal leeches, Hirudo medicinalis) {2211}, physical or chemical agents as well may induce lymphocytoma-like reactions.

Two thirds of all lesions are situated on the head, tending to occur on the ear lobes. Other predilections are the nose as well as the nipples, the inguinal area and scrotum. Usually the lesion is a solitary papule or nodule, but several disseminated lesions may occur as well {1068}.

Microscopic examination shows a nodular dermal infiltrate with reactive follicles. In addition, there is a rather diffuse infiltrate containing T cells, histiocytes, eosinophils and polyclonal plasma cells. The presence of macrophages containing ingested nuclear material (tingible body macrophages) within the follicles producing a "starry sky" pattern is a common feature in B-PSL and a hallmark of all reactive germinal centres. The infiltrate is predominantly located in the upper and mid dermis, but may extend into the deep dermis. Small groups of lymphoid cells between collagen bundles may be observed at the periphery of

the lesions. This is a helpful histological criterion in the differentiation from cutaneous B-cell lymphoma, in which the nodular infiltrate shows convex rather than concave sharply demarcated borders.

Phenotypically {428} a polyclonal B-lymphocytic infiltrate without light chain restriction of the infiltrate is found in most cases. The cells express the phenotype of mature B-cells (CD 20, CD 79a). In B-PSL, regular and sharply demarcated networks of CD21+ follicular dendritic cells are present, whereas in CBCL these networks are irregularly shaped {342}.

Acral pseudolymphomatous angiokeratoma of children (APACHE) is a rare benign pseudolymphomatous disorder occurring mainly in children {1888}.

The typical clinical presentation is multiple (up to 40), asymptomatic, small papules located unilaterally on the fingers, toes and hands. Their colour is usually red-violet, accounting for their angiomatous appearance {1887}.

Histologically the dermis contains a moderately to very dense, non-epidermotropic infiltrate composed of small well-differentiated lymphocytes admixed with a few plasma cells, histiocytes, and giant cells. Blood vessels show prominent plump endothelial cells {1165,1887}.

Immunohistochemically the cellular infiltrate represents a mixture of polyclonal mature T- and B-lymphocytes {936}.

Inflammatory pseudotumour (IPT) (plasma cell granuloma, inflammatory myofibroblastic pseudotumour) refers to a spectrum of idiopathic benign conditions with unknown etiology that can develop in various organs and deep tissues, particularly in the lung. Cutaneous IPT occurs as a solitary, slowly growing, tender nodule measuring 1-3 cm in diameter. Irrespective the anatomic location, the lesions share common histological features, showing well circumscribed proliferation of myofibroblasts/fibroblasts expressing smooth muscle actin (SMA) and vimentin, a mixed cell infiltrate containing high numbers of plasma cells with prominent germinal centres dispersed throughout the lesion. The plasma cells are polyclonal and are seen in the interfollicular areas (plasma cell granuloma) 21, {508,509}. Later stages show marked fibrosis/sclerosis with thick collagen bundles arranged in concentric whorls.

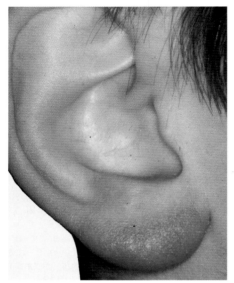

Fig. 4.74 Lymphadenosis benigna cutis (LABC, B-pseudolymphoma) following tick bite in the earlobe.

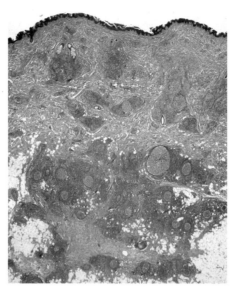

Fig. 4.75 B-PSL. Reactive follicles in lymphadenosis benigna cutis (B-pseudolymphoma).

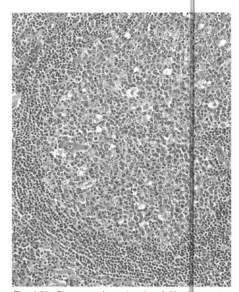

Fig. 4.76 Close up view showing follicular centre with tingible-body macrophages featuring a starry sky pattern.

Histological variations include presence of high endothelial venules, admixture of eosinophils, calcification, psammoma bodies, and presence of large polygonal myofibroblasts (vimentin+, CD15-, CD30-) {1476} with single, double or multiple nuclei and prominent eosinophilic nucleoli resembling Reed-Sternberg cells {388,1084,1476,1881,2561}.

Differential diagnosis of cutaneous IPT includes lymphoma, angiolymphoid hyperplasia with eosinophilia and Kimura and infectious dermatoses (mycobacteria, deep fungal infections). The later stages of cutaneous IPT should be distinguished from erythema elevatum diutinum, granuloma faciale and dermatofibroma with lymphoid infiltrate.

PSL with mixed and unclassified infiltrates

There are reactive lymphocytic infiltrates in the context of other skin disorders that can be referred to as pseudolymphomatous reactions in an even broader sense. Neoplasms, especially squamous cell carcinoma, basal cell carcinoma, and malignant melanoma, or naevi (halo [Sutton] naevi) may show a dense mononuclear infiltrate, composed of T cells or of B cells, sometimes with follicle formation, with polyclonal plasma cells being numerous especially in head and neck localizations.

Histogenesis

Polyclonality is the hallmark of cutaneous pseudolymphomas. Besides T-cells and B-cells, mononuclear phagocytes represent a considerable proportion of the infiltrate. Eosinophils and polytypic plasma cells as well are present in most cases of either B-cell or T-cell pseudolymphomas of the skin {342}.

Somatic genetics

No clonal rearrangement of T-cell receptor genes or of immunoglobulin heavy chain genes or light chain restriction of plasma cells is found.

Prognosis and predictive factors

The prognosis of cutaneous pseudolymphomas by definition is excellent, showing spontaneous regression of the lesions after cessation of the causative factor or due to treatment with non-aggressive treatment modalities. However there is a potential for some cutaneous pseudolymphomas to progress to cutaneous B-cell lymphoma (CBCL) {433,807,1339}, or to cutaneous T-cell lymphoma (CTCL) {2545,2546}.

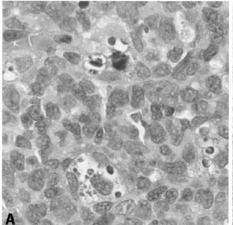
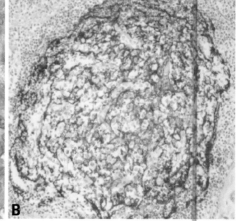

Fig. 4.77 A Tingible body macrophages containing ingested nuclear fragments. **B** Regular network of CD21+ dendritic cells.

Parapsoriasis

G. Burg   J. Guitart
M. Santucci   M Everett
B. Smoller   W. Kempf

Definition

The term "parapsoriasis" is confusing. It encompasses a number of different pathologic states clinically manifested by chronic recalcitrant erythematous scaling skin lesions.

Those diseases which have distinct clinical and histological changes do not fulfill criteria of malignancy, deserve to be labeled with a term which reflects this intermediate situation and labels them as distinct nosologic entities. This term since the days of Brocq has been "parapsoriasis" and there is no reason for changing it {311,312}. Otherwise there will be a bias in epidemiologic data on frequencies, mortality rates and other parameters.

Two groups of parapsoriasis can be differentiated. The benign form ("parapsoriasis en plaques" [Brocq's disease]), which never evolves into malignant lymphoma and large plaque forms with or without poikiloderma which after several decades may evolve into mycosis fungoides or CTCL in up to 50% of the cases. Table 4.3 summarizes criteria for differentiation of benign and premalignant forms of parapsoriasis en plaques.

Small plaque parapsoriasis

Synonyms

Parapsoriasis, small patch (digitiform) type (Brocq's disease); Parapsoriasis en plaques, benign type; digitate dermatosis, xanthoerythrodermia perstans; chronic superficial dermatitis

Epidemiology

This form preferentially occurs in young adults and affects males more frequently than females. There are no statistically reliable data on the incidence, which is estimated less than 0.1 per 100,000 per year. There is little tendency to progress. Survival is not affected since SPP never evolves into malignant lymphoma

Clinical Features

Trunk and upper extremities are preferentially involved. Small (2-5cm in diameter), mostly oval or finger-like patches, slightly erythematous, following skin lines. The color is brown red, and fine and powdery (pityriasiform) scaling may be present. The surface is slightly wrinkled resulting in a pseudoatrophic appearance.

Histopathology

The epidermis is normal or slightly spongiotic with patchy parakeratosis. Patchy loose perivascular and disseminated lymphocytic infiltrate, but no oedema, are present in the dermis. Significant epidermotropism of lymphoid cells is lacking.

Immunohistochemistry

Lymphoid cells exhibit mostly CD4+ and some CD8+ {935}.

Somatic genetics

Clonal rearrangement for the T-cell receptor genes is not detectable. However clonal rearrangement of lymphoid cells in the peripheral blood of patients has been reported {1661}.

Prognosis and predictive factors

The skin lesions are extraordinarily stable in shape and size over years and decades without spreading to extracutaneous localizations. Lymph nodes, peripheral blood, bone marrow or internal organs are not affected. Life-expectancy is normal. Progression into mycosis fungoides or other CTCL does not occur.

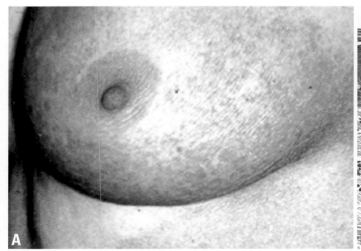
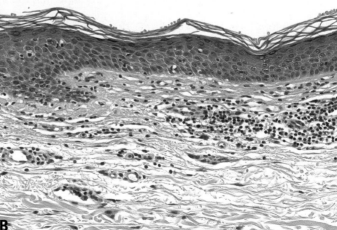

Fig. 4.78 Parapsoriasis. **A** Large plaque parapsoriasis with poikiloderma, showing large telangiectatic patches and a net-like pigmentation. **B** Flattening of the epidermal rete ridges. Band-like lichenoid infiltrate. Dilated small blood vesels in the upper dermis.

Parapsoriasis - Large patch type, with or without poikiloderma

Definition
Pre-malignant inflammatory disorder with tendency to evolve into mycosis fungoides. Some authors consider this lesion a manifestation of early cutaneous T-cell lymphoma (CTCL).

Synonyms
Non-poikilodermatous variant. Parapsoriasis en plaques, premalignant type, parapsoriasis en grandes plaques simples. Poikilodermatous variant: Prereticulotic poikiloderma, parapsoriasis en grandes plaques poikilodermiques; poikiloderma vasculare atrophicans; parapsoriasis lichenoides; parakeratosis variegata

Epidemiology
All age groups may be affected with a slight male preponderance.

Localization
Breast and buttocks are most commonly involved.

Clinical Features
Few large (more than 5 cm in diameter) patches showing pityriasiform scaling with (poikilodermatous variant), telangiectasia and net-like pigmentation are present. There is no palpable infiltration.

Tumour spread and staging
Lesions may stay unchanged over years and decades, or slowly show enlargement in a few cases. No plaques or tumours occur, except when the disease evolves into CTCL in some of the cases.

Histopathology
Under patchy parakeratosis there is a slight atrophy of the epidermis, due to loss of rete ridges, in the poikilodermatous form. The subepidermal zone is free of lymphocytes, which accumulate in a band-like arrangement in the upper dermis, sparing the papillary region. There is no significant epidermotropism as usually seen in early stages of mycosis fungoides. The poikilodermatous variant of the disease in addition shows dilated blood vessels in the upper dermis.

Somatic genetics
T-cell receptor gamma gene rearrangement, which is clonal in about half of the patients with LPP, is probably without any prognostic significance {2186}.

Increased telomerase activity and shortened telomere length was also detected in CD4+ T cells from patients with parapsoriasis {2552}.

Prognosis and predictive factors
There is no significant difference between the observed and expected survivals in patients with less than 10% skin involved. {2575}. However when skin involvement exceeds 10%, as seen in LPP, sporadic cases have an increased risk of transforming into mycosis fungoides after years or decades {2031}.

Table 4.03
Criteria for distinguishing benign and premalignant forms of parapsoriasis en plaques.

	Benign form (small patch type)	Premalignant form (large patch type) with or without poikiloderma
Age distribution	Adults	All ages
Sex incidence (m:f)	5:1	2:1
Clinical features	Small (2-5cm in diameter), mostly oval, or finger-like patches, slightly erythematous and wrinkled surface (pseudoatrophy) uniformly pinkish or yellowish with pityriasiform scaling	Few large patches (>5cm in diameter) pityriasiform scaling with or without telangiectases and netlike pigmentation, sometimes slightly hyperkeratotic (parakeratosis variegata)
Preferential localizations	Trunk and upper extremities	Breast and buttocks
Histological features	Patchy parakeratosis, slight perivascular patchy infiltrate, no oedema, no significant epidermotropism	Slight epidermal atrophy with loss of rete ridges, significant band-like dermal lymphocytic infiltrate sparing the subepidermal zone, no significant epidermotropism, no oedema; telangiectases may be prominent in the poikilodermatous variant
Prognosis	Life expectancy normal; no progression to mycosis fungoides	Life expectancy normal in most cases; progression to mycosis fungoides occurs

Langerhans cell histiocytosis

B. Zelger
R.P. Rapini
W Burgdorf
G. Burg

Definition
Langerhans cell histiocytosis (LCH) is a clonal disorder with systemic spread, characterized by proliferation of dendritic cells which bear morphologic and phenotypic markers of Langerhans cells, characterized by Birbeck granules and expression of CD1a and S-100.

ICD-O code   9751/1

Synonyms
Histiocytosis-X, Langerhans cell granulomatosis, Langerhans cell disease

Epidemiology
LCH predominantly occurs in infants. Median age at diagnosis is 3-5 years {2,299}. It has also been reported in patients up to the ninth decade of life {1551,1578,1941}, and occurs equally in men and women. The incidence has been estimated as 0.1–0.5 per 100.000 population per year. There have been reports on familiar cases with autosomal recessive inheritance.

Etiology
The etiology is unknown. Different groups have studied female patients with cutaneous LCH using a variety of x-linked polymorphisms to demonstrate clonality {2530,2574}. In some cases, association with lymphomas, leukaemias and lung tumours {666} has been observed; in others, infections and environmental factors, including El Nino, have been related to childhood LCH {455}. Many view LCH as a reactive process {716,2583} because of its tendency toward spontaneous remission and response to mild, non-toxic therapy.

Localization
Two thirds of the sites of involvement diagnosed throughout the course of the disease are present at diagnosis {2}. Initial bone involvement is found in almost all patients. Other organs involved skin (25-100%, depending on subtype), ear, liver, lung, and lymph nodes {299}.

Clinical Features
The clinical presentation of LCH is very diverse and depends on the subtype. Skin lesions may be seen either as single organ involvement or as part of a multiorgan systemic disease in 25-100% of cases. Any anatomic site can be involved including scalp, nails, palms and soles as well as mucous membranes.

Letterer-Siwe Disease
This is the most severe, disseminated form of Langerhans cell histiocytosis. It affects children in their first year of life but occurrence in adults has been reported {1731}. Tiny (0.5 mm in diameter) rose-yellow or brownish-red, translucent papules and patches are found on the scalp, diaper and seborrhoeic sites like nasolabial folds, perioral region, and on the upper trunk. In time, the papules become scaly and crusted and may coalesce into plaques. Petechial and purpuric lesions, pustules and vesicles as

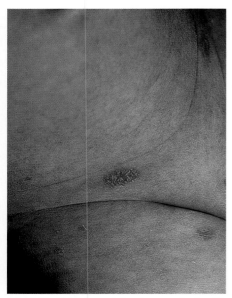

Fig. 4.79 Multiple nodules in a patient with Congenital self-healing reticulohistiocytosis (CSHRH).

Table 4.04
Langerhans cell histiocytoses and their characteristics. This classification has limitations because of the highly variable manifestations of the disease with many overlapping features {340}.

Disease	Age	Skin involvement	Clinical Features	Course	Prognosis
Letterer Siwe	First years of life	~90-100%	Fever, weight loss, lymphadenopathy, hepatosplenomegaly, pancytopenia, bone lesions	Acute	Mortality rate: 50-66%
Hand-Schüller Christian	Children adults	~30%	Osteolytic bone lesions, diabetes insipidus exophthalmos, otitis	Subacute to chronic	Mortality rate: < 50%
Eosinophilic granuloma	Mainly adults	<10%	Solitary bone or skin lesions	Chronic	Favorable
Congenital self-healing reticulohistio-cytosis (CSHR)	Congenital	100%	Skin lesions only	Self healing	Excellent*
*Both relapses and conversion to systemic disease can occur, so long-term follow-up is needed {1369}.					

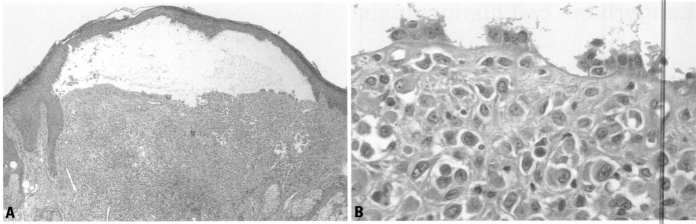

Fig. 4.80 Congenital self-healing reticulohistiocytosis (CSHRH). **A** Papule of CSHRH with **B** Characteristic kidney-shaped nuclei.

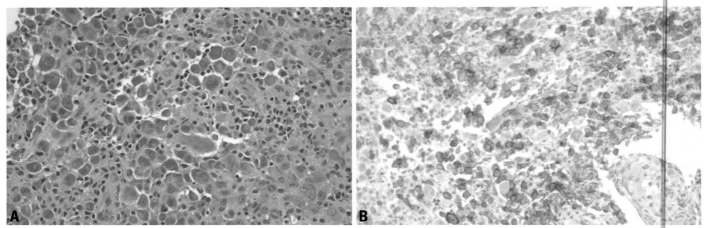

Fig. 4.81 Langerhans cell histiocytosis. **A** Typical ground glass ("reticulocytic") appearance of Langerhans cells. **B** Langerhans cells with membranous staining for CD1a .

well as small erosions can also be seen. Nodules are uncommon, but may be found on the trunk and tend to ulcerate. Additional symptoms include fever, weight loss, rash, lymphadenopathy, hepatosplenomegaly, pancytopenia and purpura.

Hand – Schüller – Christian disease

The typical triad includes osteolytic skull lesions (100%), hypopituitarism induced diabetes insipidus (50%), and exophthalmos (10%). Otitis media, generalized lymphoadenopathy, hepatosplenomegaly, and pulmonary disease may be additional findings.

Skin lesions occur in about 30% of cases, usually in the intertriginous areas, most often as papules and nodules which may be ulcerated, erosive and superinfected.

Eosinophilic granuloma

The most common site of involvement is bone. The uncommon cutaneous lesions are deep dermal or subcutaneous nodules which are not clinically distinct {818,1956}. Lesions have to be differentiated from granuloma eosinophilicum faciei, a chronic variant of leukocytoclastic vasculitis with variable presence of eosinophils, but usually no extracutaneous manifestation {452}.

Congenital self-healing reticulohistiocytosis (CSHRH)

CSHRH (synonyms: Hashimoto-Pritzker disease; congenital reticulohistiocytosis; congenital self-healing Langerhans cell histiocytosis) {981,2082} is a rare condition (5% of all LCH), initially seen at birth or in the neonatal period, with solitary, localized to generalized papules, vesicles, or nodules on the trunk, head,

palms and soles, sometimes showing central ulceration {217}. The skin lesions tend to involute spontaneously within weeks to months leaving behind hypo- or hyperpigmented macules or patches {979,1372}. Affected infants are otherwise well {1369}. Patients should be carefully followed since relapses may occur, including bone involvement, and the occasional case may progress to Letterer-Siwe disease {1445}. Some cases of CSHRH may be clinically confused with the blueberry muffin syndrome, congenital leukaemic infiltrates, xanthogranulomas or mast cell disease, but the microscopic picture brings clarity {360}.

Histopathology

The hallmark and unifying feature of all variants of LCH is a cell with large, pale, folded or lobulated, often reniform, vesicular nucleus and abundant, slightly eosinophilic or amphophilic cytoplasm. Nucleoli are not prominent. Histological variations correlate with the clinical appearance of the lesions. Features may be predominantly proliferative in Letterer-Siwe disease, xanthomatous in Hand-Schüller-Christian disease, granulomatous as in eosinophilic granuloma, or "reticulocytic" with abundant eosinophilic cytoplasm (ground glass appearance of giant cells) in Hashimoto-Pritzker disease. Fully developed papules and plaques show a dense band-like infiltrate obscuring the dermo-epidermal junction. Epidermotropism of LCs with intraepidermal microabscess formation can be found. In addition to LCs and eosinophils, the infiltrate may contain variable numbers of lymphocytes, epithelioid macrophages including foam cells and giant cells, neutrophils, plasma cells, and extravasated erythrocytes.

Immunohistochemistry

The phenotypic hallmarks in LCH are expression of CD1a, CD4 and S-100 protein, while macrophage markers, including CD68 and lysozyme, are usually negative.

Electron microscopy

Rod- or rocket-shaped granules measuring 200-400 nm (Birbeck granules, Langerhans cell granules) are the ultra-

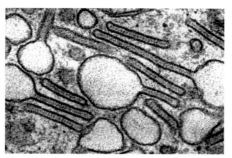

Fig. 4.82 Electron microscopy with numerous Birbeck or Langerhans cell granules. Courtesy Dr. N. Romani, University of Innsbruck, Austria

structural hallmark of LCs. The number of Birbeck granules varies, with usually greater prominence in early lesions. Coexistence of myelinoid laminated inclusions or "vermiform" bodies {1372} and Birbeck granules is common in CSHRH.

Genetics

A variety of inconsistent cytogenetic abnormalities have been found in several patients with LCH studied so far using comparitive genomic hybridization, loss of heterozygosity (LOH) and other techniques {107,227,848,1666}. Heterogeneous overexpression of TGFbeta receptor I and II, MDM2, p53, p21, p16, Rb, and BCL2 has been detected in lesional LCH cells {2097}. Familial clustering of two different manifestations of LCH support a role for genetic factor(s) in LCH

and raise the possibility of inherited mutations that promote emergence of clonal Langerhans cells {93,134,1200}. LCH may follow percursor T-cell acute lymphoblastic leukaemia, and in such cases a clonal relationship has been shown for T-cell receptor gene rearrangements {720}.

Prognosis and predictive factors

The biologic behaviour of LCH ranges from spontaneous remission to lethal dissemination, and such behaviour cannot be predicted on the basis of histologic features {1941}. The presence and degree of organ dysfunction, age less than 1 year at diagnosis (except the Hashimoto-Pritzker type), male sex, progressive episodes, and the absence of response to therapy are the most reliable indicators of prognosis {2,1019}. In general, about 10% of patients with multifocal disease die, 30% undergo complete remission, and the remaining 60% embark upon a chronic course {1065, 1425}.

Indeterminate cell histiocytosis

R. Caputo
E. Berti

Definition
Indeterminate cell histiocytosis (ICH) is a proliferative cutaneous disorder of the so-called "indeterminate cells" (IC), i.e. distinct dendritic cells of the skin that display histological, ultrastructural and antigenic features similar to those of Langerhans cells, but do not contain Birbeck granules.

Epidemiology
The disease is very rare (about 15 cases described up to 2003), usually occurs during adulthood, although two cases were in teenagers {1621,2019} and two cases in children {1413,1524}. Both sexes have been affected.

Etiology
The origin of indeterminate cells is still debated. Indeterminate cells may derivate from an arrest of Langerhans cell migration and maturation {1302}, may represent precursors of Langerhans cells which acquire Birbeck granules as they transit from dermal to epidermal sites {1499}. Furthermore it has been suggested {222} that indeterminate cells represent members of the epidermal/dermal dendritic cell system which migrate from skin to regional lymph nodes. According to this concept, indeterminate cell histiocytosis can be considered a disorder due to locally arrested dermal indeterminate cells proliferating prior to their departure for lymph nodes.

Localization
Lesions are usually restricted to the skin. Solitary lesions have been described on the trunk and arms, while multiple lesions are widespread.

Clinical features
The eruption consists of a solitary nodular lesion {222,279,1413,1621} or of multiple papulonodules {279,531,1499,2019, 2179}.
Solitary nodules are soft, red in colour and about 1 cm in diameter, and may be ulcerated. Multiple lesions are firm, asymptomatic papulonodules ranging in size from a few millimetres to 1 cm, varying in colour from dark-red to brownish, and covered by intact skin. These lesions appear in successive crops. Mucous membranes are always spared. Visceral involvement has been observed only in a child. Patients are in good general health.

Histopathology
Light-microscopic evaluation reveals an infiltration of histiocytic cells in the whole dermis and sometimes within the epidermis. The proliferating cells show an abundant pale eosinophilic cytoplasm and large irregular folded or twisted nuclei.
A few mitotic figures and multinucleated giant cells may be observed. Clusters of lymphocytes are admixed.

Immunohistochemistry
Proliferating cells are weakly positive for CD1a, CD68 (KP1), CD11c (Leu M5), CD14 (OKM1), factor XIIIa, lysozyme, α1-antitrypsin, HLA-DR, but negative for CD207 (langerin) {1302,1499,1524,1621, 2179}.

Electron microscopy
The proliferating cells reveal an indented nucleus and an abundant cytoplasm with lysosomes, phagosomes and a well-developed endoplasmic reticulum. Birbeck granules are absent {222,531, 1413}.

Prognosis and predictive factors
Most cases have exhibited complete or partial spontaneous regression of lesions without recurrences. Two cases displayed malignant behaviour {279,1524}. The prognosis is reasonably good, but leukaemia may be associated with this disease {279,1302}.

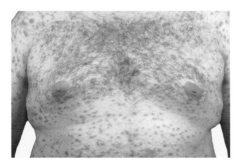

Fig. 4.83 Indeterminate cell histiocytosis. Multiple firm, asymptomatic papulonodules on the trunk, ranging in size from few millimetres to 1 cm, varying in colour from dark red to brownish.

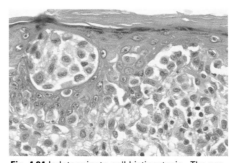

Fig. 4.84 Indeterminate cell histiocytosis. The proliferating cells show an irregular, often reniform, vesicular nucleus, surrounded by abundant pale cytoplasm. From: R. Caputo {378}.

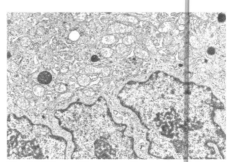

Fig. 4.85 The proliferating cells reveal an indented nucleus and an abundant cytoplasm with lysosomes, phagosomes and a well-developed endoplasmic reticulum. Birbeck granules are absent.

Sinus histiocytosis with massive lymphadenopathy (Rosai-Dorfman disease)

B. Zelger
S. Kohler
W. Burgdorf

Definition
Sinus histiocytosis with massive lymphadenopathy is a reactive condition of unknown etiology, charactericed by a poliferation of histiocytes which usually exhibit emperipolesis of lymphocytes. The disease can mimic lymphoma. Extranodal involvement is frequent.

Synonyms
Sinus histiocytosis with massive lymphadenopathy, Rosai-Dorfman disease

Epidemiology
Sinus histiocytosis is a rare non-neoplastic disease. Lymph nodes are predominantly affected in children and young male adults; the cutaneous form is particularly seen during the third and fourth decades in female patients {74,307,483}.

Etiology
The etiology is unknown. Lesions are polyclonal, probably the consequence of a cytokine dysregulation {1603}.

Localization
Cervical lymph node involvement is most characteristic. Cutaneous lesions frequently occur on the head and neck, mucous lesions {1105,2498} in the nose and paranasal sinus. Extranodal disease may also affect any other organ {2455}.

Clinical features
Children with massive cervical lymph node swellings frequently suffer from fever and malaise. Laboratory tests show leukocytosis, anemia, polyclonal hypergammaglobulinaemia and an accelerated erythrocyte sedimentation rate. Extranodal involvement is common, up to 40%. Pure cutaneous forms are rare; solitary, clustered or wide-spread, red to brownish papules, rarely plaques and nodules are seen. Regression leaves atrophic, brown macules.

Histopathology
Lymph node architecture is replaced by sheets of faintly stained ("clear") to slightly eosinophilic macrophages. In extranodal location infiltrates frequently simulate lymph node sinuses ("sinusoidal pattern").
Emperipolesis of lymphocytes, erythrocytes or other nuclear debris is prominent, but not specific; it can also be seen in, e.g., subcutaneous T-cell lymphomas. Lymphocytes, plasma cells, neutrophils and fibrosclerosis are found to a variable degree.

Immunohistochemistry
Macrophages are positive for CD68 (PGM1, KP1) and S100 protein; CD1a, factor XIIIa and CD34 are negative {1796}.

Electron microscopy
Macrophages ingest intact lymphocytes. Phagolysosomal structures, but no Birbeck granules are found.

Prognosis and predictive factors
Manifestation in children and lymph node involvement are more readily and rapidly associated with regression than in adults and spread to extranodal sites. The vast majority of lesions is self-limited and benign. Rare fatalities have been associated with immunologic disorders, lymphomas of Hodgkin and non-Hodgkin type, leukaemias {62}, and exceptional cases with solid tumours {1900}.

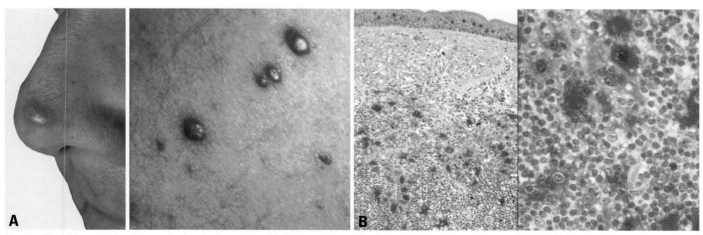

Fig. 4.86 Sinus histiocytosis with massive lymphadenopathy. **A** Left: Brownish nodule of sinus histiocytosis on the nose. 1595 Right: Clustered brownish papules of sinus histiocytosis on the trunk. **B** Left: Sheets of macrophages in sinus histiocytosis positive for S100 protein. Right: Lymphocytes within cytoplasm of histiocytes, i.e. emperipolesis.

Juvenile xanthogranuloma

R. Caputo
B. Zelger

Definition
Juvenile xanthogranuloma (JXG) is a benign, self-healing, non-Langerhans-cell (LC) histiocytosis most frequently seen in infants and children, characterized by yellowish asymptomatic papules and/or nodules located in the skin and other organs and consisting of an infiltrate of macrophages with a variable degree of lipidization in the absence of a metabolic disorder.

Synonyms
Xanthoma multiplex {33}; Nevoxanthoendothelioma {1551}.

Epidemiology
JXG is the most common form of non-LC histiocytosis {378,824}. JXG appears within the first year of life in about 75% of cases; in 15-30% it is present at birth.

Etiology
The etiology is unknown. Foamy cells constitute the main part of the mature lesions of JXG and accumulate lipids, despite normal levels of plasma lipids.
It has been suggested {208} that the uptake of low-density lipoprotein cholesterol and the biosynthesis of intracellular cholesterol are both enhanced; such enhancement might play a role in the process of accumulation of cholesterol esters in the macrophage.

Localization
Cutaneous lesions are irregularly scattered throughout the skin without a tendency to cluster, and are mainly located on the upper part of the body {378,824}. Mucous membranes may rarely be involved.
The most common extracutaneous manifestation of JXG (occurring mainly in the papular and subcutaneous {256} forms) is ocular involvement {256,614,2045, 2603}. Ocular lesions may occur in about 1-10% of affected children and are almost always unilateral and may lead to haemorrhage and glaucoma. Such lesions may precede or follow the cutaneous lesions. The nodular variant of JXG may occasionally be related to systemic lesions of lungs, bones, kidneys, pericardium, colon, ovaries, testes and central nervous system {378,824,2536}.

Clinical features
Two main clinical variants can be distinguished: a papular form and a nodular form {824}.
The *papular form* is the most frequent and is characterized by numerous (up to 100), firm hemispheric lesions, 2-5 mm in diameter, that are red-brown at first and then quickly turn yellowish. These lesions are associated in perhaps 20% of patients with café-au-lait spots of neurofibromatosis {1140} and may be related to juvenile chronic myeloid leukaemia {538,1650}.
The *nodular form* is less frequent, and is marked by one or a few lesions. The nodules are round to oval, 1-2 cm in diameter, high-domed, shiny, translucent, yellowish or red brown and sometimes show telangectasias on their surface. The term giant JXG has been used to indicate lesions larger than 2 cm. Unusual clinical variants {378,383} are the mixed form (simultaneous presence of both papules and nodules) and the form en plaque, a group of JXG lesions with a tendency to coalesce into a plaque as the only expression of the disease.

Histopathology
Early lesions are characterized by a dense infiltrate of monomorphous, non-lipid containing, macrophages with abundant, slightly eosinophilic, cytoplasm {378,824}. With time the cytoplasm of macrophages becomes laden with lipid and appears foamy.
Mature lesions contain foamy cells, for-

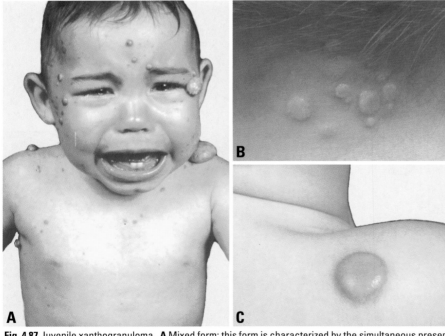

Fig. 4.87 Juvenile xanthogranuloma. **A** Mixed form: this form is characterized by the simultaneous presence of both red brown papules and nodules, irregularly scattered throughout the skin. Previously published by R. Caputo in "Text Atlas of Histiocytic Syndromes. A Dermatological Perspective", Martin Dunitz, London 1998 {378}. **B** Plaque form: this cluster of yellow nodules on the back of the neck is the only expression of the disease. **C** Nodular form: a round, high-domed, yellow brown nodule on the right shoulder.

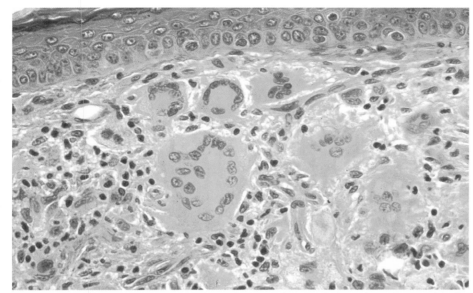

Fig. 4.88 Juvenile xanthogranuloma. Conventional microscopy. In mature lesions, giant cells are mainly distributed in the superficial dermis and on the border of the infiltrate. From: R. Caputo {378}.

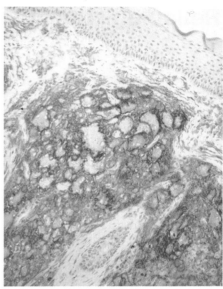

Fig. 4.89 Juvenile xanthogranuloma. Frozen section showing large macrophages stained by CD14.

eign body giant cells and Touton giant cells, mainly distributed in the superficial dermis and on the border of the infiltrate. In addition to macrophages and foamy cells, there may be lymphocytes, eosinophils, neutrophils and plasma cells scattered throughout the lesion. In older lesions fibrosis replaces the cellular infiltrate, and lipids are not present extracellularly.

Immunohistochemistry
Immunohistochemically {824,2049} macrophages and Touton cells show a uniform positive staining with CD14, CD68, HAM56 (markers with specificity for macrophages) and vimentin, frequent positive staining for factor XIII (markers of dermal dendrocytes) and for cathepsin B and occasional staining for MAC387 (a marker for monocytes and macrophages).
S100 protein, CD1a (OKT6), CD15 (Leu M1) and peanut agglutinin (PNA) are not usually expressed on the macrophages of JXG.

Electron microscopy
Under the electron microscope {378, 824}, the macrophages that characterize the early stage of the disease exhibit pleomorphic nuclei, are rich in pseudopods, and contain many elongated and irregular dense bodies.
Clusters of comma-shaped bodies, but no Langerhans granules (LG) can occasionally be observed. In older lesions there is a predominance of foamy cells, the cytoplasm of which is completely filled with lipid vacuoles, cholesterol clefts, and myeloid bodies. The cells corresponding to Touton giant cells are large (150-250 μm) and sometimes contain more than 10 nuclei. At their periphery, such cells are rich in lipid material, whereas in their centre, mitochondria and lysosomes predominate.

Genetics
JXG is not linked to any genetic locus, but the association with café-au-lait spots of neurofibromatosis (NF1) {2536} and the occasional association with neurilemmomatosis (NF2) {1115} suggests that a JXG locus could reside on

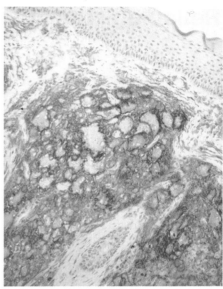

chromosome 17q11.2 or 22q12. Clinical {1115} and genetic analyses {1056} indicate that neurilemmomatosis and neurofibromatosis type 2 (NF2) genes are identical.

Prognosis and predictive factors
The papules and nodules of the skin tend to flatten with time and both the skin and most of the visceral lesions disappear spontaneously within 3-6 years. A few cases of JXG with fatal evolution, probably due to central nervous system involvement {378} or fatal liver disease {614}, have been reported. In JXG periodic complete blood count and peripheral smears would be judicious during a patient's first two years of life, which is the time of the peak incidence for juvenile chronic myeloid leukaemia.

Fig. 4.90 Juvenile xanthogranuloma. Electron microscopy. This large macrophage exhibits lipid droplets, myeloid bodies and cholesterol clefts.

Reticulohistiocytosis

E. Berti
B. Zelger
R. Caputo

Definition

Reticulohistiocytosis of the skin represents a spectrum of rare clinical entities, ranging from the solitary cutaneous form (SCR) through the generalized cutaneous form without systemic involvement (GCR), to multicentric reticulohistiocytosis with systemic involvement (MR). The skin lesions in all these conditions demonstrate an identical histological pattern, characterized by numerous mononucleated or multinucleated macrophages with abundant, eosinophilic, homogeneous to finely granular cytoplasm with a characteristic ground-glass appearance.

Synonyms

Giant cell reticulohistiocytosis, giant cell histiocytosis; cutaneous reticulohistiocytoma, reticulomatosis with giant cell histiocytes; normocholesterolemic xanthomatosis; lipoid dermatoarthritis; lipoid rheumatism; multicentric reticulohistiocytosis; non-diabetic cutaneous xanthomatosis; reticulohistiocytic granuloma; reticulohistiocytosis of the skin and synovia.

Epidemiology

Reticulohistiocytosis mostly occurs in adults over 40 years of age, but the disease may appear during adolescence: SCR and GCR have been also observed in children. In adults, the most frequent variant is MR, with about 50 and GCR with 10 patients reported in the literature.

There is no preference for either sex {167,465,1405,1462}.

Etiology

The etiopathogenesis is unknown. Reticulohistiocytosis may represent an abnormal macrophage response to different stimuli. In solitary forms, local trauma such as insect bites, folliculitis or ruptured infundibular cysts may play a role {379}, while in systemic forms the association with autoimmune disorders and internal malignancies suggests an immunological basis for the initiation of this reaction {1752}.

Localization

SCR involves mainly the head and the neck, but may be found in any cutaneous site {382,1082}. In GCR the lesions are widely scattered on the skin {381,547, 847,2363}. In MR {167,413,465,1405, 1752} skin lesions preferentially affect the fingers, the palms and the back of the hands, the juxta-articular regions of the limbs and the face. Oral, nasal and pharyngeal mucosa are involved in 50% of cases. Osteoarticular lesions involve mainly the hands (80%), knee (70%), and wrists (65%).

Clinical features

The solitary cutaneous reticulohistiocytosis (SCR) or reticulohistiocytoma cutis {382,1082} is characterized by a single, firm, rapidly growing nodule varying in colour from yellow-brown to dark-red.

The lesion is often clinically misdiagnosed, it occurs without evidence of systemic involvement, and its onset may be preceded by trauma.

Generalized cutaneous histiocytosis (GCR) {381,547,847,2363} is a purely cutaneous form characterized by the eruption of firm, smooth, asymptomatic papulonodular lesions, 3-10 mm in diameter. The colour of the recent lesions is pink-yellow, while the older lesions show a red-brown colour. Joint and visceral lesions are absent. Possibly, this purely cutaneous form could represent an early stage of multicentric reticulohistiocytosis, before the appearance of joint or visceral lesions.

The term multicentric reticulohistiocytosis {167,413,465,1405,1752} is used to indicate a form of reticulohistiocytosis characterized by the association of a cutaneous and mucous membrane papulonodular eruption with severe arthropathy and other visceral symptoms. The papulonodular lesions range in diameter from a few mm to 2 cm, and are round, translucent and yellow-rose or yellow-brown in colour. Grouping of lesions into plaques can give a cobblestone appearance, but lesions are mostly scattered and isolated. They do not tend to ulcerate, and are pruritic in about one-third of cases. Osteoarticular manifestations cause severe chronic polyarthritis with arthralgias, and are the initial sign of the disease in about 5-65% of cases {167, 465,1405}. The osteoarticular lesions

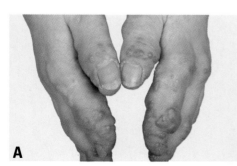
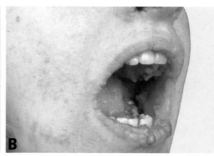
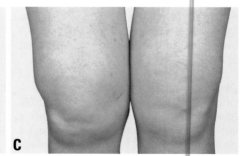

Fig. 4.91 Multicentric reticulohistiocytosis. **A** Purplish-brown, firm nodules characteristically affect the fingers. Periungual papules are arranged about the nail folds. **B** Papulonodular lesions are spread on the face, lips and oral mucosa. Mucous membranes are involved in about 50% of cases. **C** Symmetrical involvement of the knees. In this patient, osteoarticular manifestations were the initial sign of the disease. From: R. Caputo {378}

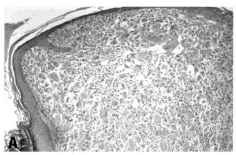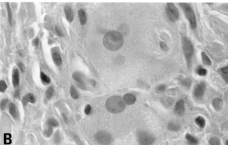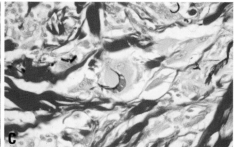

Fig. 4.92 Reticulohistiocytosis. **A** Conventional microscopy: the histological pattern of the lesions is characterized by the presence of numerous, large, mononucleated histiocytes with an abundant eosinophilic, finely granular cytoplasm. **B** Conventional microscopy: in these giant cells showing leukocyte phagocytosis, the typical ground-glass appearance of the cytoplasm is evident. **C** Conventional microscopy: Weigert-Van Gieson staining. Collagen phagocytosis is an occasional finding.

show a progressive destructive course of 6-8 years, and then become stable. Other systemic localizations, histopathologically documented are very rare. Muscular {667} (myositis, myotonia and myoatrophy), cardiopulmonary {532} (pericarditis, cardiac insufficiency, pleuritis, pulmonary infiltration), ocular {667} (exophthalmos, conjunctival infiltration), gastric (gastric ulcer), thyroid (thyroid nodules) and submandibular salivary gland involvements have occasionally been reported. Fever, weight loss and weakness can be present. In MR there is an association with a variety of autoimmune disorders such as dermatomyositis, lupus erythematosus, or Hashimoto thyroiditis as well as internal malignancies in 15-27% of cases {167,413,1405, 1752}. Solid tumours such as bronchial, breast, stomach and cervical carcinomas are most common. Lymphomas and myelodysplastic syndromes have been found less frequently.

Histopathology

The histological findings in the three types of reticulohistiocytosis and in the different tissues are identical {167,465, 1405,1462}. Early lesions are composed of macrophages and lymphocytes, and therefore may be confused with other histiocytoses of the skin. Older lesions show the characteristic histological pattern: the presence of numerous large, mononuclear or multinucleated macrophages with an abundance of eosinophilic, homogeneous to finely granular cytoplasm having a ground glass appearance. At times, phagocytosis of connective tissue and/or cellular components may be seen {379,532}. Histochemically, the granular material in macrophages and giant cells stains with periodic acid-Schiff, Sudan black and

scarlet red, indicating the presence of glycolipids and/or glycoproteins and neutral fat {167}.

Immunohistochemistry

Macrophages stain with macrophage markers KP1/PGM1 (CD68), Ki-M1p, and for the mesenchymal epitope of vimentin, and show variable reactivity with HAM56 and for factor XIIIa, lysozyme and α1-antitrypsin {381,382,424,2027,2585}. In contrast, these cells are usually negative for CD1α, S100 protein, Leu-M1 (CD15) and MAC387. Rare exceptions have been reported. According to Zelger et al. {2585}, SCR differs histopathologically and immunohistochemically from MR as lesions are better circumscribed, multinucleated giant cells more prominent, gigantic and bizarre, and macrophages regularly negative for factor XIIIa in the former entity.

Electron microscopy

The infiltrate is formed by large mononuclear to multinucleated cells exhibiting numerous peripheral villi {532,667}. Nuclei are irregular and often polylobated, with nucleoplasm of medium electron density and one or two nucleoli. The

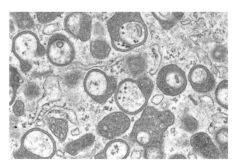

Fig. 4.93 Reticulohistiocytosis. Electron microscopy: the polymorphism of the granules is evident at higher magnification.

cytoplasm contains one or more Golgi apparatus, and is rich in mitochondria, lysosomes, dense bodies, phagosomes and myelin figures. The cytoplasm of about 5-40% of the cells of the infiltrate in many cases contains the so-called pleomorphic cytoplasmic inclusions {380-382,532}, varying in number from cell to cell. The pleomorphic cytoplasmic inclusions are unique and highly complex structures consisting mainly of unit membranes, occasionally surrounding electron-dense areas containing vesicles. Birbeck granules are absent. About 20% of all macrophages show collagenophagic activity {379,766}, but not pleomorphic cytoplasmic inclusions.

Prognosis and predictive factors

The purely cutaneous forms of reticulohistiocytosis (solitary and generalized) may involute spontaneously {382,847}. It is possible that the generalized purely cutaneous form is an early stage of MR, before the appearance of joint and visceral lesions {381,847}. In MR, there is no parallelism between the mucocutaneous and articular manifestations. The mucocutaneous lesions have an unpredictable course, and may remit spontaneously. In half of the patients, the osteoarticular manifestations become stable, while in the other half, they show a progressive destructive course {1405}. The prognosis is favourable for the cutaneous forms. The prognosis of MR is related to the importance of the osteoarticular manifestations and of the underlying immunologic disorders and neoplasms.

Mastocytosis

B.J. Longley
B.M. Henz

Definition
Mastocytosis is a heterogeneous group of disorders characterized by the abnormal growth and accumulation of a clone of mast cells in one or more organ system {1448}. Most patients have cutaneous mastocytosis (CM) with indolent disease that is confined to the skin and that may regress spontaneously.

A minority of patients, usually adults, have systemic mastocytosis (SM) that may rarely be highly aggressive and associated with multi-system involvement and short survival time, or that may be associated with non-mast-cell haematopoietic malignancies {1450, 2372,2405}.

ICD-O Codes
Cutaneous mastocytosis (CM); maculopapular or plaque type mastocytosis, formerly urticaria pigmentosa (UP); telangiectatic mastocytosis, formerly telangiectasia macularis eruptiva perstans (TMEP); diffuse cutaneous mastocytosis (DCL); solitary mastocytoma {965,2405}   9740/1
Indolent systemic mastocytosis
                                  9741/1
Aggressive systemic mastocytosis
                                  9741/3
Mastocytosis with associated haematopoietic disorder   9741/3
Mast cell leukaemia   9742/3

Synonyms
Mast cell disease; mast cell proliferative disease

Epidemiology
Cutaneous mastocytosis may be present at birth and usually first appears before six months of age. A second peak incidence is found in young adults in their 3rd and 4th decades. Paediatric mastocytosis usually regresses by adolescence. Adult mastocytosis is more likely to be persistent and may be associated with SM, rarely also with aggressive systemic mastocytosis. There is no clear gender or ethnic predominance of cases {964,1450}.

Etiology
The KIT protein is a receptor tyrosine kinase that is also known as the mast cell growth factor receptor. Adult mastocytosis and rare pediatric cases are associated with somatic mutations in the c-KIT proto-oncogene that alter the enzymatic site of the KIT protein {361,1449}. Rare kindreds with familial mastocytosis have germ line c-KIT mutations that affect regulatory portions of the KIT protein, also causing constitutive kinase activation. These patients may also have gastrointestinal stromal tumours (GISTs) which are known to be caused by regulatory type c-KIT activating mutations {189,

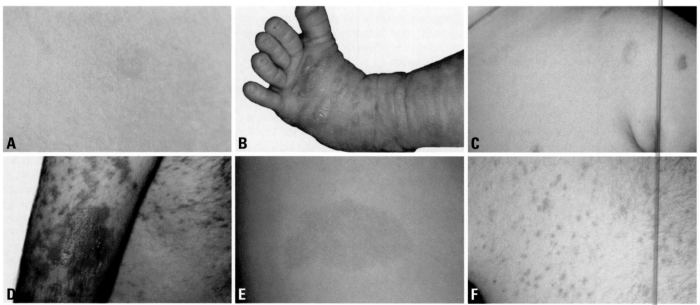

Fig. 4.94 Cutaneous mastocytosis. **A** Wheal and flare of Darier sign. The skin lesions of all forms of cutaneous mastocytosis may urticate when stroked. A palpable wheal appears a few moments after physical stimulation, due to histamine from the mast cells. **B** Tense blister containing clear fluid on skin of infant with diffuse cutaneous mastocytosis. The skin may appear thickened and reddish brown with diffuse involvement. Note the blister caused by mast cell degranulation and histamine release. Blisters may form in infants because the dermal-epidermal junction is not yet well developed. **C** Large pigmented papules of paediatric urticaria pigmentosa. **D** Reddish brown macules, patches and plaques on abdomen and arm of an adult with cutaneous and systemic mastocytosis. **E** Telangiectasia macularis eruptiva perstans form of cutaneous mastocytosis in an adult. **F** Pigmented macules of adult type urticaria pigmentosa. The number of lesions may range from a few to thousands.

1447}. In skin and bone marrow mast cells, there is also an increased expression of anti-apoptotic molecules in both paediatric and adult mastocytosis {963, 966}.

Localization
Eighty percent of patients with mastocytosis have disease confined to the skin. Conversely, of the 20% of patients with systemic mastocytosis, about half have cutaneous involvement. Essentially all patients with SM are adults and have involvement of the bone marrow, but any other organ may also be involved, most commonly the spleen, lymph nodes, or gastrointestinal tract {116,580,2224, 2372}.

Clinical features
Cutaneous mastocytosis includes several distinct clinico-pathologic entities whose morphologies include solitary tumours (Mastocytoma), maculo-papular or plaque-type lesions that are mostly symmetrically distributed (UP/TMEP), and diffuse cutaneous involvement (DCM).
Stroking of any lesion of CM may cause mast cell degranulation with localized swelling or urtication (Darier sign). Clinically normal skin may also urticate when stroked (so-called dermographism). Moderate itching is present in about half of the patients {579}. Most cutaneous lesions show an increase in epidermal melanin pigment which, combined with the tendency of these lesions to urticate, has led to the term "urticaria pigmentosa", a historic designation that has recently been proposed to be abandoned {2405}. Blistering or bullous mastocytosis is not a distinct entity but represents an exaggeration of Darier sign seen in infants whose dermo-epidermal junction is not well developed so that accumulation of oedema fluid results in the formation of localized blisters {964}.
Other symptoms of mastocytosis may be due to mast cell infiltration of specific organs or due to release of mast cell mediators into the circulation. Organs affected include: the gastrointestinal tract (peptic ulcer disease, diarrhoea and cramping) or the cardio-pulmonary and cardio-vascular systems (flushing, syncope, headache, seizures, hypertension, hypotension including anaphylaxis, tachycardia, and respiratory symptoms). Patients with extensive involvement may

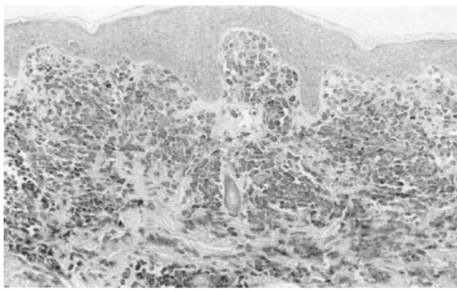

Fig. 4.95 Mastocytoma of the skin. Stains containing toluidine blue stain the mast cell cytoplasmic granules metachromatically purple.

have relatively vague constitutional symptoms including fatigue, weight loss, fever, sweats, and non-specific psychiatric symptoms {964,1450}.
Patients with SM may have also bone-related complaints such as pain, fractures, or arthralgias, secondary to direct mass effects or generalized osteoporosis.
The diagnosis of cutaneous mastocytosis is established by skin biopsy that demonstrates increased numbers of mast cells in the dermis. Imaging studies or biopsy of bone marrow or other internal organs are usually not indicated in the absence of abnormality of the peripheral blood counts or specific signs or symptoms pointing to internal organ involvement.
The clinical presentation of CM may range from subtle diffuse erythema to grossly evident, widespread doughy dermal thickening with accentuation of cutaneous surface markings, giving a so-called "grain leather" (peau chagrine) or orange skin (peau d'orange) appearance {964,1449,1450,2430,2525}. Tense blisters filled with clear fluid, occasionally slightly-tinged with blood, may be seen overlying lesions of any form of cutaneous mastocytosis in infants.
Individual lesions in young children tend to be lightly pigmented and occur as solitary nodules or multiple papules, or rarely as large heavily-pigmented macules, large plaques, or diffuse infiltration of the skin {964}. Large lesions or diffuse

involvement in children may point to the presence of c-KIT activating mutations {2405}. In adolescents and adults, the individual lesions tend to be more heavily pigmented and macular, rather than papular, like those of young children. The term TMEP has been used for these macular lesions and for larger, lightly pigmented patches with telangiectasias that may rarely occur in adults {964}. Cutaneous involvement in SM usually appears morphologically identical to CM in adults, but may also show larger plaque like lesions.

Histopathology
In haematoxylin and eosin (H&E) stained sections, normal mast cells have moderately abundant, oval or polygonal shaped cytoplasms with round to oval nuclei, sometimes giving the appearance of a "fried egg". The nuclei have clumped chromatin and indistinct or inapparent nucleoli. The cytoplasms are filled with small, faintly visible, eosinophilic or amphiphilic granules which stain metachromatically with the Giemsa or toluidine blue stains. Occasionally, mast cells may be spindle-shaped or show bi- or multi-lobated nuclei {1401,1450,1607, 2405}.
In normal skin, individual mast cells are found perivascularly and scattered throughout the dermis, without formation of clusters. Mast cells in mastocytosis also tend to accumulate perivascularly, and are most often evident in the super-

ficial dermis, within the dermal papillae {1401,1607}. In solitary mastocytomas and papular, nodular, or diffuse CM, the papillary and/or reticular dermis may show either scanty increases in mast cell numbers or heavy mast cell infiltrates, and there may be extension into the subcutaneous fat. In CM, individual mast cells may rarely be found in the lower epidermis. Unequivocal diagnosis of cutaneous mastocytosis requires the demonstration of aggregates of mast cells within the dermis, and this may be difficult and require multiple biopsies in the TMEP form of adult mastocytosis. Lesions of mastocytosis are usually composed of an infiltrate of monomorphous mast cells, and rarely observed infiltrating eosinophils should raise the possibility of dermal hypersensitivity reaction, parasitosis or an arthropod bite.

Immunohistochemistry
Mast cells are bone-marrow derived cells and therefore express CD45 (CLA). They also express CD117 (the KIT protein) and HLA-DR. Relatively specific mast cell markers include highly sulfated glycosaminoglycans like heparin (toluidine blue stain), tryptase and chymase. CD-2 and/or CD25 may be aberrantly expressed in mast cells of SM {934, 2404, 2405}.

Histogenesis
Mast cells are derived from CD34+ haematopoetic precursor cells {1982}.

Somatic genetics
Mastocytosis is a clonal disease in both adults and children {1448,1449}. The tumour cells of almost all cases of adult onset sporadic disease carry somatic point mutations of c-KIT that change the enzymatic site of the KIT protein, causing constitutive activation {361,1449}. Paediatric sporadic mastocytosis has also been shown to be clonal, but c-KIT activating mutations are rare {361,1449}. Very rare cases of familial mastocytosis, usually associated with GISTs tumours, are associated with germ line c-KIT mutations that activate KIT by affecting regulatory portions of the molecule, rather than the enzymatic site {189, 1447}.

Prognosis and predictive factors
Patients with mastocytosis confined to the skin generally have a good prognosis, and cutaneous involvement is usually an indicator of a relatively better prognosis in SM. CM in paediatric patients with solitary mastocytomas or typical papular and macular rashes usually regresses by adolescence. The presence of enzymatic site type KIT activating mutations may indicate persistent

disease in this population, and classification of mastocytosis based on both clinical and molecular genetic features may eventually prove to be both prognostically and therapeutically useful {1446, 1465}. In adults, although CM may be symptomatic and persist, overall survival is usually not adversely affected, even in the face of concomitant systemic involvement. Patients having aggressive variants of SM, however, may have a rapidly progressive downhill course with survival measured in months. In patients with associated haematologic malignancies, the prognosis is determined by the course of the related haematologic disease {964}.

CHAPTER 5

Soft Tissue Tumours

Most soft tissue tumours are benign, outnumbering malignant ones by about 100 to 1. Soft tissue sarcomas comprise over 50 histological types, many of which have more than one subtype. Their behaviour varies from indolent to very aggressive, with consequent variation in survival, according to histological type, grade, and sometimes genetic constitution, but the overall 5-year survival is about 65-75%. In general, sarcomas in skin or subcutis have a more favourable outcome than those located beneath deep fascia. Only those tumours with a predilection for the skin, and not already covered in the WHO Classification of Tumours of Soft Tissue and Bone are described in this chapter.

WHO histological classification of soft tissue tumours

Vascular tumour

Haemangioma of infancy	9131/0
Cherry haemangioma	9120/0
Sinusoidal haemangioma	9120/0
Hobnail haemangioma	9120/0
Glomeruloid haemangioma	9120/0
Microvenular haemangioma	9120/0
Angiolymphoid hyperplasia with eosinophilia	
Spindle cell haemangioma	9136/0
Tufted angioma	9161/0
Arteriovenous haemangioma	9123/0
Cutaneous angiosarcoma	9120/3

Lymphatic tumours

Lymphangioma circumscriptum	9170/0
Progressive lymphangioma	9170/0

Smooth and skeletal muscle tumours

Pilar leiomyoma	8890/0
Cutaneous leiomyosarcoma	8890/3

Fibrous, fibrohistiocytic and histiocytic tumours

Dermatomyofibroma	8824/0
Infantile myofibromatosis	8824/1
Sclerotic fibroma	8823/0
Pleomorphic fibroma	8832/0
Giant cell fibroblastoma	8834/1
Dermatofibrosarcoma protuberans	8832/3
Dermatofibroma (fibrous histiocytoma)	8832/0

____

[1] Morphology code of the International Classification of Diseases for Oncology (ICD-O) {786} and the Systematized Nomenclature of Medicine (http://snomed.org). Behaviour is coded /0 for benign tumours, /3 for malignant tumours, and /1 for borderline or uncertain behaviour.

TNM classification of soft tissue sarcomas

Primary Tumour (T)

TX:	Primary tumour cannot be assessed
T0:	No evidence of primary tumour
T1:	Tumour ≤ 5cm in greatest dimension
	T1a: superficial tumour*
	T1b: deep tumour
T2:	Tumour > 5cm in greatest dimension
	T2a: superficial tumour
	T2b: deep tumour

Regional lymph nodes (N)

NX:	regional lymph nodes cannot be assessed
N0:	no regional lymph node metastasis
N1:	regional lymph node metastasis

Notes: Regional node involvement is rare and cases in which nodal status is not assessed either clinically or pathologically could be considered N0 instead of NX or pNX.

Distant metastasis (M)

M0:	no distant metastasis
M1:	distant metastasis

G Histopathological Grading

Translation table for three and four grade to two grade (low vs. high grade) system

TNM two grade system	Three grade systems	Four grade systems
Low Grade	Grade 1	Grade 1
		Grade 2
High Grade	Grade 2	Grade 3
	Grade 3	Grade 4

Stage grouping

Stage IA	T1a	N0,NX	M0	Low grade
	T1b	N0,NX	M0	Low grade
Stage IB	T2a	N0,NX	M0	Low grade
	T2b	N0,NX	M0	Low grade
Stage IIA	T1a	N0,NX	M0	High grade
	T1b	N0,NX	M0	High grade
Stage IIB	T2a	N0,NX	M0	High grade
Stage III	T2b	N0,NX	M0	High grade
Stage IV	Any T	N1	M0	Any grade
	Any T	Any T	M1	Any grade

____

From references {892,2219}.
Superficial tumour is located exclusively above the superficial fascia without invasion of the fascia; deep tumour is located either exclusively beneath the superficial fascia, or superficial to the fascia with invasion of or through the fascia. Retroperitoneal, mediastinal and pelvic sarcomas are classified as deep tumours.

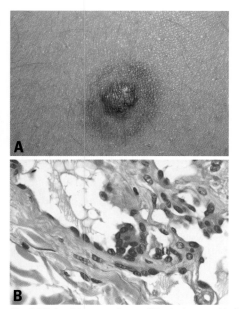

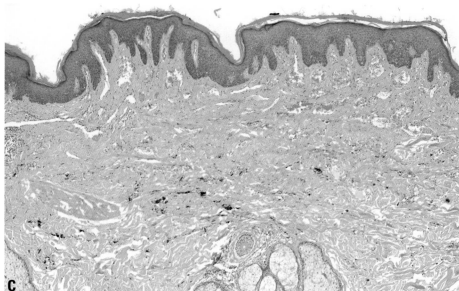

Fig. 5.2 Hobnail haemangioma. **A** Typical targetoid clinical appearance, only seen in a minority of cases. **B** Intravascular papillae lined by hobnail endothelial cells are sometimes seen. **C** Dilated irregular superficial vascular spaces and prominent haemosiderin deposition.

of these lesions {2052}. One possible origin is via trauma to lymphangiomas or angiokeratomas, resulting in dispersion of endothelial cells and erythrocytes into the surrounding dermis.

Localization
Most cases occur on the lower limbs with predilection for the thigh followed by the upper extremities and the trunk. Rare lesions have been reported in the oral cavity including the tongue and gingivae.

Clinical features
Some lesions show a characteristic targetoid clinical appearance with variably pigmented ecchymotic haloes secondary to bleeding and haemosiderin deposition within the tumour {2052}. Most often however, the clinical presentation is non-distinctive and the clinical differential diagnosis includes haemangioma, naevus or fibrous histiocytoma. HH is asymptomatic, usually less than 2 cm in diameter and increases in size very slowly. Patients usually describe cyclic changes {389}. Multiple lesions are exceptional. Similar histological changes may occur after trauma {481}.

Histopathology
The most striking low-power feature is the presence of a wedge-shaped vascular proliferation consisting of superficial, dilated and thin-walled vascular chan-

nels lined by bland endothelial cells that appear flat or have hobnail morphology. Some of the vascular channels resemble lymphatics. Focally, intraluminal small papillary projections with collagenous cores are occasionally seen. As the vascular channels descend further into the reticular dermis they gradually become smaller and disappear. Inflammation is not usually a feature. Haemorrhage and haemosiderin deposition are prominent but vary according to the stage of evolution. A Perls stain may be useful in highlighting the haemosiderin.

Immunohistochemistry
The endothelial cells in HH stain diffusely for vascular markers including CD31 and VWF (von Willebrand factor). CD34 is usually negative or very focal. A layer of alpha-smooth muscle actin pericytes surrounds some of the vascular channels. The positive staining for vascular endothelial growth factor receptor-3 (VEGFR-3) in some cases has led to the suggestion that HH displays lymphatic differentiation {1584}. VEGFR-3 is however, not entirely specific for lymphatic endothelium. Staining for human herpes virus 8 is consistently negative {932}.

Differential diagnosis
Kaposi sarcoma differs by the absence of dilated blood vessels lined by hobnail cells.

Prognosis
The lesion is entirely benign and there is no tendency for local recurrence.

Glomeruloid haemangioma

Definition
Glomeruloid haemangioma is a benign vascular proliferation that occurs inside ectatic blood vessels, producing a pattern reminiscent of renal glomeruli.

ICD-O code   9120/0

Epidemiology
This is a very rare vascular proliferation that occurs exclusively in patients with POEMS syndrome (Polyneuropathy, Organomegaly, Endocrinopathy, Monoclonal paraproteinaemia and Skin lesions), which is associated with multicentric Castleman disease {440,2562}. Multiple haemangiomas occur in 24-44% of all patients with POEMS syndrome, with most being cherry-type haemangiomas, and only some being glomeruloid haemangiomas {1301,2312,2580}. The reported cases of glomeruloid haemangiomas show female predominance, with patients ranging in age from 40-68 years {440,1278,1285,1965,2083,2380, 2562}.

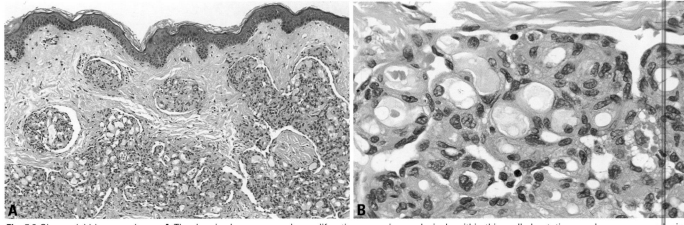

Fig. 5.3 Glomeruloid haemangioma. **A** The dermis shows a vascular proliferation occurring exclusively within thin-walled ectatic vascular spaces, producing a glomerulus-like appearance. **B** The vascular proliferation consists of aggregates of capillaries projecting as a broad tuft into a vascular space. The endothelial cells that line the vascular space and surface of the tuft have dark-staining nuclei ("sinusoidal endothelium"), while those that line the capillaries have plumper and paler nuclei. "Interstitial" cells containing eosinophilic hyaline globules are also seen.

Etiology

Glomeruloid haemangioma has so far only been found in patients with POEMS syndrome. Its development may be mediated by circulating vascular endothelial factor, which is present at high titres in the blood of most patients with POEMS syndrome {2225,2464}.

Localization

The lesions are mainly found on the trunk, face and proximal limb, and exceptionally also in the fingers and deep soft tissues {440,1278,1285, 1965,2380,2562}.

Clinical features

The lesions manifest as multiple purplish-red papules or nodules, ranging in size from a few to 15 mm {1278,1285,1965, 2380,2562}. They occur in patients already known to have POEMS syndrome, or as an early phenomenon before the full-blown syndrome develops {1278,1285,1965,2083,2380,2562}.

Histopathology

Glomeruloid haemangioma is mainly centred in the upper and mid dermis. It is characterized by tufts of proliferated, coiled capillaries projecting inside thin-walled ectatic blood vessels, mimicking renal glomeruli. The "sinusoidal" endothelial cells that line the ectatic vascular spaces and the surface the vascular tufts possess dark round nuclei. These cells also show cleft-like extensions into the cores of the vascular tufts. The capillary loops within the tufts are lined by plump

endothelium with slightly larger and paler nuclei, and supported by pericytes. Scattered "interstitial" cells that contain PAS-positive eosinophilic globules are found between the capillary loops, but similar cytoplasmic globules can also be seen in some endothelial cells.

Immunohistochemistry
On immunohistochemical staining, the endothelial cells of the capillary loops stain for CD31 and CD34, and they are well supported by actin-positive pericytes. The sinusoidal endothelial cells covering the tufts are positive for CD31 but not CD34, while those lining the ectatic vascular spaces are strongly CD31 positive but weakly CD34 positive. The eosinophilic globules probably represent immunoglobulin. The cells that contain these globules represent a mixture of histiocytes (CD68+) and endothelial cells (CD31+).

Precursor lesions

Progression from cellular immature, non-specific, vascular proliferation with slit-like canals reminiscent of tufted angioma to classical glomeruloid haemangioma has been reported {2562}. In addition, cherry-type haemangiomas with miniature glomeruloid structures formation can coexist with glomeruloid haemangiomas in patients with POEMS syndrome {440}. Thus these might represent precursor lesions of glomeruloid haemangioma.

Histogenesis

The currently favoured view is that glo-

meruloid haemangioma is a reactive vascular proliferation, perhaps representing a distinctive form of reactive angioendotheliomatosis.

Prognosis and predictive factors

Glomeruloid haemangioma per se is a totally innocuous lesion. The outcome of the patients depends on the underlying POEMS syndrome.

Microvenular haemangioma

Definition

Microvenular haemangioma is an acquired, slowly growing asymptomatic lesion with an angiomatous appearance {1080}.

ICD-O code   9120/0

Etiology

A histogenetic relationship between microvenular haemangioma and hormonal factors such as pregnancy and hormonal contraceptives has been postulated {144,2065}, but this feature has not been corroborated by other authors. An example of microvenular haemangioma has developed in a patient with Wiskott-Aldrich syndrome {1939}. Haemangiomas identical to microvenular haemangioma can be seen in patients with POEMS syndrome {25}.

Localization

It most commonly affects the upper limbs, particularly the forearms.

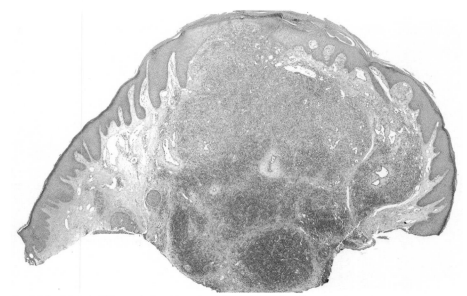

Fig. 5.4 Angiolymphoid hyperplasia with eosinophilia. Lobulated proliferation of small to medium size blood vessels with admixed inflammation and a central prominent vessel.

However, lesions on the trunk, face and lower limbs have also been recorded {65,1061}.

Clinical features
Microvenular haemangiomas appear as sharply circumscribed, bright red, solitary lesions varying in size from 0.5-2 cm.

Histopathology
Microvenular haemangioma appears as a poorly circumscribed proliferation of irregularly branched, round to oval, thin-walled blood vessels lined by a single layer of endothelial cells. They involve the entire reticular dermis and a variable degree of dermal sclerosis is present in the stroma. The lumina of the neoplastic blood vessels are inconspicuous and often collapsed with only a few erythrocytes within them.

The main differential diagnosis is with Kaposi sarcoma in the patch stage. Kaposi sarcoma shows irregular anastomosing vascular spaces, newly formed ectatic vascular channels surrounding pre-existing normal blood vessels and adnexa (promontory sign), plasma cells, hyaline (eosinophilic) globules, and small interstitial fascicles of spindle cells. All of these features are absent in microvenular haemangioma.

Immunohistochemistry
Immunohistochemically, the cells lining the lumina show positivity for factor VIII-related antigen and Ulex europaeus I lectin {144,1080,2065} which qualifies them as endothelial cells. Some smooth muscle actin positive perithelial cells have been also described surrounding this vascular space {65,1061}.

Prognosis
Microvenular haemangioma is a benign neoplasm and it is cured by simple excision.

Angiolymphoid hyperplasia with eosinophilia

Definition
Angiolymphoid hyperplasia with eosinophilia (ALHE) is a benign skin or subcutaneous tumour that is a circumscribed combined proliferation of immature blood vessels and chronic inflammatory infiltrate usually containing eosinophils. Endothelial cells have a distinctive epithelioid or histiocytoid appearance with ample eosinophilic cytoplasm.

Synonyms
Epithelioid haemangioma, cutaneous histiocytoid angioma, pseudo- or atypical pyogenic granuloma, inflammatory angiomatous nodule, intravenous atypical vascular proliferation, nodular angioblastic hyperplasia with eosinophilia and lymphofolliculosis {201,1154, 1967,1968, 2381}.

Epidemiology
ALHE was originally described as a lesion commonly found in young women on the head and neck {1011}. Recent reviews show a wide age range peaking at 20-50 years without female predominance {738,1753}. There is no predilection for Asian populations.

Etiology
Reactive vascular proliferation and inflammation {2441} in a traumatized vascular structure is a postulated cause of some ALHE lesions. History of antecedent trauma, histologic evidence of

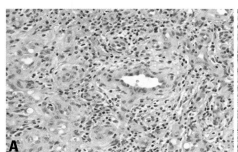
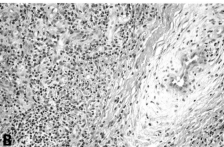
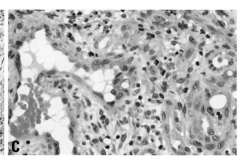

Fig. 5.5 Angiolymphoid hyperplasia with eosinophilia. **A** Epithelioid endothelial cells with abundant cytoplasms, some of which are vacuolated. **B** Proliferating immature vessels with protuberant endothelial nuclei associated with lymphoid and eosinophilic inflammation. **C** Epithelioid endothelial cells with abundant cytoplasms, some of which are vacuolated.

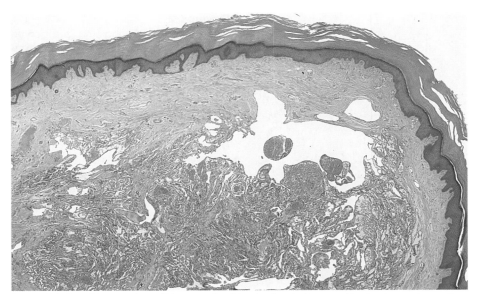

Fig. 5.6 Spindle cell haemangioma. This tumour involving the dermis shows pushing borders, and comprises cavernous vessels intimately intermingled with spindle cells.

adjacent vascular damage {738,2400} and pre-existing arteriovenous malformation {1754} are found in some cases. Although earlier reported, HHV-8 has not been consistently found in ALHE {1130,1241}.

Localization
ALHE most commonly occurs on the head and neck with a predilection for the forehead, scalp and skin around the ear {738,1011,1753}. Occurrence on distal extremities and digits is not uncommon {97}. Multiple other reported sites include trunk, breast {1676}, oral mucosa {1512, 1530,1776}, orbital tissues {145,1513}, vulva {37,2125} and penis {2240}.

Clinical features
ALHE lesions are small red or violaceous papules or plaques with an average size of 1 cm, measuring up to 10 cm. When symptomatic they can be pulsatile, painful and pruritic with scale crust {1011,1753}. When multiple they are usually grouped or zosteriform {647} and may coalesce. In contrast to Kimura disease, lymphadenopathy, eosinophilia, asthma and proteinuria are uncommon and serum IgE is usually normal {97, 441}.

Histopathology
The lobulated, circumscribed dermal or subcutaneous proliferation has a combined vascular and inflammatory compo-

nent. Sometimes an origin from a medium-sized vessel, usually a vein, is seen. There are arborizing small blood vessels that may surround a larger vascular structure. The vessel walls have smooth muscle cells or pericytes and contain mucin. The endothelial cells have distinct abundant eosinophilic (epithelioid) cytoplasms that can be vacuolated. They protrude into and can occlude vascular lumina or form solid sheets that may mimic angiosarcoma {2582}. Their nuclei have open chromatin, often with a central nucleolus and may protrude into lumina with occasional mitoses.
Multinucleate cells that are endothelial sprouts or histiocyte-like cells can be present {2020}. The density of the inflammatory component between vessels is variable with a prominence of lymphocytes and eosinophils.
Plasma cells, mast cells and lymphoid follicles with reactive germinal centres can be present. Older lesions typically become more fibrotic, less inflammatory and their vascular nature becomes less conspicuous.

Immunoprofile
The endothelial cells are positive for CD31, CD34, VWF (VIIIrAg) and are keratin negative. The proliferative index of the endothelial cells has been reported as 5% using Ki-67 with negative staining for Cyclin D1 and bcl-2. This may support a reactive rather than neoplastic

endothelial proliferation {97}. Lymphocytes are a mixture of T- and B-cells. There is no light chain restriction {97, 1753}. One series has shown T-cell clonality in ALHE that may define a subgroup of lesions with a higher incidence of recurrences {1241}.

Differential diagnosis
Kimura disease is a distinct clinicopathological entity, characterized by a more prominent lymphoid proliferation and less prominent vascular component with almost complete absence of epithelioid endothelial cells.

Prognosis and predictive factors
The lesions tend to persist if not completely excised and only rarely will they spontaneously regress. Local recurrence can occur and may be related to persistence of an underlying arteriovenous fistula that is not completely excised {97, 1753,1754}.

Spindle cell haemangioma

Definition
Spindle cell haemangioma is a benign

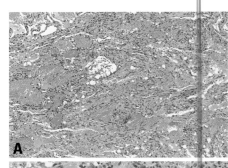

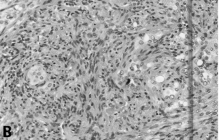

Fig. 5.7 Spindle cell haemangioma. **A** There is intricate mixing of cavernous vessels and spindly cells, with irregular branching narrow vascular spaces coursing through the latter component. **B** Short fascicles of uniform spindly cells are evident. There are interspersed small groups of epithelioid cells with lightly eosinophilic cytoplasm, sometimes with vacuolation.

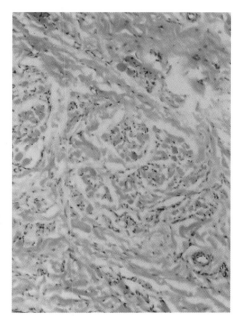

Fig. 5.23 Rhabdomyomatous mesenchymal hamartoma. In the lower part, skeletal muscle fibres among thick collagen bundles of the reticular dermis. In the upper part there are eccrine sweat coils and aggregates of smooth muscle.

was not substantiated when a number of examples were described in girls. Thus far, familial occurrence of this lesion has not been documented.

Histopathology

The most striking feature is the presence of intersecting bundles of mature skeletal muscle fibres, with demonstrable cross striations, and with a general orientation perpendicular to the surface epidermis. Varying amounts of collagen and mature fat surround these muscle fibres {2037}. They extend through the reticular dermis and become attenuated in the papillary dermis {1618}, where they appear to surround adnexal structures, particularly vellus follicles and sebaceous glands {678,713,1618}. Sebaceous and eccrine sweat glands are usually observed, and in one case there were ectopic apocrine glands {2320}. Nerve elements in these lesions vary considerably; in some cases they are not prominent {2010}, but in others there may be numerous small nerve twigs {987} or a large nerve bundle in the central core of the lesion {2037}. One example contained elastic cartilage {2037}, and calcification or ossification have also been reported {2010}. In some cases, elastic fibre distribution has been reported to be normal {1618}, while in others these fibres are markedly decreased {2037}.

Immunoprofile

Skeletal muscle fibres in RMH stain positively for actin, desmin and myoglobin {678,899}.

Differential diagnosis

Although RMH bears a resemblance to fibroepithelial polyp, naevus lipomatosus, and accessory tragus, the combination of midline location and a microscopic skeletal muscle component should permit distinction from those lesions (though small amounts of skeletal muscle have been reported in accessory tragi) {324}). Deeper or more primitive tumours such as foetal rhabdomyoma, fibrous hamartoma of infancy, or neuromuscular hamartoma (benign Triton tumour) should not be difficult to distinguish from RMH {678,2010}.

Somatic genetics

There has been speculation about a human homologue of the mouse disorganization gene (Ds), which is responsible, directly or indirectly, for the development of hamartomas and other defects {1973,2242}.

Fibrous, fibrohistiocytic and histiocytic tumours

W. Weyers
T. Mentzel
R.C. Kasper
A. Tosti
M. Iorizzo
B. Zelger
R. Caputo

H. Kamino
J. D. Harvell
P. Galinier
G.F. Kao
E.J. Glusac
E. Berti
D. Weedon
C. Rose

Keloid scar

Definition
Keloid scars are raised scars that extend beyond the confines of the original wound.

Epidemiology
Keloid scars occur with equal frequency in men and women. They affect all races, but are more common in dark-skinned individuals. In Black, Hispanic, and Asian populations, the incidence ranges between 4.5 and 16%. Keloids occur chiefly in persons under 30 years of age {1711,2149}.

Etiology
There is a genetic predisposition to the formation of keloid scars. Moreover, hormonal and immunological factors may play a role. Keloids often appear in puberty and tend to enlarge during pregnancy; they have been claimed to be more common in patients with signs of allergy and increased serum levels of IgE. Wounds subjected to great tension or which become infected are more likely to heal with a keloid scar {1711,2149}.

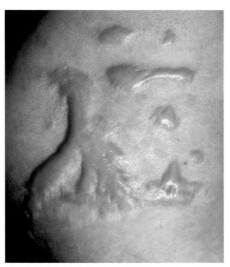

Fig. 5.25 Keloid. Raised erythematous plaques are present.

Localization
Keloids are most common on the earlobes, cheeks, upper arms, upper part of the back, and deltoid and presternal areas. They are seen only rarely on the genitalia, eyelids, and on palms and soles {1711,2149}.

Clinical features
Keloids are well-circumscribed, firm, smooth-surfaced erythematous papules or plaques that occur at the site of an injury. The preceding injury may be only minor and, therefore, not always apparent (e.g., rupture of an inflamed hair follicle). Older lesions may be pale or hyperpigmented. Especially in early stages, keloids are often itchy, tender, or painful {1711,2149}.

Histopathology
After a prolonged period of wound healing thick, homogeneous, strongly eosinophilic bundles of collagen, in haphazard array, develop {1498}. Those "keloidal" collagen bundles are the histopathologic hallmark of keloid scars, but are not seen in many cases fulfilling the clinical definition of keloids. The border of keloids is often irregular, with tongue-like extensions of bands of thickened collagen underneath normal appearing epidermis and superficial dermis.

Histogenesis
Keloid scars are characterized by an enhanced proliferation and metabolic activity of fibrocytes that seems to result, in part, from the excess of various cytokines produced by inflammatory cells, including transforming growth factor-b1 and platelet-derived growth factor. Moreover, a deficiency of cytokines that down-regulate collagen synthesis and inhibit proliferation of fibrocytes, such as interferon-α, has been noted. There is also evidence of reduced degradation of collagen caused, in part, by inhibition of collagenase activity through acid mucopolysaccharides, proteoglycans, and specific protease inhibitors {1686,1711,2149,2551}.

Genetic susceptibility
Keloidal scar formation may run in families. It is also more common in Black individuals. A relationship with various human leukocyte antigens has been reported {1711}.

Prognosis and predictive factors
The clinical and histopathologic features of keloid scars indicate a high probability of recurrence following surgical excision alone. Recurrence rates of 45-100% have been described {1711}.

Hypertrophic scar

Definition
Hypertrophic scars are raised scars that do not extend beyond the confines of the original wound. As such, they are closely related to keloids, both being examples of a disturbance of wound healing leading to the formation of exuberant fibrous tissue. Whether hypertrophic scars are simply a less severe variant of keloid scars or represent a different pathologic process is controversial.

Epidemiology
Hypertrophic scars are common. The incidence of hypertrophic scarring (including keloid scars) ranges between 39 and 68% after surgery and between 33 and 91% after burns, depending on the depth of the wound {1711}.

Localization
Hypertrophic scars are most common above the flexor aspects of joints and on the abdomen {2149}.

Clinical features
By definition, hypertrophic scars differ from keloid scars by remaining confined to the original wound. Other distinguishing features are earlier manifestation of

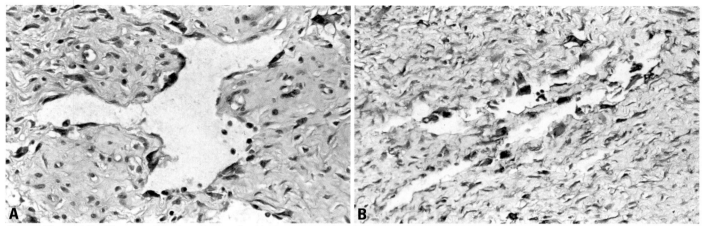

Fig. 5.31 Giant cell fibroblastoma. **A** Angiectoid space lined by hyperchromatic spindle and multinucleate giant cells. **B** CD34 highlights both the giant cells and the surrounding spindle cells.

Macroscopy
Grossly, GCF is a firm yellow or grey tumour with gelatinous or rubbery consistency and without haemorrhage or necrosis {751,2174}.

Histopathology
GCF is usually a subcutaneous tumour, but it often extends into the overlying dermis. Cellularity is variable, but for the most part, GCF is a hypocellular neoplasm composed of wavy spindle shaped cells and scattered giant cells set within a stroma that varies from myxoid to collagenous to sclerotic and contains scattered mast cells. Scattered giant cells with hyperchromatic and angulated nuclei are characteristic. Most giant cells are multinucleated, but some are mononucleated. The nuclei of multinucleate cells are either conglomerated towards the centre of the cell or arranged peripherally, in a characteristic floret pattern. Irregularly branching "angiectoid" spaces which resemble the vascular spaces of lymphangioma are characteristic but are not seen in all cases. These are lined by spindle and multinucleate cells with morphology identical to those seen in the surrounding stroma. Cellular areas representing DFSP or less often pigmented DFSP (Bednar tumour) may be present. Recurrent lesions are uncommon, but when they occur, the lesions may show a pattern of DFSP. Fibrosarcomatous transformation of GCF has been reported in a recurrent lesion originally diagnosed as DFSP {1841}.

Immunoprofile
The stromal and lining cells are CD34 positive, but negative for VWF (VIIIrAg), CD31, S100, actin, desmin, and EMA {971,2338}.

Differential diagnosis
Since CD34 can be focally positive in other soft tissue lesions, finding the characteristic giant cells is important in diagnosing GCF.

Histogenesis
GCF and DFSP are currently classified as neoplasms derived from fibroblasts, but CD34 positivity suggests possible derivation from interstitial dendritic cells {971}.

Somatic genetics
Both GCF and DFSP exhibit an identical t(17;22) (q22;q13) translocation, which in some cases results in a ring chromosome. The t(17;22) translocation fuses the collagen type I alpha 1 gene from chromosome 17q22 to the platelet-derived growth factor β chain gene from chromosome 22q13, resulting in a chimeric COL1A1-PDGFB gene that encodes for a transforming protein with biologic effects similar to normal PDGFB. The neoplastic cells not only harbour the mutation, but also have PDGFB receptors on their cell surface, resulting in an autocrine loop whereby the tumour cells stimulate their own growth {1735}.

Prognosis and predictive factors
Like DFSP, GCF is a locally aggressive tumour of intermediate malignancy, with up to 50% local recurrence in the original series. Metastases from GCF have not been reported.

Dermatofibrosarcoma protuberans

Definition
Dermatofibrosarcoma protuberans (DFSP) is a mesenchymal neoplasm of the dermis and subcutis, generally regarded as a superficial low-grade sarcoma {1605,2491}.

ICD-O code   8832/3

Synonym
Progressive and recurring dermatofibroma.

Epidemiology
DFSP typically presents during early or middle adult life, with male predominance. However, there is evidence that many tumours may have begun during childhood and become apparent during young adulthood.

Localization
The tumour occurs most commonly on the trunk, including chest, back, and abdominal wall. Less commonly, the neoplasm is located on the proximal extremities; it rarely involves the distal extremities. The head and neck, especially the scalp, are also commonly involved. The vulva {1377} and parotid gland are unusual sites of involvement.

Clinical features
DFSP typically presents as a nodular cutaneous mass, with a history of slow but persistent growth, often of several years duration. Early lesions may be sharply demarcated, and may some-

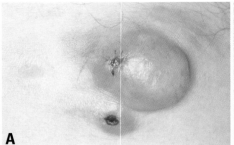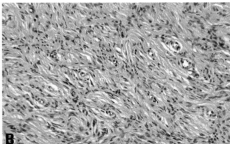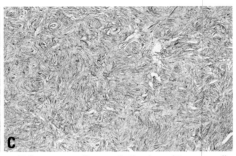

Fig. 5.32 Dermatofibrosarcoma protuberans. **A** DFSP exhibiting reddish nodular component with biopsy sites. **B** Compact, uniform, spindle-shaped tumour cells arranged in a storiform pattern. **C** Tumour cells show a strong immunoreactivity for CD34.

times be observed as plaque-like areas of induration, often with peripheral red or blue discolouration. These tumours may resemble morphoea (localized scleroderma) or a morphoeic basal cell carcinoma. The lesion expands slowly, and eventuates in the typical, fully developed protuberant appearance with single or multiple nodules on a plaque-like base. Fungating ulcerated lesions with satellite nodules characterize an advanced neoplasm.

Patients with advanced DFSPs do not exhibit signs and symptoms of chronic wasting, as seen in patients with aggressive, high-grade soft tissue sarcomas. Previous burns, surgical scars, and antecedent trauma have been reported in association with this tumour. There are reports of DFSP occurring at Bacille-Calmette-Guérin (BCG) vaccination sites {1558}, and in association with chronic arsenism {2176}, acanthosis nigricans, and acrodermatitis enteropathica {2161}. The tumour may show rapid enlargement during pregnancy {2329}.

Macroscopy

Most excised primary DFSPs are indurated plaques with one or more associated nodules. Multiple discrete, protuberant skin and subcutaneous tumours are more characteristic of recurrent neoplasms. Often, there is evidence of a surgical scar on the skin surface of the

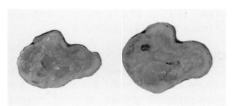

Fig. 5.33 Dermatofibroma (fibrous histiocytoma) Cut surface with distinctive yellow colour.

tumourous tissue. Ulceration may be present. The cut surface of the tumour is grey-white and firm, with occasional areas showing a gelatinous or translucent appearance, corresponding to microscopic areas of myxoid change. Haemorrhage and cystic change are sometimes seen. However, necrosis, a common feature of malignant fibrous histiocytoma, is rarely observed in DFSP. It is unusual to encounter DFSP confined solely to subcutaneous tissue without involvement of the dermis {629}.

Histopathology

DFSP diffusely infiltrates the dermis, and invades into subcutaneous tissue, especially along the fibrous septa of fat. The epidermis is usually uninvolved. A Grenz zone may be present. In a well-sampled specimen, the tumour shows some variation in histologic features. The centre of the tumour is typically composed of compact, uniform, slender, mildly atypical, spindle-shaped cells, arranged in a whorled, storiform, or cartwheel pattern. The tumour cells tightly encase skin appendages without destroying them. Nuclear pleomorphism is inconspicuous, and mitotic activity is low-to-moderate (<less than 5/10 HPF). Some tumours have a prominent myxoid matrix, and microscopic myxoid changes have been observed in both primary and recurrent tumours {368}. Superficial areas of the neoplasm are less cellular, and spindle cells are separated by dermal collagen. The deep portion of the tumour shows a proliferation of spindle cells which expand fibrous septa and interdigitate with fat lobules, resulting in a honeycomb appearance. In some tumours, giant cells similar to those of giant cell fibroblastoma are seen. At times, peculiar myoid nodules may be present, which represent a nonneoplastic myointimal or

myofibroblastic proliferation. Occasional foci may resemble a low-grade fibrosarcoma, with longitudinal fascicles of spindle cells demonstrating more prominent nuclear atypia and mitotic activity (but not greater than 5/10 HPF). Such areas have been seen in a minority of primary or recurrent lesions {853}.

Immunoprofile

DFSP cells label diffusely and strongly with antibodies to CD34 and vimentin. CD34 positivity may be lost in nodular regions. P75 (low-affinity nerve growth factor receptor) has been reported positive in DFSP cells {853}. Tumour cells are negative for S-100 protein, smooth muscle actin, desmin, keratins, and epithelial membrane antigen. Scattered Factor XIIIa positive cells may be present. Tenascin is negative at the dermoepidermal zone (DEZ) in DFSP {1180}. Stromelysin 3 is not expressed in the cells of a DFSP in contrast to dermatofibroma in which it is invariably expressed {558}.

Differential diagnosis

Benign and cellular fibrous histiocytoma or dermatofibroma (DF) can be differentiated from DFSP by the presence of epidermal (sometimes basal cell) hyperplasia, more prominent collagenous stroma, collagen trapping, and infiltration of the fibrous septa, but minimal extension into fat lobules. Immunostains are also helpful. DF contains a focally but not diffusely positive CD34 spindle cell component. P75 and stromelysin 3 are negative, and tenascin is positive at the DEZ in DF. Diffuse positivity for S-100 protein and the presence of Meissner-like corpuscles separate lesions of diffuse neurofibroma from DFSP.

Malignant fibrous histiocytoma (MFH) exhibits a higher degree of cellular atypia, pleomorphism, and mitotic activity

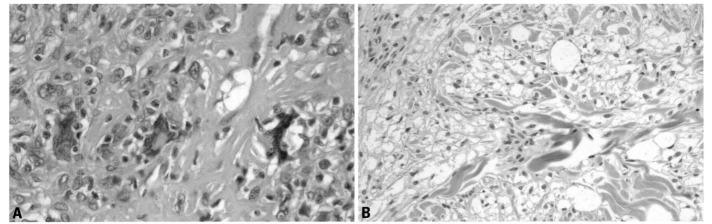

Fig. 5.34 Dermatofibroma (fibrous histiocytoma). **A** Dermatofibroma with monster cells. **B** Clear cell dermatofibroma. Typical cytology with prominent collagen bundles.

than DFSP. Necrosis is usually not a feature of DFSP, but is generally seen in MFH. Myxoid liposarcoma is distinguished from myxoid forms of DFSP by the presence of lipoblasts, negative CD34 staining, and deep soft tissue involvement.

Histogenesis
DFSP and its variant, giant cell fibroblastoma (GCF) are currently classified as neoplasms derived from fibroblasts. CD34 labelling suggests a close linkage to dermal dendrocytes.

Somatic genetics
DFSP and GCF exhibit an identical chromosomal translocation. See page 259.

Prognosis and predictive factors
As with GCF, DFSP has a significant risk of local recurrence. The average recurrence rate in reported cases treated by wide local excision (2-3 cm.) is 18%. A much higher recurrence rate (43%) is reported in tumours treated by superficial or incomplete excisions only {853} Local recurrence usually develops within three years after initial surgery. Metastasis occurs rarely.

Dermatofibroma (fibrous histiocytoma)

Definition
Dermatofibroma (fibrous histiocytoma) {21} is an ill-defined, predominantly dermal lesion characterized by a variable number of spindle and/or rounded cells. A variable admixture of inflammatory cells, coarse collagen bundles in haphazard array, and variable epidermal, melanocytic and folliculosebaceous hyperplasia are present.

ICD-O code   8832/0

Synonyms
Histiocytoma (cutis) {2134}, fibroma durum, subepidermal nodular fibrosis or sclerosis {1602}, sclerotic or sclerosing fibroma {1895}, sclerosing haemangioma {910}.

Epidemiology
Dermatofibroma is a very common lesion and may develop at any age, but particularly during the third and fourth decades. The gender distribution varies among different populations.

Etiology
The etiology has not been established unequivocally. It is controversial whether it is an inflammatory {21,2590,2591} or neoplastic process {365,518,522,919}. Dermatofibroma has been reported following local injuries such as trauma, insect bites or folliculitis, suggesting an inflammatory etiology. By contrast some examples have been reported to be clonal, supportive of a neoplastic etiology {457,1078,2422}.

Localization
Most lesions, including various clinicopathological variants, occur on the extremities {840,1081,1114,1155,1187, 1346,1786,1895,2115,2587,2592-2594} and trunk {187,370,2403}. Rare cases occur on the face {1583}.

Clinical features
Most lesions are single, round, oval to targetoid papules. Early lesions are reddish, but older ones are brown to skin coloured, frequently with a brown rim at the periphery. They usually evolve rapidly. Dermatofibromas are moderately well circumscribed; the consistency usually is hard, but may be cystic, eroded or crusted when secondary changes such as prominent haemorrhage, lipidization or trauma alter the lesions. Most lesions are flat, slightly elevated or show a shallow dell. The "dimpling" sign, when lesions are squeezed between the thumb and index finger, is characteristic.

Occasionally, there may be a few, up to several dozen, sometimes grouped ("agminated") papules. Multiple dermatofibromas are regarded as a marker of immune suppression; they have been observed in Black females with systemic lupus erythematosus; various other autoimmune disease such as Sjögren syndrome, pemphigus vulgaris, myasthenia gravis and ulcerative colitis treated with immunosuppressive drugs; occasionally in renal graft recipients or AIDS patients. Still other lesions form plaques or nodules to tumours. Dermatofibromas usually are long-standing lesions which cause no symptoms.

Macroscopy
Gross examination reveals a moderately well-circumscribed, hard papule, nodule or tumour. The cut surface reveals a skin-coloured to distinctive yellow colour, which may show areas of haemorrhage and lipidization and then become cystic.

Histopathology

Dermatofibromas show a dense infiltrate of spindle-shaped and/or round cells, some of which may be fibrocytes and/or macrophages, centred in the reticular dermis and sometimes, the upper part of the subcutis. Early lesions are rich in macrophages, some of which may be siderophages, and/or lipophages, others multinucleate, e.g. Touton or foreign body giant cells. Established lesions show prominent cellularity and coarse haphazardly arranged collagen bundles. They are frequently arranged in short fascicles that interweave ("storiform"), sometimes with a sclerotic centre.

Lesions are ill-defined and at the periphery there can be collagen trapping by lesional cells ("collagen ball formation"). Epidermal, melanocytic and folliculosebaceous hyperplasia is characteristically found above the lesions, and this can be so prominent that buds of hair follicles mimic superficial basal cell carcinoma. Rare cases show smooth muscle proliferation {1381}. Lymphocytes are often spread throughout the lesion with frequent prominence at the periphery, but may be lacking in later stages. At times foam cells may be prominent in deeper areas adjacent to subcutaneous fat.

A wide number of variants of dermatofibromas have been proposed {369}. Early lesions may show prominent proliferation of blood vessels, previously called sclerosing haemangioma {910}, more recently haemangiopericytoma-like fibrous histiocytoma {2594}. Prominent lipophages and siderophages are seen in the xanthomatous/histiocytic variant {1081,1114} and haemosiderrhotic variant {2036}, respectively. Older lesions become progressively fibrotic, with shrinkage of the lesion, particularly seen in atrophic dermatofibroma. Other variants show a heavy eosinophilic infiltrate {40} or pseudolymphomatous features {150}, respectively. Lichenoid, erosive and ulcerated variants {2034} have also been reported. Deep penetrating variants extend into the subcutis and may be easily confused with dermatofibrosarcoma protuberans {1187,2587}. Other rare variants include dermatofibroma with monster cells {2316}; ossifying dermatofibroma with osteoclast-like giant cells {1345}; granular {2403} and clear cell dermatofibromas {1786,2592}; myofibroblastic dermatofibroma with slender cytoplasmic cell extensions {2593}; myxoid dermatofibromas {2183,2588}; or combined dermatofibromas {2589}, which show a combination of several unusual histopathologic features in one lesion.

Immunoprofile

Dermatofibromas reveal a variable immunohistochemical profile: early lesions are rich in reactivity for macrophage markers such as PGM1 or KP1 (CD68), but also exhibit strong reactivity for factor XIIIa in both macrophages and fibroblasts {2590}. This reactivity is mostly seen at the periphery and continuously diminishes with the ageing of the lesion to be completely absent in atrophic variants. Actin expression is variably seen in dermatofibromas particularly in the myofibroblastic variant {2593}. Occasionally dermatofibromas are focally positive for CD34 {1840,2584}. Recently, stromelysin 3 expression has been reported. It is not expressed in DFSP {558}.

Differential diagnosis

The most important histologic differential diagnoses are dermatofibrosarcoma protuberans (particularly with the cellular variant of dermatofibroma) and Kaposi sarcoma. Dermatofibrosarcoma protuberans is poorly circumscribed, usually much broader and deeper with irregular dissection of subcutis, and shows cells with wavy nuclei in association with delicate fibrillary bundles of collagen frequently arranged in a storiform pattern. In contrast to dermatofibroma it is regularly positive for CD34. Kaposi sarcoma in nodular and tumour stage is characterized by erythrocytes extravasated into slits between interweaving fascicles of spindle-shaped cells; often, tiny pink hyaline globules that represent degenerated erythrocytes are found in these spindle-shaped endothelial cells.

Lesions are positive for CD34 and vascular markers such as CD31.

Variants

Aneurysmal fibrous histiocytoma

This is not uncommon {367,2054}, It may rapidly enlarge because of spontaneous or traumatic haemorrhage into a previously unspectacular lesion or rarely de novo development, and frequently is painful. Clinically, it may mimic nodular melanoma or nodular Kaposi sarcoma. Histology reveals extravasation of erythrocytes, pseudovascular spaces and iron deposits. This histology may occasionally also be confused with melanoma or nodular Kaposi sarcoma, yet the absence of melanocytic as well as vascular markers in the spindle cells easily excludes these simulants.

Epithelioid cell histiocytoma

This lesion {840,1155}, including a cellular variant {794} is rare. It occurs on the upper extremities and trunk as a skin-coloured to reddish-brown, hard, exophytic papule, frequently thought to be a Spitz naevus. Histology reveals a lesion mostly restricted to the papillary dermis, prominent epidermal hyperplasia ("collarette") and a sheet-like infiltrate of epithelioid to scalloped fibroblasts. These features may also closely simulate Spitz naevus, yet lesions are negative for melanocytic markers, but positive for factor XIIIa.

Cellular fibrous histiocytoma

This variant is rare {370}. It occurs on the trunk or distal extremities and has a tendency to recur when incompletely excised. Histology reveals a dense, frequently deeply infiltrating lesion of spindle cells in an otherwise typical dermatofibroma. There may be moderate nuclear atypia, occasional mitoses and bizarre giant cells and these lesions have therefore also been called pseudosarcomatous or atypical fibrous histiocytomas {794}. Exceptional cases of this variant have been reported to metastasize and, accordingly, they should always be completely excised.

Prognosis and predictive factors

The vast majority of lesions are benign. Occasionally incomplete excision may result in recurrence. The cellular and aneurysmal variants and lesions of the face may recur in a significant percentage of cases {1583}. Exceedingly rare cases of local aggressive growth or metastases to local or regional lymph nodes or even with wide spread metastases to lung have been recorded in the cellular variant.

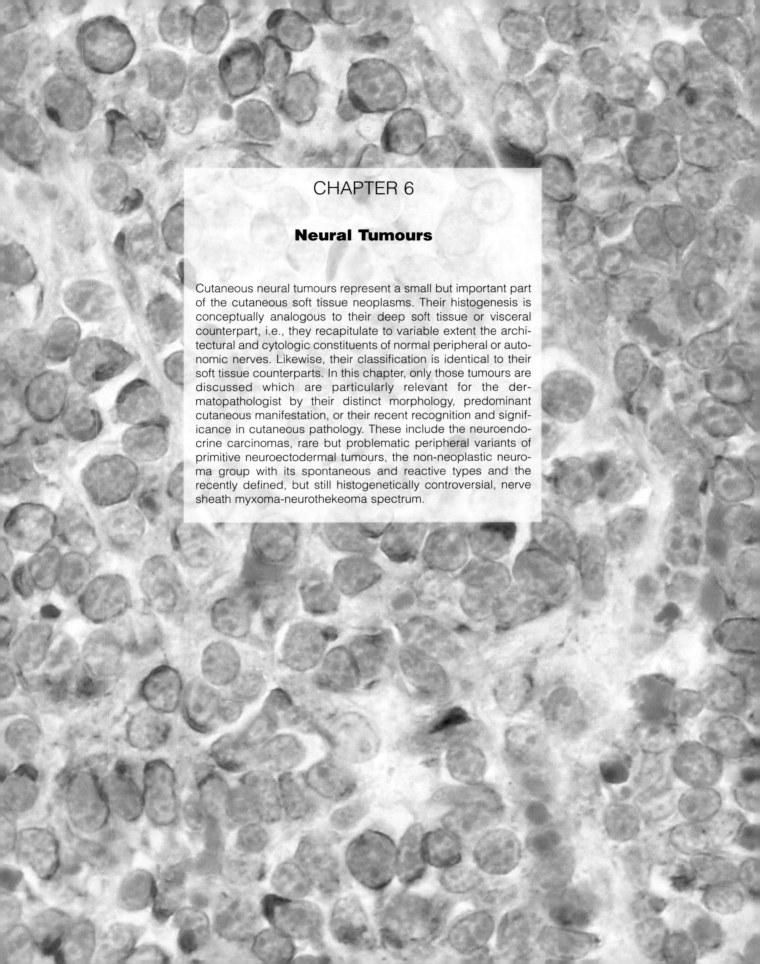

CHAPTER 6

Neural Tumours

Cutaneous neural tumours represent a small but important part of the cutaneous soft tissue neoplasms. Their histogenesis is conceptually analogous to their deep soft tissue or visceral counterpart, i.e., they recapitulate to variable extent the architectural and cytologic constituents of normal peripheral or autonomic nerves. Likewise, their classification is identical to their soft tissue counterparts. In this chapter, only those tumours are discussed which are particularly relevant for the dermatopathologist by their distinct morphology, predominant cutaneous manifestation, or their recent recognition and significance in cutaneous pathology. These include the neuroendocrine carcinomas, rare but problematic peripheral variants of primitive neuroectodermal tumours, the non-neoplastic neuroma group with its spontaneous and reactive types and the recently defined, but still histogenetically controversial, nerve sheath myxoma-neurothekeoma spectrum.

WHO histological classification of neural tumours

Primitive neuroectodermal tumour (PNET)	9364/3
Ewing sarcoma	9260/3
Nerve sheath myxoma	9562/0
Merkel cell carcinoma	8247/3
Granular cell tumour	9580/0

___

[1] Morphology code of the International Classification of Diseases for Oncology (ICD-O) {786} and the Systematized Nomenclature of Medicine (http://snomed.org). Behaviour is coded /0 for benign tumours, /3 for malignant tumours, and /1 for borderline or uncertain behaviour.

TNM classification of skin (Merkel cell) carcinomas[1]

TNM classification [2,3]

T – Primary tumour

TX	Primary tumour cannot be assessed
T0	No evidence of primary tumour
Tis	Carcinoma in situ
T1	Tumour 2 cm or less in greatest dimension
T2	Tumour more than 2 cm but no more than 5 cm in greatest dimension
T3	Tumour more than 5 cm in greatest dimension
T4	Tumour invades deep extradermal structures, i.e., cartilage, skeletal muscle, or bone

Note: In the case of multiple simultaneous tumours, the tumour with the highest T category is classified and the number of separate tumours is indicated in parentheses, e.g., T2(5).

N – Regional lymph nodes

NX	Regional lymph nodes cannot be assessed
N0	No regional lymph node metastasis
N1	Regional lymph node metastasis

M – Distant metastasis

MX	Distant metastasis cannot be assessed
M0	No distant metastasis
M1	Distant metastasis

Stage grouping

Stage 0	Tis	N0	M0
Stage I	T1	N0	M0
Stage II	T2, T3	N0	M0
Stage III	T4	N0	M0
	Any T	N1	M0
Stage IV	Any T	Any N	M1

[1] For PNET and Ewing sarcoma see TNM table of soft tissue tumours
[2] {894,2219}.
[3] A help desk for specific questions about the TNM classification is available at www.uicc.org/index.php?id=508 .

Palisaded, encapsulated neuroma and traumatic neuroma

Z.B. Argenyi

Palisaded, encapsulated neuroma

Definition
Palisaded, encapsulated neuroma (PEN) is considered a spontaneous proliferation of nerve fibres without evidence of previous trauma.

Synonyms
Solitary circumscribed neuroma, spontaneous neuroma, true neuroma

Historical annotation
The tumour was described by Reed et al. in 1972, who pointed out that despite the occasional nuclear palisading and encapsulation, the tumour is different from Schwannoma {1908}.

Epidemiology
PEN is most common in the 5th and 7th decades and occurs in an approximately equal ratio in both genders. The majority of the lesions, about 90%, are located on the face, but they can occur anywhere on the body. Mucosal involvement has also been recorded {453,752,1908}.

Clinical features
PEN usually manifests as a solitary, small (2-6 cm), skin-coloured or pink, firm or rubbery, dome-shaped, asymptomatic papule or nodule. There is no established association with neurofibromatosis {453,752,1908}.

Macroscopy
On cut sections, the tumour is a yellow-pink, firm ovoid mass in the dermis.

Histopathology
On low magnification, PEN is a well-circumscribed, round or oblong nodule located in the dermis. It is surrounded by a thin fibrous capsule, which is poorly discernible or incomplete near to the epidermal aspect of the tumour. The tumour is composed of tightly woven fascicles which are separated by cleft-like spaces. The proliferating cells are slender spindle cells with ovoid, evenly chromatic nuclei and eosinophilic cytoplasm.
A parallel arrangement of nuclei resembling a palisading pattern or rudimentary Verocay bodies is occasionally present. Mitotic figures are rare or absent. PEN lacks distinct fibrosis, inflammation or granulomatous reaction. A connection with the originating nerve usually requires serial sectioning of the tissue. Silver impregnation reveals numerous nerve fibres (axons), usually in parallel arrangement with the longitudinal axes of the fascicles {55,80,90,453,585,646, 752,1314,1908}.

Immunophenotype
The cells in the capsule stain for epithelial membrane antigen, whereas the spindle cells of the fascicles are positive for S-100 protein and collagen type IV. The axons are labeled with antibodies to neural filaments. Variable myelinization is detected by CD57 (Leu-7) and myelin basic protein {55,80,90}.

Variants
Plexiform and multinodular types
These rare variants represent unusual growth pattern, but otherwise they retain the usual internal structures and composition of PEN {81,84}.

Spontaneous, non-encapsulated neuromas
These tumours are part of the Multiple Mucosal Neuroma (MMN) syndrome, which is often part of the Multiple Endocrine Neoplasia syndrome (MEN2b), which is associated with pheochromocytoma and medullary carcinoma of the thyroid {815}. The neuromas in MMN manifest as numerous, soft-rubbery, skin-coloured or pink papules and nodules around mucosal orifices, lip, eyelids, and tongue, but scattered cutaneous involvement can also occur {835,1658,1994}. Musculoskeletal abnormalities and intestinal ganglioneuromatosis are also part of

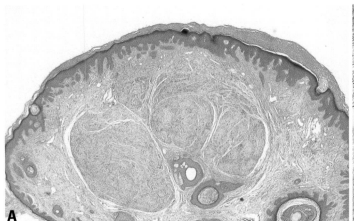
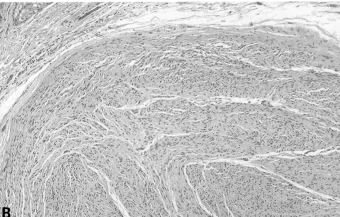

Fig. 6.1 Palisaded, encapsulated neuroma. **A** Multinodular variant of palisaded encapsulated neuroma. **B** The tumour is formed by compactly arranged fascicles separated by artificial clefts.

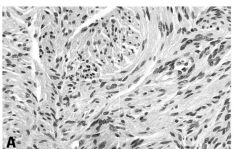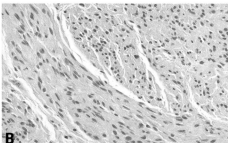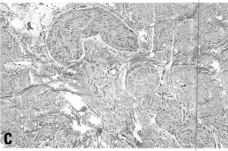

Fig. 6.2 Palisaded, encapsulated neuroma (PEN). **A** Internal structure and cytology correspond to the classical type of PEN. **B** The fascicles are composed of uniform spindle cells without cytologic atypia. Despite the term, no distinct nuclear palisading is present. **C** Spontaneous, non-encapsulated neuromas of Multiple Mucosal Neuroma Syndrome. The tumour is composed of linearly arranged hyperplastic nerve bundles infiltrating the dermis.

the syndrome {236,2504}. Histologically, the tumour is composed of numerous tortuous or fascicular arrangements of hyperplastic nerve bundles infiltrating the submucosa or the dermis, hence the term "non-encapsulated neuroma" has also been applied. The individual fascicles have a linear, elongated appearance instead of the round or oblong structure of PEN; however, the constituent cells are identical to those seen in PEN. Occasionally perineurial and endoneurial increase of mucin can be noted. The immunohistochemical profile of this variant is similar to PEN {815, 835,1658,1994}.

Genetics
Activated mutations of the RET proto-oncogene, involving the somatic or the germinal cell-lineage are found in both the inherited and acquired forms {466, 545,2310}. However, MMN without genetic abnormalities has also been reported {1863,2379}.

Prognostic factors
PEN and its variants are benign, and simple excision is a sufficient treatment. The mucosal neuromas of MEN2b often precede the manifestation of the other endocrine tumours. Therefore their correct recognition is important {1020}.

Traumatic neuroma

Definition
Traumatic neuromas represent reactive or regenerative proliferation of the nerve sheath components as an attempt to reestablish lost nerve integrity after sharp or blunt physical trauma.

Synonyms
Amputation neuroma, supernumerary digit

Epidemiology
Traumatic neuromas can occur at any age or gender. The amputation type is more common on the extremities {1535}. A special variant sometimes referred to incorrectly as "supernumerary digit" occurs on the lateral aspects of hands or feet of newborns. They represent amputation neuromas at the site of the in-utero separated extranumerary digit {487, 2152}.

Clinical features
Traumatic neuromas develop at the sites of previous trauma usually as solitary, skin-coloured, broad-based, firm papules and nodules. They are often sensitive or painful on pressure.
Lancinating pain is characteristic of amputation neuromas {351,530,2342}.

Macroscopy
Traumatic neuromas are firm, white-yellow, ill-defined dermal or subcutaneous masses often in a discernible association with the proximal nerve stump.

Histopathology
The tumour is composed of an irregular, haphazardly arranged proliferation of regenerating nerve fascicles of various sizes and shapes embedded in a fibrous stroma. Earlier lesions show acute and chronic inflammation, occasional granulomatous inflammation, whereas more established lesions are markedly fibrotic. Although the tumour is encased in the sclerotic stroma, there is no true encapsulation, and the distal end of the regenerating nerve fascicles often infiltrates the stroma {90,2084}. The individual nerve fascicles appear to recapitulate the architecture of the normal nerve fascicles, but there is considerable variation in their diameter. The constituent cells

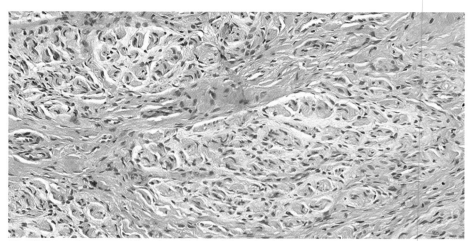

Fig. 6.3 Traumatic neuroma. There is an ill-defined dermal nodule composed of irregularly arranged proliferation of nerve fascicles embedded in a fibrotic (scarred) stroma.

are slender spindle cells (Schwann cells, perineurial cells, and endoneurial fibroblasts). Silver impregnation reveals numerous nerve fibres (axons) in the tumour in a pattern approximating the normal 1:1 ratio of Schwann cells and axons. The "supernumerary digit" is a polypoid lesion covered by thick hyperorthokeratosis with a fibrous stalk containing regenerating nerve fascicles. The morphology of the regenerating nerve fibres is identical to the ones seen in other amputation neuromas.

Immunohistochemistry

The constituent spindle cells of the nerve fascicles are positive for S-100 protein, collagen type IV, whereas the surrounding perineurial cells, when present, stain for epithelial membrane antigen. Antibodies to neural filaments highlight the axons, and myelinization can be demonstrated by antibodies to myelin basic protein and CD57 (Leu-7).

Prognostic factors

Traumatic neuroma is a reactive lesion; however, it can cause local interference with adjacent organs and is often symptomatic. The usual treatment is simple excision.

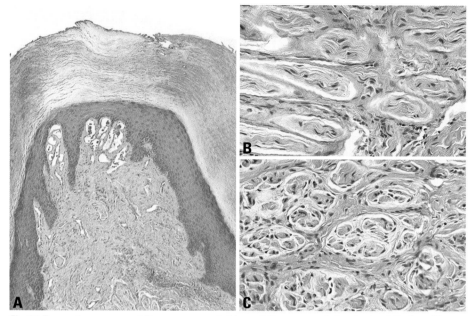

Fig. 6.4 Traumatic neuroma. **A** Supernumerary digit (amputation neuroma). Acral polypoid lesion with proliferation of nerve fascicles at the base of stalk. **B** Higher magnification of the regenerating nerve fascicles in the fibrous stroma. **C** The regenerating nerve fascicles show variation of diameter and orientation. The clear spaces correspond to increased perineurial mucin.

Primary malignant peripheral primitive neuroectodermal tumour (PNET) / Extraskeletal Ewing sarcoma (ES)

S.S. Banerjee

Definition
PNET/ES are malignant small blue round cell tumours, which exhibit varying degrees of neuroectodermal differentiation. In the past, they were regarded as separate entities, but recent cytogenetic and molecular genetic studies have proven that they represent two ends of a phenotypic spectrum of the same tumour type – Ewing sarcoma being relatively undifferentiated and PNET showing morphological (light microscopic/ultrastructural) and/or immunohistochemical features of neuroectodermal differentiation.

ICD-O codes
PNET   9364/3
Ewing sarcoma   9260/3

Synonyms
Peripheral neuroepithelioma, peripheral neuroblastoma

Epidemiology
Primary PNET/ES of skin and subcutaneous tissue are rare neoplasms. These tumours are mainly seen in children and young adults (median age 18 yrs), but they occasionally afflict elderly individuals. There is no significant sex predilection {72,82,138,449,978,1389,1791,1815, 2050,2146,2210,2295,2328,2416}.

Etiology
The etiology of this tumour is unknown.

Localization
These neoplasms have been described on the scalp, face, neck, shoulder, trunk and extremities.

Clinical features
The tumours usually present as ulcerated or non-ulcerated, often painless, but rarely tender, nodules. Occasionally, they appear polypoid {138,978}. Not infrequently, they are clinically misdiagnosed as benign tumours or cysts. A case of cutaneous PNET with numerous tumour nodules that were present for several years has been documented {2050}.

Macroscopic features
The tumours are greyish white and fleshy. Foci of haemorrhage are sometimes noted. Their sizes usually vary from 5 cm to 10 cm.

Histopathology
The tumours usually occupy the dermis with focal extension into subcutis. Some tumours are entirely subcutaneous in location. The overlying epidermis may become ulcerated. The margins may be pushing or infiltrative. The neoplastic cells are small, round to oval and contain hyperchromatic or vesicular nuclei and scanty pale eosinophilic or vacuolated cytoplasm with ill-defined borders. The nucleoli are indistinct or absent. The cells are arranged in sheets, lobules, nests and trabeculae. The mitotic activity and necrosis vary from case to case. Many dark apoptotic cells may be seen. Prominent fibrovascular septa are present in most lesions and some exhibit peritheliomatous or pseudopapillary arrangement of cells. Occasionally, the stromal blood vessels form glomeruloid tufts with prominent endothelial and myointimal cells. Microcystic, pseudoglandular and pseudovascular spaces are observed in many neoplasms. Homer Wright rosettes and neuropil are only rarely present. In atypical examples of this tumour, larger cells with prominent nucleoli, pleomorphic cells with irregular nuclei or groups of mononuclear or binucleate rhabdoid or plasmacytoid cells are seen. Prominent epidermal inclusion cysts within the tumour have been described in one case. Intracytoplasmic glycogen can be demonstrated in most cases. The reticulin stain reveals fibrils around groups of tumour cells. The differential diagnosis of this neoplasm includes deposits of lymphoma / leukaemia, Merkel cell carcinoma, metastatic small cell neuroendocrine carcinoma, metastatic neuroblastoma, primary or metastatic rhabdomyosarcoma, glomus tumour, small cell melanoma and rare types of sweat gland tumour such as eccrine spiradenoma and non-neuroendocrine small cell carcinoma. Attention to histological detail, immunohistochemistry, EM studies and genetic analysis help to reach the right diagnosis.

Immunohistochemistry
Characteristically, the neoplastic cells exhibit positivity for CD99 (MIC2 gene product), ß2 microglobulin, FLI-1 gene product, vimentin and one or more puta-

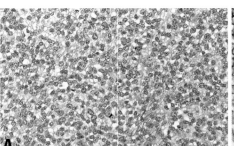 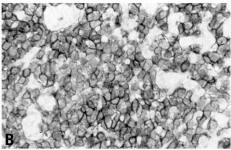 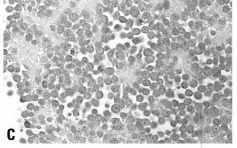

Fig. 6.5 Primary PNET/EES of skin. **A** Tumour composed of sheets of monomorphic small round cells containing hyperchromatic nuclei and scanty cytoplasm. **B** Strong membranous CD99 positivity in the neoplastic cells. **C** Homer-Wright rosettes. They are only rarely seen in these neoplasms.

tive neural/neuroendocrine markers such as NSE, PGP 9.5, neurofilament proteins, synaptophysin and Leu-7. The stain for chromogranin is usually negative. The CD99 positivity is usually strong, diffuse and membranous. The FLI-1 stains the nuclei of the neoplastic cells. Aberrant cytokeratin, desmin, GFAP, S100 protein and NKIC3 expression may be noted in scattered cells in some cases. The tumour cells are negative for LCA, B&T cell markers, myeloperoxidase, muscle specific actin, MYO-D1, myogenin, EMA and HMB 45 {138}.

Electron microscopy

At the Ewing end of the spectrum, the cells appear rather non-descript with round nuclei and scanty organelles. There is usually abundant glycogen. The PNETs show elongated interdigitating cytoplasmic processes with a few rudimentary junctions, intermediate filaments, microtubules and sparse membrane bound dense core neurosecretory granules (100-250 nm in diameter). No myofilaments, desmosomes or melanosomes are seen {138}.

Genetics

Around 90% of skeletal and extraskeletal PNET/ES exhibit a characteristic chromosomal translocation, t(11;22)(q24;q12). This results in the fusion of EWS gene on chromosome 22q12 with FLI-1 gene on chromosome 11q24. A small number of cutaneous cases have been subjected to cytogenetic/genetic studies and these have also demonstrated the typical genetic defects {978,1389}. An additional copy of chromosome 22 was detected in one case. Conventional cytogenetic study, FISH and RT-PCR techniques have been used to detect these abnormalities.

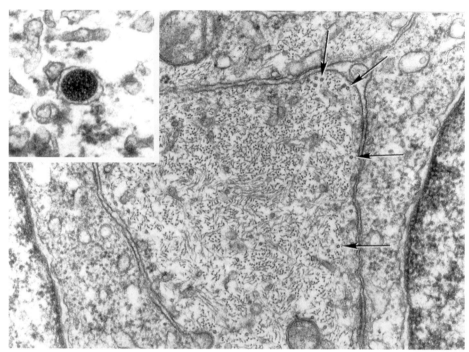

Fig. 6.6 Primary PNET of skin. Electron microscopy of a cutaneous PNET: the cytoplasmic processes of the neoplastic cells contain intermediate filaments and microtubules (arrow). The inset shows a neurosecretory granule.

Prognosis and predictive factors

These neoplasms are aggressive with metastatic potential. The usual sites of metastasis are regional lymph nodes, lung, liver and bones. However, the cutaneous PNET/ES appear to have a better prognosis than their soft tissue counterparts, probably because they are detected early and can be resected adequately. Long term survival has been recorded in a few cases with or without radiotherapy and adjuvant combination chemotherapy {138,478,978,2328}. A prognostically relevant grading or staging system is not yet available for these neoplasms.

Nerve sheath myxoma / neurothekeoma
Z.B. Argenyi

Definition
These tumours encompass a spectrum of neuromesenchymal neoplasms characterized by proliferation of nerve sheath cells in a variable myxomatous stroma. They can be further classified into "classic" and "cellular" types.

ICD-O code
9562/0

Synonyms
Cellular neurothekeoma (used exclusively for the cellular variant), cutaneous lobular neuromyxoma, myxomatous perineuroma

Epidemiology
These tumours are rare. The "classic type" has been reported in middle-aged adults (mean 48.4), with predominance in females, of the head and neck areas and upper extremities {73,1865}. The "cellular type" has been observed in younger adults (mean 24 yrs), more common in females, predominantly on the head and neck areas {88,99,161,371}. However, both types can occur at any age and at any location {229,418,479, 1222,1674,1684,2355}.

Clinical features
The "classic types" manifest as skin-coloured, pink, soft, rubbery papules and nodules, whereas the "cellular types" have a firmer, rather red-tan-brown appearance. Their size ranges between 0.5–2.0 cm. Both types are commonly asymptomatic, but may become sensitive or tender {73,88,99, 161,371,1865}.

Histopathology
The "classic type" is usually a well-defined, multilobular or fascicular tumour located in the dermis with or without extension to the subcutis. The lobules contain abundant myxomatous stroma, which appear to be confined by a thin fibrous encapsulation. The mucin is connective tissue type acidic mucopolysaccharide and stains strongly with colloidal iron, which clears after hyaluronidase treatment. Within the mucinous stroma, there are sparsely distributed spindle, stellate, and polygonal cells without appreciable cytologic atypia. Mitotic figures are rare or absent {73,88,755,1865}. The "cellular variant" shows an ill-defined, often infiltrative growth pattern involving the dermis and subcutis. The proliferating cells form fascicles and nests and are arranged in a plexiform or multilobular pattern. The constituent cells are mainly epithelioid type with ample eosinophilic cytoplasm and indistinct cytoplasmic membranes. The cells have large "bubbly nuclei" with prominent nucleoli. In a smaller percentage of the cases, the tumour is composed of spindle cells with plump or ovoid nuclei forming nests and whorls. In the "cellular type", cytologic and nuclear atypia are more common and mitotic figures can be conspicuous. Myxoid material is usually scant or present only around the individual nests {88,99,161,371}. In both the "classic" and "cellular types", associated stromal changes, such as fibrosis, hyalinization of the collagen, patchy chronic inflammation, and angioplasia can occur. Changes showing transition between the "classic" and "cellular types" within the same lesion have been documented. A direct connection with nerve twigs can be demonstrated only rarely.

Immunohistochemistry
The stromal cells in the "classic" type stains strongly for S-100 protein, collagen type IV and weakly for neuron-specific enolase and CD57 (Leu-7). The capsule, when present, may label for epithelial membrane antigen. The "cellular" type does not have a specific or consistent phenotype. The cells show variable expression of PGP9.5, collagen type IV, NK1/C3, CD34, and occasionally smooth muscle specific actin and CD57 (Leu-7). Staining for S-100 protein is rare, and

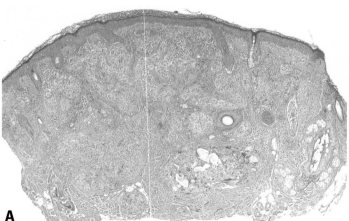
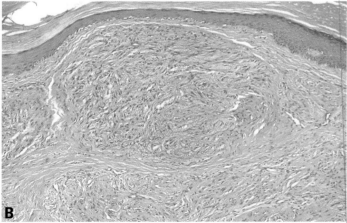

Fig. 6.7 Nerve sheath myxoma (neurothekeoma). **A** Cellular neurothekeoma (cellular variant of nerve sheath myxoma). The tumour cells form nests and strands infiltrating the dermis. **B** Nerve sheath myxoma "classical type". Lobular and fascicular dermal proliferation with myxomatous stroma.

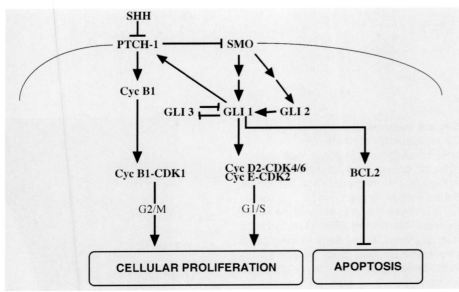

Fig. 7.10 Model of Sonic Hedgehog (SHH) signalling pathway. The function of the pathway is to stimulate cellular proliferation and inhibit apoptosis. The *PTCH-1* gene is predicted to encode a 12-transmembrane receptor with high affinity for the SHH secreted 19 kDa protein ligand. In presence of SHH, the pathway releases the 7-transmembrane protein. Smoothened (SMO) from its inhibition by PTCH-1, thus activating target genes through the glioma (GLI) family of zinc-finger transcription factors (GLI1 is the most studied of the three GLI factors). GLI1 may control the G1/S transition checkpoint through activation of the transcription of *Cyclin D2* and *E* genes, and apoptosis through activation of BCL2 expression. *PTCH-1* may also be involved in a G2/M transition checkpoint via Cyclin B1 which localizes to the nucleus upon SHH binding {152}. *PTCH-1* transcription is induced by GLI1, thus generating a negative feedback loop.
Abbreviations : Cyc, cyclin ; CDK, cyclin-dependent kinase.

involvement may give the impression that medulloblastoma has spread to bone. Histologically, the flame-like lesions are hamartomas consisting of fibrous connective tissue, nerves and blood vessels. Subcutaneous calcification of fingers and scalp has been rare. Sclerotic bone lesions have been reported occasionally. Ovarian fibromas are found in about 25% of females. They are bilateral and often calcified, at times overlapping medially. Prenatal diagnosis by sonography has been accomplished {235}.

Genetics
The first link between the Sonic Hedgehog (SHH) signalling pathway and tumour formation in humans was in famil-ial cancers, as 30-40% of NBCCS patients harbour loss-of-function muta-tions in the PATCHED1 (*PTCH1*) gene {514,939,1992}. That disruption of the SHH signalling pathway is a major deter-minant of tumour formation, particularly for BCCs, was established from the dis-covery that PTCH1 is mutated in 10-38% of sporadic BCCs {514,1992}.

Inactivation of both *PTCH1* alleles also results in the formation of cysts {1408}. Consistent with its pivotal role in embry-onic development, aberrant SHH sig-nalling is associated with a range of human developmental anomalies {2434}. In NBCCS, tumours (BCCs, keratocysts, meningiomas, ovarian fibromas, odonto-genic keratocysts) exhibit loss of het-erozygosity (LOH) in the *PTCH1* locus (9q22.3) {514}. Various physical anom-alies (bifid rib, macrocephaly, cleft lip, etc.) apparently need but one-hit {1407}. LOH in the *PTCH1* locus was observed in 89% of hereditary BCCs. The majority (61-71%) of germline *PTCH1* mutations are rearrangements. Most mutations (>80%) are likely to represent null muta-tions since they are predicted to result in truncation of the *PTCH1* protein {133, 514,1408,1992}.

The *PTCH1* tumour suppressor gene comprises 23 exons which encode 12 putative transmembrane domains and two large extracellular loops. The func-tion of PTCH1 is to silence the SHH sig-nalling pathway in absence of active SHH ligand {2308}. In presence of SHH, the pathway acts in at least two ways to regulate target genes. One is to activate GLI 1/2 transcription factors and the other is to inhibit the formation of GLI repressors, mostly from GLI3, to dere-press target genes {1992}.

Prognosis and predictive factors
New keratocystic odontogenic tumours (odontogenic keratocysts) and basal cell carcinomas continue for life. Limitation of sun exposure reduces the appearance of the skin cancers. The medulloblastoma appears before the age of 4 years, the ovarian fibromas after puberty.
Therapeutic radiation should be avoided whenever possible due to the high occurrence of basal cell carcinomas in the radiation field.

Cowden syndrome

D. V. Kazakov
G. Burg
C. Eng

Definition

Cowden syndrome (CS) is an autosomal-dominant disorder with age-related penetrance and variable expression, characterized by multiple hamartomas arising in tissues derived from all three embryonic germ cell layers and with a high risk of developing benign and malignant neoplasms in many organ systems, especially in the skin, breast, and thyroid gland. The condition was described in 1963 by Lloyd and Dennis {1439}. It is caused by germline mutations in the tumour suppressor gene *PTEN* located on chromosome 10q23 {1424}.

OMIM number   158350

Synonyms

Multiple hamartoma syndrome, Cowden disease

Epidemiology

Incidence

The incidence of CS, after *PTEN* was identified as the gene, was found to be 1 in 200 000 {1693}. The latter may be an underestimate, since CS has variable expression and often manifests itself only with subtle skin changes, so that this condition may be difficult to recognize {688}. Although the exact proportion of isolated and familial cases is not known, previous and on-going observations suggest that 40-60% are familial {1521, 2448,688A}.

Clinical features

CS is classically characterized as a multiple hamartoma syndrome with a high risk of breast and thyroid cancers. Although the reported age at onset varies from 4–75 years {1451}, CS usually manifests in the second or third decade. More than 90% of individuals affected with CS are likely to manifest a phenotype by the age of 20 years, and 99% develop at least mucocutaneous lesions by the age of 30 years {1694,2448}. CS is characterized by the development of hamartomas, benign and malignant tumours in multiple organ systems including the skin, soft tissues, breast, thyroid gland, gastrointestinal tract, genitourinary tract, and central nervous system. The most common lesions are trichilemmomas (90-100%), breast fibroadenomas (70%), thyroid adenomas (40-60%), multinodular goiter (40–60%), and multiple gastrointestinal polyps (35–40%) {688,1451}. Macrocephaly is seen in 35-40% of cases. Malignant neoplasms develop in the breast in 25–50% of CS females, in the thyroid gland in 3–10% (usually follicular adenocarcinoma) and in the uterus in 3-6%. The most common malignant neoplasm in the breast is ductal adenocarcinoma, which is bilateral in one third of cases {2098}. The average age of CS patients at diagnosis of breast cancer is 10 years younger than in those with sporadic disease {2252}. Male breast cancers also occur, but with unknown fre-

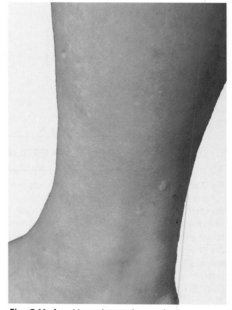

Fig. 7.11 Acral hyperkeratotic papules.

quency {704,1519}. A feature that distinguishes CS from other breast cancer susceptibility syndromes is the occurrence of benign breast disease prior to the development of breast cancer {2098,2099}.

Many other internal malignancies have been reported to occur in individuals affected with CS. There are no data to state whether they are true components of this syndrome or merely coincidental.

Bannayan–Riley–Ruvalcaba syndrome (BRRS)

This pediatric disorder characterized by congenital macrocephaly, multiple lipomatosis and angiomatosis involving the skin and visceral tissues, intestinal hamartomatous polyposis, and pigmented penile lesions, shows a partial clinical overlap with CS {711,1519}.

Diagnostic criteria

The International Cowden Consortium originally proposed a set of operational diagnostic criteria in 1996 {1694}. Because of new data, the Consortium revised the criteria in 2000 {688}, which

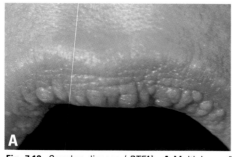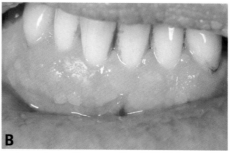

Fig. 7.12 Cowden disease (*PTEN*). **A** Multiple confluent papules on the upper lip. **B** Multiple wart-like lesions on the gingivae.

have also been adopted by the United States' National Comprehensive Cancer Center (NCCN) Practice Guidelines Panel.

Cutaneous and mucosal lesions

Cutaneous lesions are the most important hallmarks for CS, since they are present in almost every patient and frequently appear prior to the development of any internal disease {1030}. Facial papules are the most frequent lesions (85-90%). They are mainly located in periorificial regions, sometimes extending into the nostrils. Histopathologically, the papules frequently show non-specific verrucous acanthomas, trichilemmomas, perifollicular fibromas or may reveal lesions with features intermediate between trichilemmomas, inverted follicular keratosis, and tumour of follicular infundibulum {322, 2249-2251}. Although human papilloma virus has not been consistently found in these lesions, some experts believe that trichilemmomas in CS represent verrucae vulgaris with trichilemmal differentiation {28}. Acral verrucous hyperkeratosis on the extensor sides of the extremities and palmoplantar translucent keratoses are seen in approximately 20-30% of cases. Histopathologically, they show wart-like changes, with prominent compact orthokeratosis, hypergranulosis, and acanthosis, in some cases with trichilemmal differentiation. Involvement of the oral mucosa is present in over 80% of cases. Coalescent lesions produce the characteristic cobblestone-like pattern in 40% of patients. Histopathologically, these lesions are composed of acellular collagen fibres, with a predominantly whorl-like arrangement {2251}. Mucosal papules and nodules with trichilemmoma-like histopathological features are also common. A scrotal tongue is another common finding. Usually mucocutaneous lesions are present in multiple locations, and extension to the oropharynx, larynx, tongue, and nasal mucosa may occur.

Other cutaneous lesions reported to occur in individuals affected with CS include lipoma, angiolipoma, multiple sclerotic fibromas, squamous cell carcinoma, melanoma, basal cell carcinoma, Merkel cell carcinoma, haemangiomas, xanthoma, vitiligo, neuroma, apocrine hidrocystoma, café au lait spots, periorificial and acral lentigines and acanthosis nigricans (reviewed in {748,1030})

Genetics

PTEN/MMAC1/TEP1 on 10q23.3, is the susceptibility gene for CS {1424,1694}.

Gene structure and function

PTEN comprises 9 exons spanning 120-150 kb of genomic distance. It encodes a 1.2 kb transcript and a 403 amino acid lipid dual-specificity phosphatase (it dephosphorylates both protein and lipid substrates) {1419,1421,2256,2448}. A classic phosphatase core motif is encoded within exon 5, which is the largest exon, constituting 20% of the coding region {1419,1421,1519,2256}.

PTEN is the major 3-phosphatase acting in the phosphatidylinositol-3-kinase (PI3K)/Akt pathway {1478,2241}. To date, virtually all naturally occurring missense mutations tested abrogate both lipid and protein phosphatase activity, and one mutant, G129E, affects only lipid phosphatase activity. Overexpression of *PTEN* results, for the most part, in phosphatase-dependent cell cycle arrest at G1 and/or apoptosis, depending on cell type (reviewed in {687,2448}). There is also growing evidence that *PTEN* can mediate growth arrest independent of the PI3K/Akt pathway and perhaps independent of the lipid phosphatase activity {460,1564,2448,2495,2496}.

Mutation spectrum

Approximately 70-85% of CS cases, as strictly defined by the Consortium Criteria, have a germline *PTEN* mutation {1424,1519,2599}. If the diagnostic criteria are relaxed, then mutation frequencies drop to 10-50% {1464,1695,2382}. A formal study which ascertained 64 unre-

Table 7.5
International Cowden Consortium operational criteria for the diagnosis of Cowden syndrome 2000 {688}.

Pathognomonic criteria
Mucocutaneous lesions
    Trichilemmomas, facial
    Acral keratoses
    Papillomatous papules
    Mucosal lesions

Major criteria
    Breast carcinoma
    Thyroid carcinoma (nonmedullary), especially follicular thyroid carcinoma
    Macrocephaly (megalencephaly) (~95th percentile or more)
    Lhermitte-Duclos disease
    Endometrial carcinoma

Minor criteria
    Other thyroid lesions (eg, adenoma or multinodular goitre)
    Mental retardation (IQ~75 or less)
    Gastrointestinal hamartomas
    Fibrocystic disease of the breast
    Lipomas
    Fibromas
    Genitourinary tumours (eg, renal cell carcinoma, uterine fibroids) or malformation

Operational diagnosis in an individual
1. Mucocutaneous lesions alone if there are:
    (a) 6 or more facial papules, of which 3 or more are trichilemmoma, or
    (b) cutaneous facial papules and oral mucosal papillomatosis, or
    (c) oral mucosal papillomatosis and acral keratoses, or
    (d) 6 or more palmoplantar keratoses,
2. Two major criteria, one of which is macrocephaly or Lhermitte-Duclos disease
3. One major and three minor criteria
4. Four minor criteria

Operational diagnosis in a family where one individual is diagnosed with Cowden syndrome
1. The pathognomonic criterion or criteria
2. Any one major criterion with or without minor criteria
3. Two minor criteria

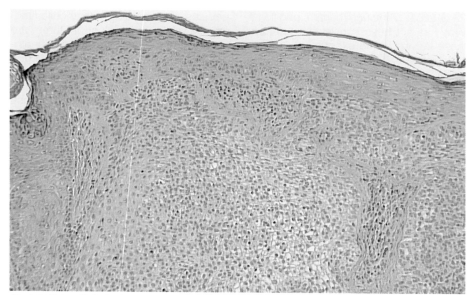
Fig. 7.13 Histopathological appearance of trichilemmoma in a patient with Cowden syndrome (Courtesy of Carl D. Morrison, MD, Ohio State University, USA).

lated CS-like cases revealed a mutation frequency of 2% if the criteria are not met, even if the diagnosis is made short of one criterion {1519}. A single research centre study involving 37 unrelated CS families, ascertained according to the strict diagnostic criteria of the Consortium, revealed a mutation frequency of 80% {1519}.

As with most other tumour suppressor genes, the mutations found in *PTEN* are scattered throughout all 9 exons. They comprise loss-of-function mutations including missense, nonsense, frameshift and splice-site mutations {1519, 1521,2448}. Approximately 30-40% of germline *PTEN* mutations are found in exon 5. Further, approximately 65% of all mutations can be found in one of exons 5, 7 or 8 {1519,1521}.

Although *PTEN* is the major susceptibility gene for CS, one CS family, without *PTEN* mutations, was found to have a germline mutation in the bone morphogenic protein receptor type 1A gene (*BMPR1A*, MIM 601299), which is one of the susceptibility genes for juvenile polyposis syndrome {1066,2600}.

Whether *BMPR1A* is a minor CS susceptibility gene or whether this family with CS features actually has occult juvenile polyposis is yet unknown.

Genotype-phenotype associations

Clinically useful genotype–phenotype correlations are being intensively investigated. Exploratory genotype-phenotype analyses revealed that the presence of a germline mutation was associated with a familial risk of developing a malignant breast disease. Further, missense mutations and/or mutations 5' of the phos-phatase core motif seem to be associated with a surrogate for disease severity (multiorgan involvement) {1519}.

Previously thought to be clinically distinct, BRRS is likely allelic to CS {1519}. Approximately 65% of BRRS families and isolated cases combined carry a germline *PTEN* mutation {420,1520,1521, 2599}. Interestingly, there were 11 cases classified as true CS-BRR overlap families in this cohort, and 10 of the 11 had a *PTEN* mutation. The overlapping mutation spectrum, the existence of true overlap families and the genotype-phenotype associations which suggest that the presence of germline *PTEN* mutation is associated with cancer, strongly indicate that CS and BRR are allelic and are along a single spectrum at the molecular level. The aggregate term "*PTEN* hamartoma tumour syndrome" (PHTS) has therefore been proposed {688,1521}. The clinical spectrum of PHTS has recently been expanded to include also subsets of Proteus syndrome and Proteus-like (non-CS, non-BRR) syndromes {2203,2598}.

Genetics of Cowden syndrome is also reviewed in detail in the WHO Classification of Tumours of the Nervous System, Tumours of the Digestive System, as well as in the WHO Classification of Tumours of the Breast and Female Genital Organs.

Carney complex

W.H.C. Burgdorf
J.A. Carney

Definition
Carney complex (CNC) is a lentiginosis-multiple endocrine neoplasia syndrome caused by at least two distinct mutations and characterized by multiple often unique tumours including myxomas and schwannomas, endocrine abnormalities, and cutaneous pigmentary lesions {397}.

OMIM numbers
CNC1 160980; CNC2 605244

Synonyms
NAME syndrome {111}, LAMB syndrome {1926}.

Epidemiology
Carney complex is an uncommon disorder, inherited in an autosomal dominant fashion. More than 350 cases are known involving more than 65 families.
The penetrance is high but the expressivity is highly variable. Patients may present with cutaneous, cardiac, or endocrine lesions; often the diagnosis is delayed until multiple manifestations are present.

Localization
The most commonly involved organs are the skin (75%), heart (50%) and adrenal glands (25%).

Clinical features
The cutaneous findings in CNC are often most dramatic. Patients may have multiple flat pigmented lesions that have been described both as ephelides (freckles) with an increased amount of melanin {111} and as lentigines with an increased number of melanocytes {1926}. Blue naevi are another marker of the syndrome; many exhibit epithelioid features on microscopic examination {396}. Pigmented lesions are also common on mucosal surfaces, such as the lips, mouth, conjunctiva and genital mucosa {1244}. Some patients have no pigmentary changes. Another highly specific cutaneous finding is myxomas, especially when they affect the eyelids and the external ear canal {734}. Histologically, these benign tumours often feature strands of lacy epithelium {398}.
The most dramatic systemic finding is cardiac myxoma(s). The CNC-associated myxomas have important differences from sporadic cardiac myxomas; they are more likely to be familial, multiple, occur at a younger age, involve the ventricles and recur {2433}. Recurrent cardiac myxoma(s) may require multiple surgical resections that may result in postoperative arrhythmias and increased mortality.

The most common endocrine finding is primary pigmented nodular adrenal disease, a very rare ACTH-independent cause of Cushing syndrome (25%) {2164}. The adrenal glands show bilateral small, pigmented nodules with internodular cortical atrophy {881,2571}. One of Cushing's first patients, Minnie G., may well have had CNC {395}. Acromegaly and thyroid tumours {2275} are each seen in around 10% of patients. About one-third of male patients have large-cell calcifying Sertoli cell tumours of the testes, often bilateral and sometimes leading to precocious puberty {1734}.
Two other uncommon tumours which should suggest the presence of CNC are psammomatous melanotic schwannomas (20%) of the GI tract, sympathetic chain and skin {394}, and myxoid mammary fibroadenomas (25% of women) {400}.

Diagnostic procedures
Both epithelioid blue naevi and myxomas (the latter sometimes with a characteristic epithelial component) may be identified on skin biopsies and suggest the diagnosis of CNC. When investigation for Cushing syndrome reveals low or undetectable ACTH levels and no adrenal tumour, a diagnosis of primary pigment-

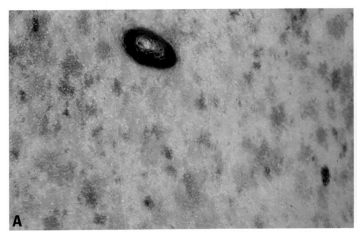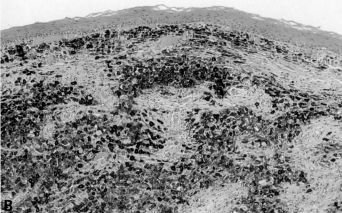

Fig. 7.14 A Spotty pigmentation and blue naevus in CNC. Courtesy of Dr. David J. Atherton, London, UK, and reference {111}. **B** Histological specimen of blue naevus showing large epithelioid melanocytes. Courtesy of Dr. Luis Requena, Madrid, Spain.

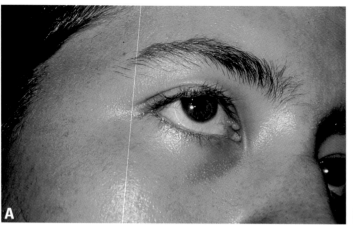 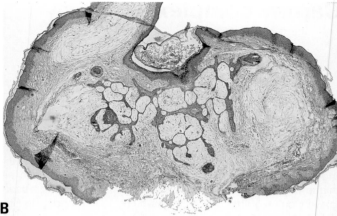

Fig. 7.15 A Eyelid myxoma in a young man with CNC and no cutaneous pigmentary changes. **B** Microscopic view of the same lesion, showing lacy epithelial strands amidst deposits of mucin.

ed nodular adrenal disease should be considered and the patient evaluated for CNC, particularly if the patient is young or has multiple pigmented skin spots or lumps. Echocardiography is particularly important {2276}.

Differential diagnosis
When multiple pigmented lesions are present, LEOPARD syndrome should be considered but myxomas are absent in this condition and the systemic manifestations more protean. Mucosal pigmentation strongly resembles that of Peutz-Jeghers syndrome, but intestinal polyps are not part of the usual spectrum of Carney complex.

Genetics
Carney complex is inherited in an autosomal dominant fashion. The gene for CNC1, known as *PRKAR1A*, normally encodes the protein kinase A regulatory subunit R1a {408,1284}. When the mutat-

ed gene is present, the regulatory subunit is no longer produced. The patients are heterozygous for the mutation: the tumours tend to have LOH of the wild type allele for this regulatory gene. The *CNC2* gene is less well characterized but appears to be involved in regulating genomic stability, perhaps via the telomeres.

Prognosis and predictive factors
The prognosis depends on detecting cardiac myxoma, the most serious complex of CNC. The average age of 22 patients who died as the result of cardiac causes (cardiac failure from myxoma, cardiac myxoma emboli or cardiac arrhythmia) was 31 years. Timely diagnosis of the neoplasms requires an awareness of the possible significance of the pigmented skin spots, skin tumours, primary pigmented nodular adrenal disease and psammomatous melanotic schwannoma. Patients with lesions sug-

gestive of CNC should be advised to have a general medical evaluation and an echocardiogram. Primary relatives of CNC patients should be similarly advised.

WHO Classification of Skin Tumours
Consensus Conference, International Agency for Research on Cancer,
22-25 September 2003   Lyon, France

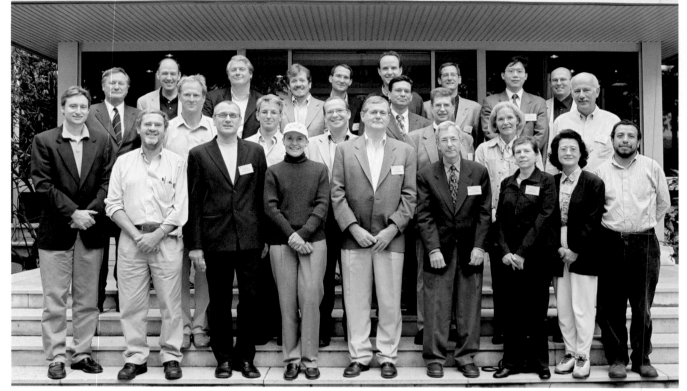

Rein Willemze   Chris Meijer   Philip LeBoit   Werner Kempf   Boris Bastian   Richard Kasper   Lawrence Yu   Wojciech Biernat
Paul Kleihues   Jan Lübbe   Eduardo Calonje   Alain Spatz   Earl Glusac   Günther Burg   Elizabeth Ralfkiaer   Walter Burgdorf
Michael Kurrer   David Elder   Bernhard Zelger   Sabine Kohler   David Weedon   Steven Sverdlow   Elain Jaffe   Grace Kao   Omar Sangueza

Dr. Daniel Jose SANTA CRUZ
Cutaneous Pathology
2326 Millpark Dr
St Louis, MO 63043-3530
USA
Tel. +1 314 991 4470
Fax. +1 314 991 4309
dsantacruz@aol.com

Dr. Marco SANTUCCI
Dept of Human Pathology and Oncology
University of Florence Medical
School
Viale G.B. Morgagni, 85
50134 Florence, ITALY
Tel. +39 055 4478105
Fax. +39 055 432144
marco.santucci@unifi.it

Dr. Alain SARASIN
Institut Gustave Roussy PR2
UPR 2169 CNRS
39, rue Camille Desmoulins
94805 Villejuif cedex
FRANCE
Tel. +33 1 42 11 63 28
Fax. +33 1 42 11 50 08
sarasin@igr.fr

Dr. Ulrico SCHMID
Department of Pathology
Kantonsspital St. Gallen
Rorschacherstrasse 95
9007 St. Gallen
SWITZERLAND
Tel. +41 71 494 21 02
Fax. +41 71 494 28 94
ulrico.schmid@kssg.ch

Dr. Tilman SCHULZ
Institute for Pathology
Escherichstrasse 6
91522 Ansbach
GERMANY
Fax. +49 0981 4888310
schulz@pathologie-ansbach.com

Dr. Richard SCOLYER
Department of Anatomical Pathology
Royal Prince Alfred Hospital
Missenden Road
NSW 2050 Camperdown
AUSTRALIA
Tel. +61 9515 7011
Fax. +61 9515 8405
richard.scolyer@email.cs.nsw.gov.au

Dr. Ratnam K. SHANMUGARATNAM
Department of Pathology
National University Hospital
Lower Kent Ridge Road
119074 Singapore
SINGAPORE
Tel. +65 6772 43 12
Fax. +65 6778 06 71
patshanm@nus.eud.sg

Dr. Henry G. SKELTON
Dept of Anatomic Pathology
Quest Diagnostics
Tucker, GA 30084
USA
Tel. +1 678 406 1509
henry.g.skelton@questdiagnostics.com

Dr. Kathleen J. SMITH
Dept of Anatomic Pathology
Quest Diagnostics
Tucker, GA 30084
USA
Tel. +1 678 406 1509
ksmith@path.uab.edu

Dr. Bruce R. SMOLLER
Department of Pathology
UAMS Medical Center
4301 West Markham Street, Slot 517
Little Rock, AR 72205
USA
Tel. +1 501 686 5170
Fax. +1 501 296 1184
smollerbrucer@uams.edu

Dr. Leslie H. SOBIN
Department of Hepatic and
Gastrointestinal Pathology
Armed Forces Institute of Pathology
14th Street and Alaska Avenue
Washington, DC 20306-6000, USA
Tel. +1 202 782 2880
Fax. +1 202 782 9020
sobin@afip.osd.mil

Dr. Alan SPATZ*
Department of Pathology
Institut Gustave-Roussy IGR
39, rue Camille Desmoulins
94805 Villejuif Cedex
FRANCE
Tel. +33 1 42 11 44 62 or 53
Fax. +33 1 42 11 52 63
spatz@igr.fr

Dr. Wolfram STERRY
Clinic for Dermatology, Allergology
and Venerology
Humboldt University
Schumannstr. 20/21
10117 Berlin, GERMANY
Tel. +49 30 450 518 061
Fax. +49 30 450 518 911
wolfram.sterry@charite.de

Dr. Geoffrey STRUTTON
Anatomical Pathology,
Princess Alexandra Hospital
Ipswich Road
Qld 4102 Woolloongabba, Brisbane
AUSTRALIA
Tel. +617 3240 2480
Fax. +617 3240 2930
geoff_strutton@health.qld.gov.au

Dr. Daniel W.P. SU
Department of Dermatology
Mayo Medical School
200 First St. SW
Rochester, MN 55905-0001
USA
Tel. +1 507 284 2511
Fax. +1 507 284 0161
su.daniel@mayo.edu

Dr. Steven H. SWERDLOW*
University of Pittsburgh
UPMC Presbyterian Pathology Dept
Room C606.1
200 Lothrop Street
Pittsburgh, PA 15213, USA
Tel. +1 412 647 5191
Fax. +1 412 647 4008
swerdlowsh@upmc.edu

Dr. John F. THOMPSON
Sydney Cancer Centre
Royal Prince Alfred Hospital
Missenden Road, Camperdown
NSW 2050 Sydney
AUSTRALIA
Tel. +61 2 9515 7185
Fax. + 61 2 9550 6316
john@mel.rpa.cs.nsw.gov.au

Dr. Yoshiki TOKURA
Department of Dermatology
University of Occupational and
Environmental Health
1-1 Iseigaoka, Yahatanishi-ku
Kitakyushu 807-8555, JAPAN
Tel. +81 93 691 7445
Fax. +81 93 691 0907
tokuray@hama-med.ac.jp

Dr. Massimo TOMMASINO
Infection and Cancer Biology Group
International Agency for Research
on Cancer
150, cours Albert Thomas
69008 Lyon, FRANCE
Tel. +33 4 72 73 81 91
Fax. +33 4 72 73 84 42
tommasino@iarc.fr

Dr. Jorge TORO
Genetics and Epidemiology Branch
National Cancer Institute, EPS
6120 Executive Bld., MSC, Room 7125
Rockville, MD 20852-7236
USA
Tel. +1 301 451-4562
Fax +1 301 402-4489
toroj@mail.nih.gov

Dr. Antonella TOSTI
Department of Dermatology
S Orsola Hospital
University of Bologna
Via Massarenti 1
40138 Bologna, ITALY
Tel. +39 051 341820
Fax. +39 051 347847
tosti@almadns.unibo.it

Dr. Goos N.P. VAN MUIJEN
Dept. of Pathology
University Medical Center St. Radboud
P.O. Box 9101
6500 HB Nijmegen
THE NETHERLANDS
Tel. +31 24 3614399
Fax. +31 24 3540520
g.vanmuijen@pathol.umcn.nl

Dr. James VARDIMAN
Department of Pathology
University of Chicago Medical Center
5841 South Maryland Ave.MC0008 /
TW-055
Chicago, IL 60637-1470, USA
Tel. +1 773 702 6196
Fax. +1 773 702 1200
jvardima@mcis.bsd.uchicago.edu

Dr. Camilla VASSALLO
Department of Dermatology
University of Pavia Policlinico S
Matteo-IRCCS
Piazzale Golgi 2
27100 Pavia, ITALY
Tel. +39 0382 503813
Fax. +39 0382 526379
cvassallo@yahoo.com

Dr. Janine WECHSLER
Departement d'Anatomie
Pathologique
Hopital Henri Mondor
51 av Mar de Lattre de Tassigny
94010 Creteil Cedex, FRANCE
Tel. +33 1 49 81 27 38
Fax. +33 1 49 81 27 33
janine.wechsler@hmn.ap-hop-paris.fr

Dr. David WEEDON*
134 Whitmore Street
Taringa, P.O. Box 344
Indooroopilly, Queensland 4068
AUSTRALIA
Tel. +61 7 3377 8776
Fax. +61 7 3371 6563
d_weedon@snp.com.au

Dr. Wolfgang WEYERS
Zentrum für Dermatopathologie
Center for Dermatopathology
Engelbergerstr. 19
79106 Freiburg
GERMANY
Tel. +49 761 31696
Fax. +49 761 39772
ww@zdpf.de

Dr. Wain L. WHITE
Greensboro Pathology Associates
Suite 104
706 Green Valley Road
Greensboro NC 27415-3508
USA
Tel. +1 336 387-2544
Fax. +1 3336 387-2501

Dr. Sean J. WHITTAKER
Head of Service
St. John's Institute of Dermatology
St. Thomas' Hospital
Lambeth Palace Rd
London SE1 7EM, UK
Tel. +44 207 188 6396
Fax. +44 207 118 6257
sean.whittaker@kcl.ac.uk

Dr. Mark R. WICK
Division of Surgical Pathology and
Cytopathology, University Hospital
University of Virginia Health System
1215 Lee Street
Charlottesville, VA 22908-0214, USA
Tel. +1 434 924 9038
Fax. +1 434 924 0217
mrwick1@usa.net

Dr. Robb E. WILENTZ
Department of Dermatology and
Cutraneous Surgery
University of Miami School of
Medicine
1444 N.W. 9th Avenue, 3rd Floor
Miami, FL 33136
USA

Dr. Rein WILLEMZE*
Department of Dermatology, B1-Q-93
Leiden University Medical Center
Albinusdreef 2, PO Box 9600
2300 RC Leiden
THE NETHERLANDS
Tel. +31 71 5262421
Fax. +31 71 5248106
willemze.dermatology@lumc.nl

Dr. Richard M. WILLIAMSON
Sullivan Nicolaides Pathology
134 Whitmore Street
Taringa, QLD 4068
AUSTRALIA
Tel. +61 7 3377 9765
Fax. +61 7 3377 8724
richard_williamson@snp.com.au

Dr. Wyndham H. WILSON
Metabolism Branch, CCR, NCI
NIH, Bldg 10, Rm 4-B-54
9000 Rockville Pike
Bethesda, MD 20892
USA
Tel. +1 301 435-2415
Fax +1 301 432-4359
wilsonw@mail.nih.gov

Dr. Xiaowei XU
Dept of Pathology and Laboratory
Medicine
University of Pennsylvania
3400 Spruce Street
Philadelphia, PA 19104, USA
Tel. +1 215 662 6503
Fax. +1 215 349 5910
xug@mail.med.upenn.edu

Dr. Lawrence L. YU*
School of Surgery and Pathology
University of Western Australia
Queen Elizabeth II Medical Centre
Hospital Avenue
Nedlands, WA 6009, AUSTRALIA
Tel. +61 8 9346 3329
Fax. +61 8 9346 2891
lawrence@cyllene.uwa.edu.au

Dr. Bernhard ZELGER*
Department of Dermatology
University of Innsbruck
Anichstrasse 35
6020 Innsbruck
AUSTRIA
Tel. +43 512 504 2971
Fax. +43 512 504 2990
bernhard.zelger@uibk.ac.at

321. Brownstein MH, Arluk DJ (1981). Proliferating trichilemmal cyst: a simulant of squamous cell carcinoma. Cancer 48: 1207-1214.
322. Brownstein MH, Mehregan AH, Bikowski JB, Lupulescu A, Patterson JC (1979). The dermatopathology of Cowden's syndrome. Br J Dermatol 100: 667-673.
323. Brownstein MH, Shapiro L (1973). Trichilemmoma. Analysis of 40 new cases. Arch Dermatol 107: 866-869.
324. Brownstein MH, Wanger N, Helwig EB (1971). Accessory tragi. Arch Dermatol 104: 625-631.
325. Brownstein MH, Wolf M, Bikowski JB (1978). Cowden's disease: a cutaneous marker of breast cancer. Cancer 41: 2393-2398.
326. Buccheri V, Mihaljevic B, Matutes E, Dyer MJ, Mason DY, Catovsky D (1993). mb-1: a new marker for B-lineage lymphoblastic leukemia. Blood 82: 853-857.
327. Buchner A, Hansen LS (1987). Pigmented nevi of the oral mucosa: a clinicopathologic study of 36 new cases and review of 155 cases from the literature. Part I: A clinicopathologic study of 36 new cases. Oral Surg Oral Med Oral Pathol 63: 566-572.
328. Buchner A, Hansen LS (1987). Pigmented nevi of the oral mucosa: a clinicopathologic study of 36 new cases and review of 155 cases from the literature. Part II: Analysis of 191 cases. Oral Surg Oral Med Oral Pathol 63: 676-682.
329. Buechner SA, Li CY, Su WP (1985). Leukemia cutis. A histopathologic study of 42 cases. Am J Dermatopathol 7: 109-119.
330. Buettner PG, Raasch BA (1998). Incidence rates of skin cancer in Townsville, Australia. Int J Cancer 78: 587-593.
331. Bulliard JL (2000). Site-specific risk of cutaneous malignant melanoma and pattern of sun exposure in New Zealand. Int J Cancer 85: 627-632.
332. Bulliard JL, Cox B (2000). Cutaneous malignant melanoma in New Zealand: trends by anatomical site, 1969-1993. Int J Epidemiol 29: 416-423.
333. Bunn PA, Jr., Lamberg SI (1979). Report of the Committee on Staging and Classification of Cutaneous T-Cell Lymphomas. Cancer Treat Rep 63: 725-728.
334. Bunn PAJr, Lamberg SI (1979). Report of the Committee on Staging and Classification of Cutaneous T-Cell Lymphomas. Cancer Treat Rep 63: 725-728.
335. Bunton TE, Wolfe MJ (1996). N-methyl-N'-nitro-N-nitrosoguanidine-induced neoplasms in medaka (Oryzias latipes). Toxicol Pathol 24: 323-330.
336. Burg G (1977). Pagetoid reticulosis-a cutaneous T-cell lymphoma. J Invest Dermatol 68: 249.
336A. Burg G, Kempf W, Cozzio A, Feit J, Willemze R, Jaffe E, Dummer R, Cerroni L, Berti E, Swerdlow S, Ralfkiaer E, Chimenti S, Diaz-Perez JL,. Duncan LM, Grange F, Harris NL, Kerl H, Kazakov DV, Kurrer M, Knobler R, Meijer CJLM, Pimpinelli N, Russel Jones R, Sander C, Santucci M, Sterry W, Wechsler J, Whittaker S (2005) WHO/EORTC Classification of Cutaneous Lymphomas 2005. Histological and Molecular Aspects. J Cutan Pathol 32 (in press)
337. Burg G, Braun-Falco M (1983). Cutaneous Lymphomas, Pseudolymphomas and Related Disorders. Springer Verlag: Berlin.
338. Burg G, Dummer R, Wilhelm M, Nestle F, Ott MM, Feller A, Hefner H, Lanz U, Schwinn A, Wiede J (1991). A subcutaneous delta-positive T-cell lymphoma that produces interferon gamma. N Engl J Med 325: 1078-1081.
339. Burg G, Kaudewitz P, Klepzig K, Przybilla B, Braun-Falco O (1985). Cutaneous B-cell lymphoma. Dermatol Clin 3: 689-704.
340. Burg G, Kempf W (2005). Cutaneous Lymphomas (Basic and Clinical Dermatology). Marcel Dekker: New York.
341. Burg G, Kempf W, Kazakov DV, Dummer R, Frosch PJ, Lange-Ionescu S, Nishikawa T, Kadin ME (2003). Pyogenic lymphoma of the skin: a peculiar variant of primary cutaneous neutrophil-rich CD30+ anaplastic large-cell lymphoma. Clinicopathological study of four cases and review of the literature. Br J Dermatol 148: 580-586.
342. Burg G, Schmid MH, Kung E, Dommann S, Dummer R (1994). Semi-malignant ("pseudolymphomatous") cutaneous B-cell lymphomas. Dermatol Clin 12: 399-407.
343. Burg G, Schmockel C (1992). Syringolymphoid hyperplasia with alopecia – a syringotropic cutaneous T-cell lymphoma? Dermatology 184: 306-307.
344. Burg G, Sterry W (1987). EORTC/BMFI Cutaneous Lymphoma Project Group. Recommendations for staging and therapy of cutaneous lymphomas.
345. Burg G, Wursch T, Fah J, Elsner P (1994). Eruptive hamartomatous clear-cell acanthomas. Dermatology 189: 437-439.
346. Burgdorf WH, Mukai K, Rosai J (1981). Immunohistochemical identification of factor VIII-related antigen in endothelial cells of cutaneous lesions of alleged vascular nature. Am J Clin Pathol 75: 167-171.
347. Burgdorf WH, Pitha J, Fahmy A (1986). Muir-Torre syndrome. Histologic spectrum of sebaceous proliferations. Am J Dermatopathol 8: 202-208.
348. Burkhardt A (1986). [Verrucous carcinoma and carcinoma cuniculatum-forms of squamous cell carcinoma?]. Hautarzt 37: 373-383.
349. Burkitt DP (1970). General features and facial tumours. In: Burkitt's Lymphoma, Burkitt DP, ed., Livingstone: Edinburgh , pp. 6-15.
350. Burnet NG, Jefferies SJ, Benson RJ, Hunt DP, Treasure FP (2005). Years of life lost (YLL) from cancer is an important measure of population burden – and should be considered when allocating research funds. Br J Cancer 92: 241-245.
351. Burtner DD, Goodman M (1977). Traumatic neuroma of the nose. Arch Otolaryngol 103: 108-109.
352. Burton JL, Holden CA (1998). Eczema, lichenification and prurigo. In: Textbook of Dermatology, Champion RH, Burton RT, Burns DA, Breathnach SM, eds., 6th ed. Blackwell Science: Malden, Massachusetts , p. 665.
353. Burton RC, Armstrong BK (1994). Recent incidence trends imply a non-metastasizing form of invasive melanoma. Melanoma Res 4: 107-113.
354. Busam KJ (1999). Metastatic melanoma to the skin simulating blue nevus. Am J Surg Pathol 23: 276-282.
355. Busam KJ, Barnhill RL (1995). Pagetoid Spitz nevus. Intraepidermal Spitz tumor with prominent pagetoid spread. Am J Surg Pathol 19: 1061-1067.
356. Busam KJ, Iversen K, Coplan KC, Jungbluth AA (2001). Analysis of microphthalmia transcription factor expression in normal tissues and tumors, and comparison of its expression with S-100 protein, gp100, and tyrosinase in desmoplastic malignant melanoma. Am J Surg Pathol 25: 197-204.
357. Busam KJ, Mentzel T, Colpaert C, Barnhill RL, Fletcher CD (1998). Atypical or worrisome features in cellular neurothekeoma: a study of 10 cases. Am J Surg Pathol 22: 1067-1072.
358. Busam KJ, Woodruff JM, Erlandson RA, Brady MS (2000). Large plaque-type blue nevus with subcutaneous cellular nodules. Am J Surg Pathol 24: 92-99.
358A. Busam KJ, Mujumdar U, Hummer AJ, Nobrega J, Hawkins WG, Coit DG, Brady MS (2004). Cutaneous desmoplastic melanoma: reappraisal of morphologic heterogeneity and prognostic factors. Am J Surg Pathol 28: 1518-1525.
358B. Busam KJ, Zhao H, Coit DG, Kucukgol D, Jungbluth AA, Nobrega J, Viale A (2005). Distinction of desmoplastic melanoma from non-desmoplastic melanoma by gene expression profiling. J Invest Dermatol 124: 412-418.
359. Buschke A, Löwenstein L (1925). Über carcinomähnliche Condylomata acuminata des Penis. Klin Wochenschr 4: 1726-1728.
360. Butler DF, Ranatunge BD, Rapini RP (2001). Urticating Hashimoto-Pritzker Langerhans cell histiocytosis. Pediatr Dermatol 18: 41-44.
361. Buttner C, Henz BM, Welker P, Sepp NT, Grabbe J (1998). Identification of activating c-kit mutations in adult-, but not in childhood-onset indolent mastocytosis: a possible explanation for divergent clinical behavior. J Invest Dermatol 111: 1227-1231.
362. Caglar H, Tamer S, Hreshchyshyn MM (1982). Vulvar intraepithelial neoplasia. Obstet Gynecol 60: 346-349.
363. Calduch L, Ortega C, Navarro V, Martinez E, Molina I, Jorda E (2000). Verrucous hemangioma: report of two cases and review of the literature. Pediatr Dermatol 17: 213-217.
364. Calista D, Schianchi S, Landi C (1998). Malignant blue nevus of the scalp. Int J Dermatol 37: 126-127.
365. Calonje E (1998). Is cutaneous benign fibrous histiocytoma (dermatofibroma) a reactive inflammatory process or a neoplasm? Histopathology 37: 278-280.
366. Calonje E, Fletcher CD (1991). Sinusoidal hemangioma. A distinctive benign vascular neoplasm within the group of cavernous hemangiomas. Am J Surg Pathol 15: 1130-1135.
367. Calonje E, Fletcher CD (1995). Aneurysmal benign fibrous histiocytoma: clinicopathological analysis of 40 cases of a tumour frequently misdiagnosed as a vascular neoplasm. Histopathology 26: 323-331.
368. Calonje E, Fletcher CD (1996). Myoid differentiation in dermatofibrosarcoma protuberans and its fibrosarcomatous variant: clinicopathologic analysis of 5 cases. J Cutan Pathol 23: 30-36.
369. Calonje E, Fletcher CDM (1994). Cutaneous fibrohistiocytic tumors: an update. Adv Anat Pathol 1: 2-15.
370. Calonje E, Mentzel T, Fletcher CD (1994). Cellular benign fibrous histiocytoma. Clinicopathologic analysis of 74 cases of a distinctive variant of cutaneous fibrous histiocytoma with frequent recurrence. Am J Surg Pathol 18: 668-676.
371. Calonje E, Wilson-Jones E, Smith NP, Fletcher CD (1992). Cellular 'neurothekeoma': an epithelioid variant of pilar leiomyoma'? Morphological and immunohistochemical analysis of a series. Histopathology 20: 397-404.
372. Calzavara Pinton P, Carlino A, Manganoni AM, Donzelli C, Facchetti F (1990). [Epidermal nevus syndrome with multiple vascular hamartomas and malformations]. G Ital Dermatol Venereol 125: 251-254.
373. Camacho FM, Burg G, Moreno JC, Campora RG, Villar JL (1997). Granulomatous slack skin in childhood. Pediatr Dermatol 14: 204-208.
374. Camp RDR (1998). Psoriasis: Psoralen photochemotherapy. In: Textbook of Dermatology, Champion RH, Burton JL, Burns DA, Breathnach SM, eds., 6th ed. Blackwell Science Ltd.: Oxford , pp. 1616-1622.
375. Campbell C, Quinn AG, Ro YS, Angus B, Rees JL (1993). p53 mutations are common and early events that precede tumor invasion in squamous cell neoplasia of the skin. J Invest Dermatol 100: 746-748.
376. Campo E, Raffeld M, Jaffe ES (1999). Mantle-cell lymphoma. Semin Hematol 36: 115-127.
377. Caporaso N, Greene MH, Tsai S, Pickle LW, Mulvihill JJ (1987). Cytogenetics in hereditary malignant melanoma and dysplastic nevus syndrome: is dysplastic nevus syndrome a chromosome instability disorder? Cancer Genet Cytogenet 24: 299-314.
378. Caputo R (1998). Juvenile Xanthogranuloma. In: Text Atlas of Histiocytic Syndromes. A Dermatological Perspective., Text Atlas of Histiocytic Syndromes. A Dermatological Perspective., Martin Dunitz: London , pp. 39-58.
379. Caputo R, Alessi E, Berti E (1981). Collagen phagocytosis in multicentric reticulohistiocytosis. J Invest Dermatol 76: 342-346.
380. Caputo R, Crosti C, Cainelli T (1977). A unique cytoplasmic structure in papular histiocytoma. J Invest Dermatol 68: 98-104.
381. Caputo R, Ermacora E, Gelmetti C (1988). Diffuse cutaneous reticulohistiocytosis in a child with tuberous sclerosis. Arch Dermatol 124: 567-570.
382. Caputo R, Grimalt R (1992). Solitary reticulohistiocytosis (reticulohistiocytoma) of the skin in children: report of two cases. Arch Dermatol 128: 698-699.
383. Caputo R, Grimalt R, Gelmetti C, Cottoni F (1993). Unusual aspects of juvenile xanthogranuloma. J Am Acad Dermatol 29: 868-870.
384. Carapeto FJ, Armijo M (1978). [Acral arteriovenous tumor]. Ann Dermatol Venereol 105: 977-979.
385. Carapeto FJ, Garcia-Perez A, Winkelmann RK (1977). Acral arteriovenous tumor. Acta Derm Venereol 57: 155-158.
386. Carless MA, Lea RA, Curran JE, Appleyard B, Gaffney P, Green A, Griffiths LR (2002). The GSTM1 null genotype confers an increased risk for solar keratosis development in an Australian Caucasian population. J Invest Dermatol 119: 1373-1378.
387. Carli P, de Giorgi V, Salvini C, Mannone F, Chiarugi A (2002). The gold standard for photographing pigmented skin lesions for diagnostic purposes: contact versus distant imaging. Skin Res Technol 8: 255-259.
388. Carlson JA, Ackerman AB, Fletcher CD, Zelger B (2001). A cutaneous spindle-cell lesion. Am J Dermatopathol 23: 62-66.

389. Carlson JA, Daulat S, Goodheart HP (1999). Targetoid hemosiderotic hemangioma- a dynamic vascular tumor: report of 3 cases with episodic and cyclic changes and comparison with solitary angiokeratomas. J Am Acad Dermatol 41: 215-224.
390. Carlson JA, Mihm MC (1997). Vulvar nevi, lichen sclerosus et atrophicus, and vitiligo. Arch Dermatol 133: 1314-1316.
391. Carlson JA, Mu XC, Slominski A, Weismann K, Crowson AN, Malfetano J, Prieto VG, Mihm MCJr (2002). Melanocytic proliferations associated with lichen sclerosus. Arch Dermatol 138: 77-87.
392. Carlson JA, Slominski A, Linette GP, Mihm MCJr, Ross JS (2003). Biomarkers in melanoma: staging, prognosis and detection of early metastases. Expert Rev Mol Diagn 3: 303-330.
393. Carlson KC, Gibson LE (1991). Cutaneous signs of lymphomatoid granulomatosis. Arch Dermatol 127: 1693-1698.
394. Carney JA (1990). Psammomatous melanotic schwannoma. A distinctive, heritable tumor with special associations, including cardiac myxoma and the Cushing syndrome. Am J Surg Pathol 14: 206-222.
395. Carney JA (1995). The search for Harvey Cushing's patient, Minnie G., and the cause of her hypercortisolism. Am J Surg Pathol 19: 100-108.
396. Carney JA, Ferreiro JA (1996). The epithelioid blue nevus. A multicentric familial tumor with important associations, including cardiac myxoma and psammomatous melanotic schwannoma. Am J Surg Pathol 20: 259-272.
397. Carney JA, Gordon H, Carpenter PC, Shenoy BV, Go VL (1985). The complex of myxomas, spotty pigmentation, and endocrine overactivity. Medicine (Baltimore) 64: 270-283.
398. Carney JA, Headington JT, Su WP (1986). Cutaneous myxomas. A major component of the complex of myxomas, spotty pigmentation, and endocrine overactivity. Arch Dermatol 122: 790-798.
399. Carney JA, Stratakis CA (1998). Epithelioid blue nevus and psammomatous melanotic schwannoma: the unusual pigmented skin tumors of the Carney complex. Semin Diagn Pathol 15: 216-224.
400. Carney JA, Toorkey BC (1991). Myxoid fibroadenoma and allied conditions (myxomatosis) of the breast. A heritable disorder with special associations including cardiac and cutaneous myxomas. Am J Surg Pathol 15: 713-721.
401. Caro WA, Helwig HB (1969). Cutaneous lymphoid hyperplasia. Cancer 24: 487-502.
402. Carr S, See J, Wilkinson B, Kossard S (1997). Hypopigmented common blue nevus. J Cutan Pathol 24: 494-498.
403. Carrasco L, Izquierdo MJ, Farina MC, Martin L, Moreno C, Requena L (2000). Strawberry glans penis: a rare manifestation of angiokeratomas involving the glans penis. Br J Dermatol 142: 1256-1257.
404. Carson HJ, Gattuso P, Raslan WF, Reddy V (1995). Mucinous carcinoma of the eyelid. An immunohistochemical study. Am J Dermatopathol 17: 494-498.
405. Carson KF, Wen DR, Li PX, Lana AM, Bailly C, Morton DL, Cochran AJ (1996). Nodal nevi and cutaneous melanomas. Am J Surg Pathol 20: 834-840.
406. Carter DK, Batts KP, de Groen PC, Kurtin PJ (1996). Angiotropic large cell lymphoma (intravascular lymphomatosis) occurring after follicular small cleaved cell lymphoma. Mayo Clin Proc 71: 869-873.
407. Casas JG, Woscoff A (1980). Giant pilar tumor of the scalp. Arch Dermatol 116: 1395.
408. Casey M, Vaughan CJ, He J, Hatcher CJ, Winter JM, Weremowicz S, Montgomery K, Kucherlapati R, Morton CC, Basson CT (2000). Mutations in the protein kinase A R1alpha regulatory subunit cause familial cardiac myxomas and Carney complex. J Clin Invest 106: R31-R38.
409. Cassileth BR, Temoshok L, Frederick BE, Walsh WP, Hurwitz S, Guerry D, Clark WHJr, DiClemente RJ, Sweet DM, Blois MS, Sagebiel RW (1988). Patient and physician delay in melanoma diagnosis. J Am Acad Dermatol 18: 591-598.
410. Castilla EA, Bergfeld WF, Ormsby A (2002). Trichilemmoma and syringocystadenoma papilliferum arising in naevus sebaceous. Pathology 34: 196-197.
411. Castilla EE, da Graca Dutra M, Orioli-Parreiras IM (1981). Epidemiology of congenital pigmented naevi: II. Risk factors. Br J Dermatol 104: 421-427.
412. Catteau B, Enjolras O, Delaporte E, Friedel J, Breviere G, Wassef M, Lecomte-Houcke M, Piette F, Bergoend H (1998). [Sclerosing tufted angioma. Apropos of 4 cases involving lower limbs]. Ann Dermatol Venereol 125: 682-687.
413. Catterall MD (1980). Multicentric reticulohistiocytosis: a review of eight cases. Clin Exp Dermatol 5: 267-279.
414. Cavalieri R, Macchini V, Mostaccioli S, Sonego G, Ferranti G, Corona R, Fucci M, Marzolini F, Rosmini F, Pasquini P (1993). Time trends in features of cutaneous melanoma at diagnosis: central-south Italy, 1962-1991. Ann Ist Super Sanita 29: 469-472.
415. Cavalli F (1998). Rare syndromes in Hodgkin's disease. Ann Oncol 9 Suppl 5: S109-S113.
416. Caylor HD (1925). Epitheliomas in sebaceous cysts. Ann Surg 82: 164-176.
Ceballos PI, Penneys NS, Acosta R (1990).
417. Aggressive digital papillary adenocarcinoma. J Am Acad Dermatol 23: 331-334.
417A. Ceballos PI, Ruiz-Maldonado R, Mihm MCJr (1995). Melanoma in children. N Engl J Med 332: 656-662.
418. Cecchi A, Giomi A, Rapicano V, Apicella P (2000). Cellular neurothekeoma on the left auricle. J Eur Acad Dermatol Venereol 14: 314-315.
419. Cecchi R, Bartoli L, Brunetti L, Pavesi M, Giomi A (1995). Lymphangioma circumscriptum of the vulva of late onset. Acta Derm Venereol 75: 79-80.
420. Celebi JT, Tsou HC, Chen FF, Zhang H, Ping XL, Lebwohl MG, Kezis J, Peacocke M (1999). Phenotypic findings of Cowden syndrome and Bannayan-Zonana syndrome in a family associated with a single germline mutation in PTEN. J Med Genet 36: 360-364.
421. Centeno JA, Mullick FG, Martinez L, Page NP, Gibb H, Longfellow D, Thompson C, Ladich ER (2002). Pathology related to chronic arsenic exposure. Environ Health Perspect 110 Suppl 5: 883-886.
422. Cerez-Pham H, Bertrand G, Tigori J, Simard C (1984). [Association of a malignant vaginal melanoma with vaginal melanosis and a blue nevus of the cervix. Apropos of a case]. Arch Anat Cytol Pathol 32: 48-51.
423. Cerio R, Oliver GF, Jones EW, Winkelmann RK (1990). The heterogeneity of Jessner's lymphocytic infiltration of the skin. Immunohistochemical studies suggesting one form of perivascular lymphocytoma. J Am Acad Dermatol 23: 63-67.
424. Cerio R, Spaull J, Oliver GF, Jones WE (1990). A study of factor XIIIa and MAC 387 immunolabeling in normal and pathological skin. Am J Dermatopathol 12: 221-233.
425. Cerroni L, Arzberger E, Putz B, Hofler G, Metze D, Sander CA, Rose C, Wolf P, Rutten A, McNiff JM, Kerl H (2000). Primary cutaneous follicle center cell lymphoma with follicular growth pattern. Blood 95: 3922-3928.
426. Cerroni L, Beham-Schmid C, Kerl H (1995). Cutaneous Hodgkin's disease: an immunohistochemical analysis. J Cutan Pathol 22: 229-235.
427. Cerroni L, Hofler G, Back B, Wolf P, Maier G, Kerl H (2002). Specific cutaneous infiltrates of B-cell chronic lymphocytic leukemia (B-CLL) at sites typical for Borrelia burgdorferi infection. J Cutan Pathol 29: 142-147.
428. Cerroni L, Kerl H (1999). Diagnostic immunohistology: cutaneous lymphomas and pseudolymphomas. Semin Cutan Med Surg 18: 64-70.
429. Cerroni L, Kerl H (2001). Primary cutaneous follicle center cell lymphoma. Leuk Lymphoma 42: 891-900.
430. Cerroni L, Volkenandt M, Rieger E, Soyer HP, Kerl H (1994). bcl-2 protein expression and correlation with the interchromosomal 14;18 translocation in cutaneous lymphomas and pseudolymphomas. J Invest Dermatol 102: 231-235.
431. Cerroni L, Zenahlik P, Hofler G, Kaddu S, Smolle J, Kerl H (1996). Specific cutaneous infiltrates of B-cell chronic lymphocytic leukemia: a clinicopathologic and prognostic study of 42 patients. Am J Surg Pathol 20: 1000-1010.
432. Cerroni L, Zenahlik P, Kerl H (1995). Specific cutaneous infiltrates of B-cell chronic lymphocytic leukemia arising at the site of herpes zoster and herpes simplex scars. Cancer 76: 26-31.
433. Cerroni L, Zochling N, Putz B, Kerl H (1997). Infection by Borrelia burgdorferi and cutaneous B-cell lymphoma. J Cutan Pathol 24: 457-461.
434. Cesarman E, Knowles DM (1997). Kaposi's sarcoma-associated herpesvirus: a lymphotropic human herpesvirus associated with Kaposi's sarcoma, primary effusion lymphoma, and multicentric Castleman's disease. Semin Diagn Pathol 14: 54-66.
435. Ceyhan M, Erdem G, Kotiloglu E, Kale G, Talim B, Kanra G, Basaran I (1997). Pyogenic granuloma with multiple dissemination in a burn lesion. Pediatr Dermatol 14: 213-215.
436. Chamberlain AJ, Fritschi L, Kelly JW (2003). Nodular melanoma: patients' perceptions of presenting features and implications for earlier detection. J Am Acad Dermatol 48: 694-701.
437. Chamberlain RS, Huber K, White JC, Travaglino-Parda R (1999). Apocrine gland carcinoma of the axilla: review of the literature and recommendations for treatment. Am J Clin Oncol 22: 131-135.
438. Chan EF, Gat U, McNiff JM, Fuchs E (1999). A common human skin tumour is caused by activating mutations in beta-catenin. Nat Genet 21: 410-413.
439. Chan GS, Choy C, NG WK, Chan KW (1999). Desmoplastic malignant melanoma on the buttock of an 18-year-old girl: differentiation from desmoplastic nevus. Am J Dermatopathol 21: 170-173.
440. Chan JK, Fletcher CD, Hicklin GA, Rosai J (1990). Glomeruloid hemangioma. A distinctive cutaneous lesion of multicentric Castleman's disease associated with POEMS syndrome. Am J Surg Pathol 14: 1036-1046.
441. Chan JK, Hui PK, Ng CS, Yuen NW, Kung IT, Gwi E (1989). Epithelioid haemangioma (angiolymphoid hyperplasia with eosinophilia) and Kimura's disease in Chinese. Histopathology 15: 557-574.
442. Chan JK, Lewin KJ, Lombard CM, Teitelbaum S, Dorfman RF (1991). Histopathology of bacillary angiomatosis of lymph node. Am J Surg Pathol 15: 430-437.
443. Chan JK, Sin VC, Wong KF, Ng CS, Tsang WY, Chan CH, Cheung MM, Lau WH (1997). Nonnasal lymphoma expressing the natural killer cell marker CD56: a clinicopathologic study of 49 cases of an uncommon aggressive neoplasm. Blood 89: 4501-4513.
444. Chan JKC, Tsang WYW, Calonje E, Fletcher CDM (1995). Verrucous hemangioma. A distinct but neglected variant of cutaneous hemangioma. Int J Surg Pathol 2: 171-176.
445. Chang H, Shih LY, Kuo TT (2003). Primary aleukemic myeloid leukemia cutis treated successfully with combination chemotherapy: report of a case and review of the literature. Ann Hematol 82: 435-439.
446. Chang SE, Ahn SJ, Choi JH, Sung KJ, Moon KC, Koh JK (1999). Primary adenoid cystic carcinoma of skin with lung metastasis. J Am Acad Dermatol 40: 640-642.
447. Chang SE, Kim KJ, Kim ES, Choi JH, Sung KJ, Moon KC, Koh JK (2002). Two cases of late onset Ota's naevus. Clin Exp Dermatol 27: 202-204.
448. Chao AN, Shields CL, Krema H, Shields JA (2001). Outcome of patients with periocular sebaceous gland carcinoma with and without conjunctival intraepithelial invasion. Ophthalmology 108: 1877-1883.
449. Chao TK, Chang YL, Sheen TS (2000). Extraskeletal Ewing's sarcoma of the scalp. J Laryngol Otol 114: 73-75.
450. Chaperot L, Bendriss N, Manches O, Gressin R, Maynadie M, Trimoreau F, Orfeuvre H, Corront B, Feuillard J, Sotto JJ, Bensa JC, Briere F, Plumas J, Jacob MC (2001). Identification of a leukemic counterpart of the plasmacytoid dendritic cells. Blood 97: 3210-3217.
451. Chapman MS, Quitadamo MJ, Perry AE (2000). Pigmented squamous cell carcinoma. J Cutan Pathol 27: 93-95.
452. Chatelain R, Bell SA, Konz B, Rocken M (1998). [Granuloma eosinophilicum faciei simulating rhinophyma. Therapeutic long-term outcome after surgical intervention]. Hautarzt 49: 496-498.
452A. Chaudru V, Chompret A, Bressac-de Paillerets B, Spatz A, Avril MF, Demenais F (2004). Influence of genes, nevi, and sun sensitivity on melanoma risk in a family sample unselected by family history and in melanoma-prone families. J Natl Cancer Inst 96: 785-795
453. Chauvin PJ, Wysocki GP, Daley TD, Pringle GA (1992). Palisaded encapsulated neuroma of oral mucosa. Oral Surg Oral Med Oral Pathol 73: 71-74.
454. Chen KR, Tanaka M, Miyakawa S (1998). Granulomatous mycosis fungoides with small intestinal involvement and a fatal outcome. Br J Dermatol 138: 522-525.
455. Chen RL, Lin KS, Chang WH, Hsieh YL, Chen BW, Jaing TH, Yang CP, Hung IJ, Peng CT, Shu SG, Lu MY, Jou ST, Lin KH, Lin DT, Lin MT, Chen JS, Liu HC, Chen SH, Liang DC, Chiou SS, Chang TT, Sheen JM, Hsiao CC, Cheng SN, Lin JC (2003).

Childhood Langerhans cell histiocytosis increased during El Nino 1997-98: a report from the Taiwan Pediatric Oncology Group. Acta Paediatr Taiwan 44: 14-20.

456. Chen S, Palay D, Templeton SF (1998). Familial eccrine syringofibroadenomatosis with associated ophthalmologic abnormalities. J Am Acad Dermatol 39: 356-358.

457. Chen TC, Kuo T, Chan HL (2000). Dermatofibroma is a clonal proliferative disease. J Cutan Pathol 27: 36-39.

458. Chen TM, Purohit SK, Wang AR (2002). Pleomorphic sclerotic fibroma: a case report and literature review. Am J Dermatopathol 24: 54-58.

459. Chen YT, Zheng T, Holford TR, Berwick M, Dubrow R (1994). Malignant melanoma incidence in Connecticut (United States): time trends and age-period-cohort modeling by anatomic site. Cancer Causes Control 5: 341-350.

460. Cheney IW, Neuteboom ST, Vaillancourt MT, Ramachandra M, Bookstein R (1999). Adenovirus-mediated gene transfer of MMAC1/PTEN to glioblastoma cells inhibits S phase entry by the recruitment of p27Kip1 into cyclin E/CDK2 complexes. Cancer Res 59: 2318-2323.

461. Cherpelis BS, Marcusen C, Lang PG (2002). Prognostic factors for metastasis in squamous cell carcinoma of the skin. Dermatol Surg 28: 268-273.

462. Chesser RS, Bertler DE, Fitzpatrick JE, Mellette JR (1992). Primary cutaneous adenoid cystic carcinoma treated with Mohs micrographic surgery toluidine blue technique. J Dermatol Surg Oncol 18: 175-176.

463. Cheuk W, Kwan MY, Suster S, Chan JK (2001). Immunostaining for thyroid transcription factor 1 and cytokeratin 20 aids the distinction of small cell carcinoma from Merkel cell carcinoma, but not pulmonary from extrapulmonary small cell carcinomas. Arch Pathol Lab Med 125: 228-231.

464. Cheung DS, Warman ML, Mulliken JB (1997). Hemangioma in twins. Ann Plast Surg 38: 269-274.

465. Chevrant-Breton J (1977). La reticulo-histiocytose multicentrique: revue de la litterature recente (depuis 1969). Ann Dermatol Venereol 104: 745-753.

466. Chiefari E, Russo D, Giuffrida D, Zampa GA, Meringolo D, Arturi F, Chiodini I, Bianchi D, Attard M, Trischitta V, Bruno R, Giannasio P, Pontecorvi A, Filetti S (1998). Analysis of RET proto-oncogene abnormalities in patients with MEN 2A, MEN 2B, familial or sporadic medullary thyroid carcinoma. J Endocrinol Invest 21: 358-364.

467. Child FJ, Russell-Jones R, Woolford AJ, Calonje E, Photiou A, Orchard G, Whittaker SJ (2001). Absence of the t(14;18) chromosomal translocation in primary cutaneous B-cell lymphoma. Br J Dermatol 144: 735-744.

468. Child FJ, Scarisbrick JJ, Calonje E, Orchard G, Russell-Jones R, Whittaker SJ (2002). Inactivation of tumor suppressor genes p15(INK4b) and p16(INK4a) in primary cutaneous B cell lymphoma. J Invest Dermatol 118: 941-948.

469. Chiller K, Passaro D, Scheuller M, Singer M, McCalmont T, Grekin RC (2000). Microcystic adnexal carcinoma: forty-eight cases, their treatment, and their outcome. Arch Dermatol 136: 1355-1359.

470. Chimenti S, Fink-Puches R, Peris K, Pescarmona E, Putz B, Kerl H, Cerroni L (1999). Cutaneous involvement in lymphoblastic lymphoma. J Cutan Pathol 26: 379-385.

471. Cho KH, Kim CW, Lee DY, Sohn SJ, Kim DW, Chung JH (1996). An Epstein-Barr virus-associated lymphoproliferative lesion of the skin presenting as recurrent necrotic papulovesicles of the face. Br J Dermatol 134: 791-796.

472. Cho KJ, Khang SK, Koh JS, Chung JH, Lee SS (2000). Sebaceous carcinoma of the eyelids: frequent expression of c-erbB-2 oncoprotein. J Korean Med Sci 15: 545-550.

473. Choi YS, Park SH, Bang D (1989). Pilar sheath acanthoma – report of a case with review of the literature. Yonsei Med J 30: 392-395.

474. Choonhakarn C, Ackerman AB (2001). Keratoacanthomas: a new classification based on morphologic findings and on anatomic site. Dermatopathology, practical & conceptual 7: 7-16.

475. Chopra A, Maitra B, Korman NJ (1998). Decreased mRNA expression of several basement membrane components in basal cell carcinoma. J Invest Dermatol 110: 52-56.

476. Chorny JA, Barr RJ (2002). S100-positive spindle cells in scars: a diagnostic pitfall in the re-excision of desmoplastic melanoma. Am J Dermatopathol 24: 309-312.

477. Chow CW, Campbell PE, Burry AF (1984). Sweat gland carcinomas in children. Cancer 53: 1222-1227.

478. Chow E, Merchant TE, Pappo A, Jenkins JJ, Shah AB, Kun LE (2000). Cutaneous and subcutaneous Ewing's sarcoma: an indolent disease. Int J Radiat Oncol Biol Phys 46: 433-438.

479. Chow LT, Ma TK, Chow WH (1997). Cellular neurothekeoma of the hypopharynx. Histopathology 30: 192-194.

480. Christensen WN, Friedman KJ, Woodruff JD, Hood AF (1987). Histologic characteristics of vulvar nevocellular nevi. J Cutan Pathol 14: 87-91.

481. Christenson LJ, Stone MS (2001). Trauma-induced simulator of targetoid hemosiderotic hemangioma. Am J Dermatopathol 23: 221-223.

482. Chu P, LeBoit PE (1992). An eruptive vascular proliferation resembling acquired tufted angioma in the recipient of a liver transplant. J Am Acad Dermatol 26: 322-325.

483. Chu P, LeBoit PE (1992). Histologic features of cutaneous sinus histiocytosis (Rosai-Dorfman disease): study of cases both with and without systemic involvement. J Cutan Pathol 19: 201-206.

484. Chuang TY, Reizner GT (1988). Bowen's disease and internal malignancy. A matched case-control study. J Am Acad Dermatol 19: 47-51.

485. Chung CK, Heffernan AH (1971). Clear cell hidradenoma with metastasis. Case report with a review of the literature. Plast Reconstr Surg 48: 177-180.

486. Chung EB, Enzinger FM (1981). Infantile myofibromatosis. Cancer 48: 1807-1818.

487. Chung J, Nam IW, Ahn SK, Lee SH, Kim JG, Sung YO (1994). Rudimentary polydactyly. J Dermatol 21: 54-55.

488. Ciotti P, Struewing JP, Mantelli M, Chompret A, Avril MF, Santi PL, Tucker MA, Bianchi-Scarra G, Bressac de Paillerets B, Goldstein AM (2000). A single genetic origin for the G101W CDKN2A mutation in 20 melanoma-prone families. Am J Hum Genet 67: 311-319.

489. Civatte J, Belaich S, Lauret P (1979). [Tubular apocrine adenoma (4 cases)

(author's transl)]. Ann Dermatol Venereol 106: 665-669.

490. Clarijs M, Poot F, Laka A, Pirard C, Bourlond A (2003). Granulomatous slack skin: treatment with extensive surgery and review of the literature. Dermatology 206: 393-397.

491. Clark WH, Jr., Elder DE, Guerry D, Braitman LE, Trock BJ, Schultz D, Synnestvedt M, Halpern AC (1989). Model predicting survival in stage I melanoma based on tumor progression. J Natl Cancer Inst 81: 1893-1904.

492. Clark WHJr (1967). A classification of malignant melanoma in men correlated with histogenesis and biological behavior. In: Advances in Biology of the Skin. The Pigmentary System, Montagna W, Hu F, eds., 1st ed. Pergamon: London , pp. 621-647.

493. Clark WH Jr, Elder DE, Van Horn M (1986). The biologic forms of malignant melanoma. Hum Pathol 17: 443-450.

494. Clark WHJr, From L, Bernardino EA, Mihm MC (1969). The histogenesis and biologic behavior of primary human malignant melanomas of the skin. Cancer Res 29: 705-727.

495. Clark WHJr, Hood AF, Tucker MA, Jampel RM (1998). Atypical melanocytic nevi of the genital type with a discussion of reciprocal parenchymal-stromal interactions in the biology of neoplasia. Hum Pathol 29: S1-24.

496. Clark WHJr, Reimer RR, Greene M, Ainsworth AM, Mastrangelo MJ (1978). Origin of familial malignant melanomas from heritable melanocytic lesions. 'The B-K mole syndrome'. Arch Dermatol 114: 732-738.

497. Clarke JT, Knaack J, Crawhall JC, Wolfe LS (1971). Ceramide trihexosidosis (fabry's disease) without skin lesions. N Engl J Med 284: 233-235.

498. Clarke LE, Ioffreda M, Abt AB (2003). Eccrine syringofibroadenoma arising in peristomal skin: a report of two cases. Int J Surg Pathol 11: 61-63.

499. Claudy AL, Garcier F, Kanitakis J (1984). Eccrine porocarcinoma. Ultrastructural and immunological study. J Dermatol 11: 282-286.

500. Cleaver JE, Thompson LH, Richardson AS, States JC (1999). A summary of mutations in the UV-sensitive disorders: xeroderma pigmentosum, Cockayne syndrome, and trichothiodystrophy. Hum Mutat 14: 9-22.

501. Clemente C, Zurrida S, Bartoli C, Bono A, Collini P, Rilke F (1995). Acral-lentiginous naevus of plantar skin. Histopathology 27: 549-555.

502. Clemente CG, Mihm MC, Jr., Bufalino R, Zurrida S, Collini P, Cascinelli N (1996). Prognostic value of tumor infiltrating lymphocytes in the vertical growth phase of primary cutaneous melanoma. Cancer 77: 1303-1310.

503. Clever HW, Sahl WJ (1991). Multiple eccrine hidrocystomas: a nonsurgical treatment. Arch Dermatol 127: 422-424.

504. Cline MS, Cummings OW, Goldman M, Filo RS, Pescovitz MD (1999). Bacillary angiomatosis in a renal transplant recipient. Transplantation 67: 296-298.

505. Cobb MW (1990). Human papillomavirus infection. J Am Acad Dermatol 22: 547-566.

506. Cockerell CJ (2000). Histopathology of incipient intraepidermal squamous cell carcinoma ("actinic keratosis"). J Am Acad Dermatol 42: 11-17.

507. Cockerell CJ, LeBoit PE (1990). Bacillary angiomatosis: a newly characterized, pseudoneoplastic, infectious, cutaneous vascular disorder. J Am Acad Dermatol 22: 501-512.

508. Coffin CM, Dehner LP, Meis-Kindblom JM (1998). Inflammatory myofibroblastic tumor, inflammatory fibrosarcoma, and related lesions: an historical review with differential diagnostic considerations. Semin Diagn Pathol 15: 102-110.

509. Coffin CM, Humphrey PA, Dehner LP (1998). Extrapulmonary inflammatory myofibroblastic tumor: a clinical and pathological survey. Semin Diagn Pathol 15: 85-101.

510. Cohen AD, Cagnano E, Vardy DA (2001). Cherry angiomas associated with exposure to bromides. Dermatology 202: 52-53.

511. Cohen C, Guarner J, DeRose PB (1993). Mammary Paget's disease and associated carcinoma. An immunohistochemical study. Arch Pathol Lab Med 117: 291-294.

512. Cohen LM (1996). The starburst giant cell is useful for distinguishing lentigo maligna from photodamaged skin. J Am Acad Dermatol 35: 962-968.

513. Cohen LM, Bennion SD, Johnson TW, Golitz LE (1997). Hypermelanotic nevus: clinical, histopathologic, and ultrastructural features in 316 cases. Am J Dermatopathol 19: 23-30.

514. Cohen MMJr (1999). Nevoid basal cell carcinoma syndrome: molecular biology and new hypotheses. Int J Oral Maxillofac Surg 28: 216-223.

515. Cohen PR, Ulmer R, Theriault A, Leigh IM, Duvic M (1997). Epidermolytic acanthomas: clinical characteristics and immunohistochemical features. Am J Dermatopathol 19: 232-241.

516. Cohn-Cedermark G, Mansson-Brahme E, Rutqvist LE, Larsson O, Johansson H, Ringborg U (2000). Trends in mortality from malignant melanoma in Sweden, 1970-1996. Cancer 89: 348-355.

517. Coit DG (2001). Merkel cell carcinoma. Ann Surg Oncol 8: 99S-102S.

518. Colby TV (1997). Metastasizing dermatofibroma. Am J Surg Pathol 21: 976.

519. Coleman WPI, Gately LEI, Krementz AB, Reed RJ, Krementz ET (1980). Nevi, lentigines, and melanomas in blacks. Arch Dermatol 116: 548-551.

520. Collina G, Deen S, Cliff S, Jackson P, Cook MG (1997). Atypical dermal nodules in benign melanocytic naevi. Histopathology 31: 97-101.

521. Collins GL, Somach S, Morgan MB (2002). Histomorphologic and immunophenotypic analysis of fibrofolliculomas and trichodiscomas in Birt-Hogg-Dube syndrome and sporadic disease. J Cutan Pathol 29: 529-533.

522. Colome-Grimmer MI, Evans HL (1996). Metastasizing cellular dermatofibroma. A report of two cases. Am J Surg Pathol 20: 1361-1367.

523. Colome MI, Sanchez RL (1994). Dermatomyofibroma: report of two cases. J Cutan Pathol 21: 371-376.

524. Colomo L, Loong F, Rives S, Pittaluga S, Martinez A, Lopez-Guillermo A, Ojanguren J, Romagosa V, Jaffe ES, Campo E (2004). Diffuse large B-cell lymphomas with plasmablastic differentiation represent a heterogeneous group of disease entities. Am J Surg Pathol 28: 736-747.

525. Cong P, Raffeld M, Jaffe ES (2001). Blastic NK cell lymphoma/leukemia: a clinicopathological study of 23 cases. Mod

Pathol 14: 160A.
526. Conley J, Lattes R, Orr W (1971). Desmoplastic malignant melanoma (a rare variant of spindle cell melanoma). Cancer 28: 914-936.
527. Connelly J, Smith JLJr (1991). Malignant blue nevus. Cancer 67: 2653-2657.
528. Connelly MG, Winkelmann RK (1985). Acral arteriovenous tumor. A clinicopathologic review. Am J Surg Pathol 9: 15-21.
529. Connelly TJ, Cribier B, Brown TJ, Yanguas I (2000). Complete spontaneous regression of Merkel cell carcinoma: a review of the 10 reported cases. Dermatol Surg 26: 853-856.
530. Conolly WB, Goulston E (1973). Problems of digital amputations: a clinical review of 260 patients and 301 amputations. Aust N Z J Surg 43: 118-123.
530A. Conti EM, Cercato MC, Gatta G, Ramazzotti V, Roscioni S (2001). Childhood melanoma in Europe since 1978: a population-based survival study. Eur J Cancer 37: 780-784.
531. Contreras F, Fonseca E, Gamallo C, Burgos E (1990). Multiple self-healing indeterminate cell lesions of the skin in an adult. Am J Dermatopathol 12: 396-401.
532. Coode PE, Ridgway H, Jones DB (1980). Multicentric reticulohistiocytosis: report of two cases with ultrastructure, tissue culture and immunology studies. Clin Exp Dermatol 5: 281-293.
533. Cooke KR, Fraser J (1985). Migration and death from malignant melanoma. Int J Cancer 36: 175-178.
534. Cooke KR, Skegg DC, Fraser J (1983). Trends in malignant melanoma of skin in New Zealand. Int J Cancer 31: 715-718.
535. Cooke KR, Spears GF, Elder DE, Greene MH (1989). Dysplastic naevi in a population-based survey. Cancer 63: 1240-1244.
536. Cooper PH (1987). Carcinomas of sweat glands. Pathol Annu 22 Pt 1: 83-124.
537. Cooper PH (1992). Deep penetrating (plexiform spindle cell) nevus. A frequent participant in combined nevus. J Cutan Pathol 19: 172-180.
538. Cooper PH, Frierson HF, Kayne AL, Sabio H (1984). Association of juvenile xanthogranuloma with juvenile myeloid leukemia. Arch Dermatol 120: 371-375.
539. Cooper PH, Frierson HFJr, Morrison AG (1985). Malignant transformation of eccrine spiradenoma. Arch Dermatol 121: 1445-1448.
540. Cooper PH, McAllister HA, Helwig EB (1979). Intravenous pyogenic granuloma. A study of 18 cases. Am J Surg Pathol 3: 221-228.
541. Cooper PH, Mills SE, Leonard DD, Santa Cruz DJ, Headington JT, Barr RJ, Katz DA (1985). Sclerosing sweat duct (syringomatous) carcinoma. Am J Surg Pathol 9: 422-433.
542. Coppeto JR, Jaffe R, Gillies CG (1978). Primary orbital melanoma. Arch Ophthalmol 96: 2255-2258.
543. Cordova A (1981). The Mongolian spot: a study of ethnic differences and a literature review. Clin Pediatr (Phila) 20: 714-719.
544. Cossman J, Fend F, Staudt L, Raffel M (2001). Application of molecular genetics to the diagnosis and classification of malignant lymphoma. In: Neoplastic Hematopathology, Knowles DM, ed., Lippincott, Williams and Wilkins: Philadelphia , pp. 365-390.
545. Cote GJ, Wohllk N, Evans D, Goepfert H, Gagel RF (1995). RET proto-oncogene mutations in multiple endocrine neoplasia type 2 and medullary thyroid carcinoma. Baillieres Clin Endocrinol Metab 9: 609-630.
546. Cotton DW, Slater DN, Rooney N, Goepel JR, Mills PM (1986). Giant vascular eccrine spiradenomas: a report of two cases with histology, immunohistology and electron microscopy. Histopathology 10: 1093-1099.
547. Coupe MO, Whittaker SJ, Thatcher N (1987). Multicentric reticulohistiocytosis. Br J Dermatol 116: 245-247.
548. Couperus M, Rucker R (1953). Early diagnosis of malignant melanoma of the skin. California Med 78: 21-24.
549. Cox NH, Aitchison TC, MacKie RM (1998). Extrafacial lentigo maligna melanoma: analysis of 71 cases and comparison with lentigo maligna melanoma of the head and neck. Br J Dermatol 139: 439-443.
550. Cox NH, Long ED (1993). Pseudoangiosarcomatous squamous cell carcinoma of skin. Histopathology 22: 295-296.
551. Creamer D, Black MM, Calonje E (2000). Reactive angioendotheliomatosis in association with the antiphospholipid syndrome. J Am Acad Dermatol 42: 903-906.
552. Creamer D, Macdonald A, Griffiths WA (1999). Unilateral linear syringomata. A case report. Clin Exp Dermatol 24: 428-430.
553. Crespo M, Bosch F, Villamor N, Bellosillo B, Colomer D, Rozman M, Marce S, Lopez-Guillermo A, Campo E, Montserrat E (2003). ZAP-70 expression as a surrogate for immunoglobulin-variable-region mutations in chronic lymphocytic leukemia. N Engl J Med 348: 1764-1775.
554. Cress RD, Holly EA (1997). Incidence of cutaneous melanoma among non-Hispanic whites, Hispanics, Asians, and blacks: an analysis of california cancer registry data, 1988-93. Cancer Causes Control 8: 246-252.
555. Cribier B, Asch P, Grosshans E (1999). Differentiating squamous cell carcinoma from keratoacanthoma using histopathological criteria. Is it possible? A study of 296 cases. Dermatology 199: 208-212.
556. Cribier B, Asch PH, Regnier C, Rio MC, Grosshans E (1999). Expression of human hair keratin basic 1 in pilomatrixoma. A study of 128 cases. Br J Dermatol 140: 600-604.
557. Cribier B, Grosshans E (1995). Tumor of the follicular infundibulum: a clinicopathologic study. J Am Acad Dermatol 33: 979-984.
558. Cribier B, Noacco G, Peltre B, Grosshans E (2002). Stromelysin 3 expression: a useful marker for the differential diagnosis dermatofibroma versus dermatofibrosarcoma protuberans. J Am Acad Dermatol 46: 408-413.
559. Crijns MB, Bergman W, Berger MJ, Hermans J, Sober AJ (1993). On naevi and melanomas in dysplastic naevus syndrome patients. Clin Exp Dermatol 18: 248-252.
560. Crocetti E, Carli P (2003). Changes from mid-1980s to late 1990s among clinical and demographic correlates of melanoma thickness. Eur J Dermatol 13: 72-75.
561. Crocker HR (1889). Paget's disease affecting the scrotum and penis. Trans Pathol Soc London 40: 187-191.
562. Crotty CP, Winkelmann RK (1981). Cytophagic histiocytic panniculitis with fever, cytopenia, liver failure, and terminal hemorrhagic diathesis. J Am Acad Dermatol 4: 181-194.
563. Crotty KA, McCarthy SW, McCarthy WH, Quinn MJ (2003). Alopecia neoplastica caused by desmoplastic malignant melanoma. Australas J Dermatol .
564. Crovato F, Nazzari G, Gambini C, Massone L (1989). Meyerson's naevi in pityriasis rosea. Br J Dermatol 120: 318-319.
565. Crovato F, Rebora A (1985). Angiokeratoma corporis diffusum and normal enzyme activities. J Am Acad Dermatol 12: 885-886.
566. Crowley NJ, Seigler HF (1990). Late recurrence of malignant melanoma. Analysis of 168 patients. Ann Surg 212: 173-177.
567. Crowson AN, Magro CM, Mihm MCJr (1999). Malignant melanoma with prominent pigment synthesis: "animal type" melanoma – a clinical and histological study of six cases with a consideration of other melanocytic neoplasms with prominent pigment synthesis. Hum Pathol 30: 543-550.
568. Crowson AN, Magro CM, Mihm MCJr (2001). The Melanocytic Proliferations: A Comprehensive Textbook of Pigmented Lesions. First ed. John Wiley & Sons: New York.
569. Croxatto JO, Charles DE, Malbran ES (1981). Neurofibromatosis associated with nevus of Ota and choroidal melanoma. Am J Ophthalmol 92: 578-580.
570. Crum CP, Liskow A, Petras P, Keng WC, Frick HC (1984). Vulvar intraepithelial neoplasia (severe atypia and carcinoma in situ). A clinicopathologic analysis of 41 cases. Cancer 54: 1429-1434.
571. Crutcher WA, Sagebiel RW (1984). Prevalence of dysplastic naevi in a community practice. Lancet 1: 729.
572. Cubilla AL, Ayala MT, Barreto JE, Bellasai JG, Noel JC (1996). Surface adenosquamous carcinoma of the penis. A report of three cases. Am J Surg Pathol 20: 156-160.
573. Cubilla AL, Reuter VE, Gregoire L, Ayala G, Ocampos S, Lancaster WD, Fair W (1998). Basaloid squamous cell carcinoma: a distinctive human papilloma virus-related penile neoplasm: a report of 20 cases. Am J Surg Pathol 22: 755-761.
574. Cullen SL (1962). Incidence of nevi: report of palms, soles and genitalia of 10.000 young men. Arch Dermatol 86: 40-43.
575. Culpepper KS, Granter SR, McKee PH (2004). My approach to atypical melanocytic lesions. J Clin Pathol 57: 1121-1131.
576. Cunningham JA, Hardy J (1947). Hidradenomas of the vulva. South Surg 13: 831-838.
577. Curtis BV, Calcaterra TC, Coulson WF (1997). Multiple granular cell tumor: a case report and review of the literature. Head Neck 19: 634-637.
578. Czarnecki DB, Aarons I, Dowling JP, Lauritz B, Wallis P, Taft EH (1982). Malignant clear cell hidradenoma: a case report. Acta Derm Venereol 62: 173-176.
579. Czarnetzki BM, Behrendt H (1981). Urticaria pigmentosa: clinical picture and response to oral disodium cromoglycate. Br J Dermatol 105: 563-567.
580. Czarnetzki BM, Kolde G, Schoemann A, Urbanitz S, Urbanitz D (1988). Bone marrow findings in adult patients with urticaria pigmentosa. J Am Acad Dermatol 18: 45-51.
581. D'Addario SF, Morgan M, Talley L, Smoller BR (2002). h-Caldesmon as a specific marker of smooth muscle cell differentiation in some soft tissue tumors of the skin. J Cutan Pathol 29: 426-429.
582. Dabora SL, Jozwiak S, Franz DN, Roberts PS, Nieto A, Chung J, Choy YS, Reeve MP, Thiele E, Egelhoff JC, Kasprzyk-Obara J, Domanska-Pakiela D, Kwiatkowski DJ (2001). Mutational analysis in a cohort of 224 tuberous sclerosis patients indicates increased severity of TSC2, compared with TSC1, disease in multiple organs. Am J Hum Genet 68: 64-80.
583. Dabska M (1971). Giant hair matrix tumor. Cancer 28: 701-706.
584. Dabski K, Stoll HLJr (1987). Granulomatous reactions in mycosis fungoides. J Surg Oncol 34: 217-229.
585. Dakin MC, Leppard B, Theaker JM (1992). The palisaded, encapsulated neuroma (solitary circumscribed neuroma). Histopathology 20: 405-410.
586. Damle RN, Ghiotto F, Valetto A, Albesiano E, Fais F, Yan XJ, Sison CP, Allen SL, Kolitz J, Schulman P, Vinciguerra VP, Budde P, Frey J, Rai KR, Ferrarini M, Chiorazzi N (2002). B-cell chronic lymphocytic leukemia cells express a surface membrane phenotype of activated, antigen-experienced B lymphocytes. Blood 99: 4087-4093.
587. Danaee H, Nelson HH, Karagas MR, Schned AR, Ashok TD, Hirao T, Perry AE, Kelsey KT (2002). Microsatellite instability at tetranucleotide repeats in skin and bladder cancer. Oncogene 21: 4894-4899.
588. Danforth WC (1949). Sweat gland tumors of the vulva. Am J Obstet Gynecol 58: 326-334.
589. Daoud MS, Snow JL, Gibson LE, Daoud S (1996). Aleukemic monocytic leukemia cutis. Mayo Clin Proc 71: 166-168.
590. Darling TN, Kamino H, Murray JC (1993). Acquired cutaneous smooth muscle hamartoma. J Am Acad Dermatol 28: 844-845.
591. Darlington S, Siskind V, Green L, Green A (2002). Longitudinal study of melanocytic nevi in adolescents. J Am Acad Dermatol 46: 715-722.
592. Dave VK, Main RA (1972). Angiokeratoma of Mibelli with necrosis of the fingertips. Arch Dermatol 106: 726-728.
593. Davidson LL, Frost ML, Hanke CW, Epinette WW (1989). Primary leiomyosarcoma of the skin.Case report and review of the literature. J Am Acad Dermatol 21: 1156-1160.
594. Davis MD, Gostout BS, McGovern RM, Persing DH, Schut RL, Pittelkow MR (2000). Large plantar wart caused by human papillomavirus-66 and resolution by topical cidofovir therapy. J Am Acad Dermatol 43: 340-343.
595. Davis TH, Morton CC, Miller-Cassman R, Balk SP, Kadin ME (1992). Hodgkin's disease, lymphomatoid papulosis, and cutaneous T-cell lymphoma derived from a common T-cell clone. N Engl J Med 326: 1115-1122.
596. Davison JM, Rosenbaum E, Barrett TL, Goldenberg D, Hoque MO, Sidransky D, Westra WH (2005). Absence of V599E BRAF mutations in desmoplastic melanomas. Cancer 103: 788-792.
597. Dawe RS, Wainwright NJ, Evans AT, Lowe JG (1998). Multiple widespread eruptive Spitz naevi. Br J Dermatol 138: 872-874.
598. De Aloe G, Rubegni P, Pacenti L, Miracco C, Fimiani M (2001). Human herpesvirus type 8 is not associated with pyogenic granulomas with satellite recurrence. Br J Dermatol 144: 202-203.
599. de Berker D, Lawrence C (2001). Ganglion of the distal interphalangeal joint (myxoid cyst): therapy by identification and repair of the leak of joint fluid. Arch

Dermatol 137: 607-610.

600. De Bruin PC, Beljaards RC, van Heerde P, Van D, V, Noorduyn LA, van Krieken JH, Kluin-Nelemans JC, Willemze R, Meijer CJ (1993). Differences in clinical behaviour and immunophenotype between primary cutaneous and primary nodal anaplastic large cell lymphoma of T-cell or null cell phenotype. Histopathology 23: 127-135.

601. De Coninck A, Willemsen M, De Dobbeleer G, Roseeuw D (1986). Vulvar localisation of epidermolytic acanthoma. A light- and electron-microscopic study. Dermatologica 172: 276-278.

602. de Gruijl FR, Longstreth J, Norval M, Cullen AP, Slaper H, Kripke ML, Takizawa Y, van der Leun JC (2003). Health effects from stratospheric ozone depletion and interactions with climate change. Photochem Photobiol Sci 2: 16-28.

603. de Leval L, Harris NL, Longtine J, Ferry JA, Duncan LM (2001). Cutaneous b-cell lymphomas of follicular and marginal zone types: use of Bcl-6, CD10, Bcl-2, and CD21 in differential diagnosis and classification. Am J Surg Pathol 25: 732-741.

604. de Sa BC, Rezze GG, Scramim AP, Landman G, Neves RI (2004). Cutaneous melanoma in childhood and adolescence: retrospective study of 32 patients. Melanoma Res 14: 487-492.

605. de Villiers EM (2001). Taxonomic classification of papillomaviruses. Papillomavirus Report 12: 57-63.

606. de Viragh PA (1995). The 'mantle hair of Pinkus'. A review on the occasion of its centennial. Dermatology 191: 82-87.

607. de Viragh PA, Szeimies RM, Eckert F (1997). Apocrine cystadenoma, apocrine hidrocystoma, and eccrine hidrocystoma: three distinct tumors defined by expression of keratins and human milk fat globulin 1. J Cutan Pathol 24: 249-255.

608. de Vries E, Boniol M, Dore JF, Coebergh JW (2004). Lower incidence rates but thicker melanomas in Eastern Europe before 1992: a comparison with Western Europe. Eur J Cancer 40: 1045-1052.

609. de Vries E, Bray FI, Coebergh JW, Parkin DM (2003). Changing epidemiology of malignant cutaneous melanoma in Europe 1953-1997: rising trends in incidence and mortality but recent stabilizations in western Europe and decreases in Scandinavia. Int J Cancer 107: 119-126.

610. de Vries E, Coebergh JW (2004). Cutaneous malignant melanoma in Europe. Eur J Cancer 40: 2355-2366.

611. de Vries TJ, Smeets M, de Graaf R, Hou-Jensen K, Brocker EB, Renard N, Eggermont AM, Van Muijen GN, Ruiter DJ (2001). Expression of gp100, MART-1, tyrosinase, and S100 in paraffin-embedded primary melanomas and locoregional, lymph node, and visceral metastases: implications for diagnosis and immunotherapy. A study conducted by the EORTC Melanoma Cooperative Group. J Pathol 193: 13-20.

612. de Wit PE, van't Hof-Grootenboer B, Ruiter DJ, Bondi R, Brocker EB, Cesarini JP, Hastrup N, Hou-Jensen K, MacKie RM, Scheffer E, Suter L, Urso C (1993). Validity of the histopathological criteria used for diagnosing dysplastic naevi. An interobserver study by the pathology subgroup of the EORTC Malignant Melanoma Cooperative Group. Eur J Cancer 29A: 831-839.

613. DeCoteau JF, Butmarc JR, Kinney

MC, Kadin ME (1996). The t(2;5) chromosomal translocation is not a common feature of primary cutaneous CD30+ lymphoproliferative disorders: comparison with anaplastic large-cell lymphoma of nodal origin. Blood 87: 3437-3441.

614. Dehner P (2003). Juvenile xanthogranuloma in the first two decades. Am J Surg Pathol 27: 579-593.

615. Dekio S, Koike S, Jidoi J (1989). Nevus of ota with nevus of Ito – report of a case with cataract. J Dermatol 16: 164-166.

616. del Rio E, Vazquez Veiga HA, Suarez Penaranda JM (2000). Blue nevus with satellitosis mimicking malignant melanoma. Cutis 65: 301-302.

617. Delecluse HJ, Anagnostopoulos I, Dallenbach F, Hummel M, Marafioti T, Schneider U, Huhn D, Schmidt-Westhausen A, Reichart PA, Gross U, Stein H (1997). Plasmablastic lymphomas of the oral cavity: a new entity associated with the human immunodeficiency virus infection. Blood 89: 1413-1420.

618. Dennis LK (1999). Analysis of the melanoma epidemic, both apparent and real: data from the 1973 through 1994 surveillance, epidemiology, and end results program registry. Arch Dermatol 135: 275-280.

619. Dennis LK (1999). Melanoma incidence by body site: effects of birth-cohort adjustment. Arch Dermatol 135: 1553-1554.

620. Dennis LK, White E, Lee JA (1993). Recent cohort trends in malignant melanoma by anatomic site in the United States. Cancer Causes Control 4: 93-100.

621. Deroo M, Eeckhout I, Naeyaert JM (1997). Eruptive satellite vascular malformations after removal of a melanocytic naevus. Br J Dermatol 137: 292-295.

622. Derre J, Lagace R, Nicolas A, Mairal A, Chibon F, Coindre JM, Terrier P, Sastre X, Aurias A (2001). Leiomyosarcomas and most malignant fibrous histiocytomas share very similar comparative genomic hybridization imbalances: an analysis of a series of 27 leiomyosarcomas. Lab Invest 81: 211-215.

623. Derrick EK, Darley CR, Burge S (1995). Comedonal Darier's disease. Br J Dermatol 132: 453-455.

624. Desmond RA, Soong SJ (2003). Epidemiology of malignant melanoma. Surg Clin North Am 83: 1-29.

625. Dessoukey MW, Omar MF, Abdel-Dayem H (1997). Eruptive keratoacanthomas associated with immunosuppressive therapy in a patient with systemic lupus erythematosus. J Am Acad Dermatol 37: 478-480.

626. Dhillon AP, Rode J (1982). Patterns of staining for neurone specific enolase in benign and malignant melanocytic lesions of the skin. Diagn Histopathol 5: 169-174.

627. Di Tommaso L, Magrini E, Consales A, Poppi M, Pasquinelli G, Dorji T, Benedetti G, Baccarini P (2002). Malignant granular cell tumor of the lateral femoral cutaneous nerve: report of a case with cytogenetic analysis. Hum Pathol 33: 1237-1240.

628. Diaz-Cascajo C, Borghi S, Weyers W, Retzlaff H, Requena L, Metze D (1999). Benign lymphangiomatous papules of the skin following radiotherapy: a report of five new cases and review of the literature. Histopathology 35: 319-327.

629. Diaz-Cascajo C, Weyers W, Rey-Lopez A, Borghi S (1998). Deep dermatofibrosarcoma protuberans: a subcutaneous variant. Histopathology 32: 552-555.

630. Diebold J, Jaffe ES, Raphael M, Warnke RA (2001). Burkitt lymphoma. In: World Health Organization Classification of Tumours. Pathology and Genetics of Tumours of Haematopoietic and Lymphoid Tissues, Jaffe ES, Harris NL, Stein H, Vardiman J, eds., IARC Press: Lyon , pp. 181-184.

631. DiGiuseppe JA, Hartmann DP, Freter C, Cossman J, Mann RB (1997). Molecular detection of bone marrow involvement in intravascular lymphomatosis. Mod Pathol 10: 33-37.

632. DiGiuseppe JA, Louie DC, Williams JE, Miller DT, Griffin CA, Mann RB, Borowitz MJ (1997). Blastic natural killer cell leukemia/lymphoma: a clinicopathologic study. Am J Surg Pathol 21: 1223-1230.

633. DiGiuseppe JA, Nelson WG, Seifter EJ, Boitnott JK, Mann RB (1994). Intravascular lymphomatosis: a clinicopathologic study of 10 cases and assessment of response to chemotherapy. J Clin Oncol 12: 2573-2579.

634. DiLeonardo M (1997). Sebaceous adenoma vs. sebaceoma vs. sebaceous carcinoma. Dermatopathology, practical & conceptual 3: 11.

634A. Dimson OG, Drolet BA, Southern JF, Rock A, Winthrop AL, Esterly NB (2000). Congenital generalized myofibromatosis in a neonate. Arch Dermatol 136: 597-600.

635. Dinehart SM (2000). The treatment of actinic keratoses. J Am Acad Dermatol 42: 25-28.

636. Dinneen AM, Mehregan DR (1996). Sebaceous epithelioma: a review of twenty-one cases. J Am Acad Dermatol 34: 47-50.

637. Dissanayake RV, Salm R (1980). Sweat-gland carcinomas: prognosis related to histological type. Histopathology 4: 445-466.

638. Dixon AY, Lee SH, McGregor DH (1989). Factors predictive of recurrence of basal cell carcinoma. Am J Dermatopathol 11: 222-232.

639. Dixon AY, Lee SH, McGregor DH (1993). Histologic features predictive of basal cell carcinoma recurrence: results of a multivariate analysis. J Cutan Pathol 20: 137-142.

640. Djawari D, Cremer H (1989). [Malignant blue nevus]. Z Hautkr 64: 51-53.

641. Dodson JM, DeSpain J, Hewett JE, Clark DP (1991). Malignant potential of actinic keratoses and the controversy over treatment. A patient-oriented perspective. Arch Dermatol 127: 1029-1031.

642. Dogru M, Matsuo H, Inoue M, Okubo K, Yamamoto M (1997). Management of eyelid sebaceous carcinomas. Ophthalmologica 211: 40-43.

643. Dohner H, Stilgenbauer S, Benner A, Leupolt E, Krober A, Bullinger L, Dohner K, Bentz M, Lichter P (2000). Genomic aberrations and survival in chronic lymphocytic leukemia. N Engl J Med 343: 1910-1916.

644. Domingo J, Helwig EB (1979). Malignant neoplasms associated with nevus sebaceus of Jadassohn. J Am Acad Dermatol 1: 545-556.

645. Dommann SN, Dommann-Scherrer CC, Zimmerman D, Dours-Zimmermann MT, Hassam S, Burg G (1995). Primary cutaneous T-cell-rich B-cell lymphoma. A case report with a 13-year follow-up. Am J Dermatopathol 17: 618-624.

646. Dover JS, From L, Lewis A (1989). Palisaded encapsulated neuromas: a clinicopathologic study. Arch Dermatol 125: 386-389.

647. Dowlati B, Nabai H, Mehregan DR, Mehregan DA, Khaleel J (2002). Zosteriform angiolymphoid hyperplasia with eosinophilia. J Dermatol 29: 178-179.

648. Drake LA, Ceilley RI, Cornelison RL, Dobes WL, Dorner W, Goltz RW, Lewis CW, Salasche SJ, Turner ML, Lowery BJ, Shama SK, Androphy EJ, Galen WK, Heaton CL, Lynch PJ (1995). Guidelines of care for warts: human papillomavirus. Committee on Guidelines of Care. J Am Acad Dermatol 32: 98-103.

649. Dreizen S, McCredie KB, Keating MJ, Luna MA (1983). Malignant gingival and skin "infiltrates" in adult leukemia. Oral Surg Oral Med Oral Pathol 55: 572-579.

650. Drews R, Samel A, Kadin ME (2000). Lymphomatoid papulosis and anaplastic large cell lymphomas of the skin. Semin Cutan Med Surg 19: 109-117.

651. Dubin N, Kopf AW (1983). Multivariate risk score for recurrence of cutaneous basal cell carcinomas. Arch Dermatol 119: 373-377.

652. Dubreuilh MW (1912). De la melanose circonscrite precancereuse. Ann Dermatol Syphilol 3: 129-151.

653. Dubreuilh W (1912). Le naevus bléu. Ann Dermatol 2: 552.

654. Dubus P, Young P, Beylot-Barry M, Belaud-Rotureau MA, Courville P, Vergier B, Parrens M, Lenormand B, Joly P, Merlio JP (2002). Value of interphase FISH for the diagnosis of t(11:14)(q13;q32) on skin lesions of mantle cell lymphoma. Am J Clin Pathol 118: 832-841.

655. Duke WH, Sherrod TT, Lupton GP (2000). Aggressive digital papillary adenocarcinoma (aggressive digital papillary adenoma and adenocarcinoma revisited). Am J Surg Pathol 24: 775-784.

656. Dummer R, Kohl O, Gillessen J, Kagi M, Burg G (1993). Peripheral blood mononuclear cells in patients with non-leukemic cutaneous T-cell lymphoma. Reduced proliferation and preferential secretion of a T helper-2-like cytokine pattern on stimulation. Arch Dermatol 129: 433-436.

657. Dummer R, Nestle FO, Niederer E, Ludwig E, Laine E, Grundmann H, Grob P, Burg G (1999). Genotypic, phenotypic and functional analysis of CD4+CD7+ and CD4+CD7- T lymphocyte subsets in Sezary syndrome. Arch Dermatol Res 291: 307-311.

658. Dunwell P, Rose A (2003). Study of the skin disease spectrum occurring in an Afro-Caribbean population. Int J Dermatol 42: 287-289.

659. Dupre A, Viraben R (1985). Congenital smooth muscle nevus with follicular spotted appearance. J Am Acad Dermatol 13: 837-838.

660. Dutton JJ, Anderson RL, Schelper RL, Purcell JJ, Tse DT (1984). Orbital malignant melanoma and oculodermal melanocytosis: report of two cases and review of the literature. Ophthalmology 91: 497-507.

661. Dwyer PK, MacKie RM, Watt DC, Aitchison TC (1993). Plantar malignant melanoma in a white Caucasian population. Br J Dermatol 128: 115-120.

662. Eckert F, Betke M, Schmoeckel C, Neuweiler J, Schmid U (1992). Myoepithelial differentiation in benign sweat gland tumors. Demonstrated by a monoclonal antibody to alpha-smooth muscle actin. J Cutan Pathol 19: 294-301.

663. Eckert F, Nilles M, Altmannsberger M (1992). Eccrine syringofibroadenoma: a case report with analysis of cytokeratin expression. Br J Dermatol 126: 257-261.

664. Eckert F, Schmid U, Hardmeier T, Altmannsberger M (1992). Cytokeratin expression in mucinous sweat gland carcinomas: an immunohistochemical analysis of four cases. Histopathology 21: 161-165.

665. Egawa K, Honda Y, Ono T, Kuroki M (1998). Immunohistochemical demonstration of carcinoembryonic antigen and related antigens in various cutaneous keratinous neoplasms and verruca vulgaris. Br J Dermatol 139: 178-185.

666. Egeler RM, Neglia JP, Puccetti DM, Brennan CA, Nesbit ME (1993). Association of Langerhans cell histiocytosis with malignant neoplasms. Cancer 71: 865-873.

667. Ehrlich GE, Young I, Nosheny SZ, Katz WA (1972). Multicentric reticulohistiocytosis (lipoid dermatoarthritis). A multisystem disorder. Am J Med 52: 830-840.

668. Eichhorn M, Jungkunz W, Worl J, Marsch WC (1994). Carbonic anhydrase is abundant in fenestrated capillaries of cherry hemangioma. Acta Derm Venereol 74: 51-53.

669. Eichmuller S, Usener D, Dummer R, Stein A, Thiel D, Schadendorf D (2001). Serological detection of cutaneous T-cell lymphoma-associated antigens. Proc Natl Acad Sci U S A 98: 629-634.

670. Eisen D, Voorhees JJ (1991). Oral melanoma and other pigmented lesions of the oral cavity. J Am Acad Dermatol 24: 527-537.

671. Elder D, Elenitsas R, Ragsdale BD (1977). Eccrine hidrocystoma. In: Lever's Histopathology of the Skin, Elder D, Elenitsas R, Jaworsky C, Johnson BJr, eds., Lippincott Williams & Wilkins: Philadelphia .

672. Elder DE, Elenitsas R, Jaworsky C, Johnson BLJr (1997). Lever's Histopathology of the Skin. 8th ed. Lippincott-Raven: Philadelphia.

673. Elder DE, Goldman LI, Goldman SC, Greene MH, Clark WHJr (1980). Dysplastic nevus syndrome: a phenotypic association of sporadic cutaneous melanoma. Cancer 46: 1787-1794.

674. Elder DE, Guerry D, Epstein MN, Zehngebot L, Lusk E, Van Horn M, Clark WHJr (1984). Invasive malignant melanomas lacking competence for metastasis. Am J Dermatopathol 6 Suppl: 55-61.

675. Elder DE, Murphy GF (1991). Atlas of Tumor Pathology. Melanocytic Tumors of the Skin. 3rd Series ed. AFIP: Washington.

675A. Elder DE, Rodeck U, Thurin J, Cardillo F, Clark WH, Stewart R, Herlyn M (1989). Antigenic profile of tumor progression stages in human melanocytic nevi and melanomas. Cancer Res 49: 5091-5096.

676. Elenitsas R, Halpern AC (1996). Eczematous halo reaction in atypical nevi. J Am Acad Dermatol 34: 357-361.

677. Elgart GW (2001). Seborrheic keratoses, solar lentigines and lichenoid keratoses. Dermatoscopic features and correlation to histology and clinical signs. Dermatol Clin 19: 347-357.

678. Elgart GW, Patterson JW (1990). Congenital midline hamartoma: case report with histochemical and immunohistochemical findings. Pediatr Dermatol 7: 199-201.

679. Elleder M, Ledvinova J, Vosmik F, Zeman J, Stejskal D, Lageron A (1990). An atypical ultrastructural pattern in Fabry's disease: a study on its nature and incidence in 7 cases. Ultrastruct Pathol 14: 467-474.

680. Elston DM, Bergfeld WF, Petroff N (1993). Basal cell carcinoma with monster

cells. J Cutan Pathol 20: 70-73.

681. Elston DM, James WD, Rodman OG, Graham GF (1986). Multiple hamartoma syndrome (Cowden's disease) associated with non-Hodgkin's lymphoma. Arch Dermatol 122: 572-575.

682. Elwood JM, Gallagher RP (1998). Body site distribution of cutaneous malignant melanoma in relationship to patterns of sun exposure. Int J Cancer 78: 276-280.

683. Elwood JM, Jopson J (1997). Melanoma and sun exposure: an overview of published studies. Int J Cancer 73: 198-203.

684. Emura I, Naito M, Wakabayashi M, Yoshizawa H, Arakawa M, Chou T (1998). Detection of circulating tumor cells in a patient with intravascular lymphomatosis: a case study examined by the cytology method. Pathol Int 48: 63-66.

685. Endo H, Mikami Y, Sano T (2003). Cervical polyp with eccrine syringofibroadenoma-like features. Histopathology 42: 301-304.

686. Eng A, Lebel RR, Elejalde BR, Anderson C, Bennett L (1994). Linear facial skin defects associated with microphthalmia and other malformations, with chromosome deletion Xp22.1. J Am Acad Dermatol 31: 680-682.

687. Eng C (1998). Genetics of Cowden syndrome: through the looking glass of oncology. Int J Oncol 12: 701-710.

688. Eng C (2000). Will the real Cowden syndrome please stand up: revised diagnostic criteria. J Med Genet 37: 828-830.

688A. Eng C (2003). PTEN: one gene, many syndromes. Hum Mutat 22: 183-198.

689. English DR, Armstrong BK, Kricker A, Fleming C (1997). Sunlight and cancer. Cancer Causes Control 8: 271-283.

690. English JCI, McCollough ML, Grabski WJ (1996). A pigmented scalp nodule: malignant blue nevus. Cutis 58: 40-42.

691. Enjolras O, Mulliken JB, Wassef M, Frieden IJ, Rieu PN, Burrows PE, Salhi A, Leaute-Labreze C, Kozakewich HP (2000). Residual lesions after Kasabach-Merritt phenomenon in 41 patients. J Am Acad Dermatol 42: 225-235.

692. Enjolras O, Wassef M, Mazoyer E, Frieden IJ, Rieu PN, Drouet L, Taieb A, Stalder JF, Escande JP (1997). Infants with Kasabach-Merritt syndrome do not have "true" hemangiomas. J Pediatr 130: 631-640.

693. Enzinger FM (1979). Angiomatoid malignant fibrous histiocytoma: a distinct fibrohistiocytic tumor of children and young adults simulating a vascular neoplasm. Cancer 44: 2147-2157.

694. Epstein JH (1983). Photocarcinogenesis, skin cancer, and aging. J Am Acad Dermatol 9: 487-502.

695. Epstein JI, Erlandson RA, Rosen PP (1984). Nodal blue nevi. A study of three cases. Am J Surg Pathol 8: 907-915.

696. Eros N, Karolyi Z, Kovacs A, Takacs I, Radvanyi G, Kelenyi G (2002). Intravascular B-cell lymphoma. J Am Acad Dermatol 47: S260-S262.

697. Estalilla OC, Koo CH, Brynes RK, Medeiros LJ (1999). Intravascular large B-cell lymphoma. A report of five cases initially diagnosed by bone marrow biopsy. Am J Clin Pathol 112: 248-255.

698. Evans DG, Ladusans EJ, Rimmer S, Burnell LD, Thakker N, Farndon PA (1993). Complications of the naevoid basal cell carcinoma syndrome: results of a population based study. J Med Genet 30: 460-464.

699. Evans HL, Su D, Smith JL,

Winkelmann RK (1979). Carcinoma arising in eccrine spiradenoma. Cancer 43: 1881-1884.

700. Evans HL, Winkelmann RK, Banks PM (1979). Differential diagnosis of malignant and benign cutaneous lymphoid infiltrates: a study of 57 cases in which malignant lymphoma had been diagnosed or suspected in the skin. Cancer 44: 699-717.

701. Evans MJ, Gray ES, Blessing K (1998). Histopathological features of acral melanocytic nevi in children: study of 21 cases. Pediatr Dev Pathol 1: 388-392.

702. Evans RW (1956). Histologic appearance of tumours. Med J Edinb London 1: 230.

703. Everett MA (1989). Histopathology of congenital pigmented nevi. Am J Dermatopathol 11: 11-12.

704. Fackenthal JD, Marsh DJ, Richardson AL, Cummings SA, Eng C, Robinson BG, Olopade OI (2001). Male breast cancer in Cowden syndrome patients with germline PTEN mutations. J Med Genet 38: 159-164.

705. Falck VG, Jordaan HF (1986). Papillary eccrine adenoma. A tubulopapillary hidradenoma with eccrine differentiation. Am J Dermatopathol 8: 64-72.

706. Falini B, Mason DY (2002). Proteins encoded by genes involved in chromosomal alterations in lymphoma and leukemia: clinical value of their detection by immunocytochemistry. Blood 99: 409-426.

707. Fallowfield ME, Collina G, Cook MG (1994). Melanocytic lesions of the palm and sole. Histopathology 24: 463-467.

708. Fan H, Oro AE, Scott MP, Khavari PA (1997). Induction of basal cell carcinoma features in transgenic human skin expressing Sonic Hedgehog. Nat Med 3: 788-792.

709. Fanburg JC, Meis-Kindblom JM, Rosenberg AE (1995). Multiple enchondromas associated with spindle-cell hemangioendotheliomas. An overlooked variant of Maffucci's syndrome. Am J Surg Pathol 19: 1029-1038.

710. Fanning J, Lambert HC, Hale TM, Morris PC, Schuerch C (1999). Paget's disease of the vulva: prevalence of associated vulvar adenocarcinoma, invasive Paget's disease, and recurrence after surgical excision. Am J Obstet Gynecol 180: 24-27.

711. Fargnoli MC, Orlow SJ, Semel-Concepcion J, Bolognia JL (1996). Clinicopathologic findings in the Bannayan-Riley-Ruvalcaba syndrome. Arch Dermatol 132: 1214-1218.

712. Farrier S, Morgan M (1997). bcl-2 expression in pilomatricoma. Am J Dermatopathol 19: 254-257.

713. Farris PE, Manning S, Vuitch F (1994). Rhabdomyomatous mesenchymal hamartoma. Am J Dermatopathol 16: 73-75.

714. Fauci AS, Haynes BF, Costa J, Katz P, Wolff SM (1982). Lymphomatoid Granulomatosis. Prospective clinical and therapeutic experience over 10 years. N Engl J Med 306: 68-74.

715. Faulhaber D, Worle B, Trautner B, Sander CA (2000). Clear cell hidradenoma in a young girl. J Am Acad Dermatol 42: 693-695.

716. Favara BE (2001). Langerhans cell histiocytosis: an identity crisis. Med Pediatr Oncol 37: 545.

717. Feal-Cortizas C, Vargas-Diez E, Buezo GF, Aragues M (1997). Meyerson's nevus immunohistochemical findings in two cases. Australas J Dermatol 38: 222.

718. Feinmesser M, Tsabari C, Fichman S, Hodak E, Sulkes J, Okon E (2003).

Differential expression of proliferation- and apoptosis-related markers in lentigo maligna and solar keratosis keratinocytes. Am J Dermatopathol 25: 300-307.

719. Feit NE, Dusza SW, Marghoob AA (2004). Melanomas detected with the aid of total cutaneous photography. Br J Dermatol 150: 706-714.

720. Feldman AL, Berthold F, Arceci RJ, Abramowsky C, Shehata BM, Mann KP, Lauer SJ, Pritchard J, Raffeld M, Jaffe ES (2005). Clonal relationship between precursor T-lymphoblastic leukaemia/lymphoma and Langerhans-cell histiocytosis. Lancet Oncol 6: 435-437.

721. Fendt H (1900). Beiträge zur Kenntnis der sogenannten sarcoiden Geschwülste der Haut. Arch Dermatol Syphilol 53: 212-242.

722. Fenske C, Banerjee P, Holden C, Carter N (2000). Brooke-Spiegler syndrome locus assigned to 16q12-q13. J Invest Dermatol 114: 1057-1058.

723. Ferguson JW, Hutchison HT, Rouse BM (1984). Ocular, cerebral and cutaneous malformations: confirmation of an association. Clin Genet 25: 464-469.

724. Ferlay J, Bray FI, Pisani P, Parkin DM (2001). Globocan 2000: Cancer incidence, mortality and prevalence worldwide. 1 ed. IARC Press: Lyon.

725. Fernandez-Acenero MJ, Manzarbeitia F, Mestre de Juan MJ, Requena L (2001). Malignant spiradenoma: report of two cases and literature review. J Am Acad Dermatol 44: 395-398.

726. Fernandez-Acenero MJ, Manzarbeitia F, Mestre MJ, Requena L (2000). p53 expression in two cases of spiradenocarcinomas. Am J Dermatopathol 22: 104-107.

727. Fernandez-Acenero MJ, Sanchez TA, Sanchez MC, Requena L (2003). Ectopic hidradenoma papilliferum: a case report and literature review. Am J Dermatopathol 25: 176-178.

728. Fernandez-Pugnaire MA, Delgado-Florencio V (1995). Familial multiple cutaneous leiomyomas. Dermatology 191: 295-298.

729. Fernandez Herrera JM, Aragues Montanes M, Fraga Fernandez J, Diez G (1988). Halo eczema in melanocytic nevi. Acta Derm Venereol 68: 161-163.

730. Fernandez EM, Helm KF (2004). The diameter of melanomas. Dermatol Surg 30: 1219-1222.

731. Fernandez M, Raimer SS, Sanchez RL (2001). Dysplastic nevi of the scalp and forehead in children. Pediatr Dermatol 18: 5-8.

732. Fernando SS, Johnson S, Bate J (1994). Immunohistochemical analysis of cutaneous malignant melanoma: comparison of S-100 protein, HMB-45 monoclonal antibody and NKI/C3 monoclonal antibody. Pathology 26: 16-19.

733. Ferrara G, Argenziano G, Zgavec B, Bartenjev I, Staibano S, De Rosa G, Soyer HP (2002). "Compound blue nevus": a reappraisal of "superficial blue nevus with prominent intraepidermal dendritic melanocytes" with emphasis on dermoscopic and histopathologic features. J Am Acad Dermatol 46: 85-89.

734. Ferreiro JA, Carney JA (1994). Myxomas of the external ear and their significance. Am J Surg Pathol 18: 274-280.

735. Ferreiro JA, Nascimento AG (1995). Hyaline-cell rich chondroid syringoma. A tumor mimicking malignancy. Am J Surg Pathol 19: 912-917.

736. Ferreri AJ, Campo E, Ambrosetti A,

Ilariucci F, Seymour JF, Willemze R, Arrigoni G, Rossi G, Lopez-Guillermo A, Berti E, Eriksson M, Federico M, Cortelazzo S, Govi S, Frungilo N, Dell'Oro S, Lestani M, Asioli S, Pedrinis E, Ungari M, Motta T, Rossi R, Artusi T, Iuzzolino P, Zucca E, Cavalli F, Ponzoni M (2004). Anthracycline-based chemotherapy as primary treatment for intravascular lymphoma. Ann Oncol 15: 1215-1221.

737. Ferry JA, Harris NL, Picker LJ, Weinberg DS, Rosales RK, Tapia J, Richardson EPJr (1988). Intravascular lymphomatosis (malignant angioendotheliomatosis). A B-cell neoplasm expressing surface homing receptors. Mod Pathol 1: 444-452.

738. Fetsch JF, Weiss SW (1991). Observations concerning the pathogenesis of epithelioid hemangioma (angiolymphoid hyperplasia). Mod Pathol 4: 449-455.

739. Feuillard J, Jacob MC, Valensi F, Maynadie M, Gressin R, Chaperot L, Arnoulet C, Brignole-Baudouin F, Drenou B, Duchayne E, Falkenrodt A, Garand R, Homolle E, Husson B, Kuhlein E, Le Calvez G, Sainty D, Sotto MF, Trimoreau F, Bene MC (2002). Clinical and biologic features of CD4(+)CD56(+) malignancies. Blood 99: 1556-1563.

740. Filie AC, Lage JM, Azumi N (1996). Immunoreactivity of S100 protein, alpha-1-antitrypsin, and CD68 in adult and congenital granular cell tumors. Mod Pathol 9: 888-892.

741. Filipowicz E, Adegboyega P, Sanchez RL, Gatalica Z (2002). Expression of CD95 (Fas) in sun-exposed human skin and cutaneous carcinomas. Cancer 94: 814-819.

742. Finch TM, Tan CY (2000). Clear cell acanthoma developing on a psoriatic plaque: further evidence of an inflammatory aetiology? Br J Dermatol 142: 842-844.

743. Fine SW, Li M (2003). Expression of calretinin and the alpha-subunit of inhibin in granular cell tumors. Am J Clin Pathol 119: 259-264.

744. Fink-Puches R, Zenahlik P, Back B, Smolle J, Kerl H, Cerroni L (2002). Primary cutaneous lymphomas: applicability of current classification schemes (European Organization for Research and Treatment of Cancer, World Health Organization) based on clinicopathologic features observed in a large group of patients. Blood 99: 800-805.

745. Finley RKI, Driscoll DL, Blumenson LE, Karakousis CP (1994). Subungual melanoma: an eighteen-year review. Surgery 116: 96-100.

746. Finn MC, Glowacki J, Mulliken JB (1983). Congenital vascular lesions: clinical application of a new classification. J Pediatr Surg 18: 894-900.

747. Firooz A, Komeili A, Dowlati Y (1999). Eruptive melanocytic nevi and cherry angiomas secondary to exposure to sulfur mustard gas. J Am Acad Dermatol 40: 646-647.

748. Fistarol SK, Anliker MD, Itin PH (2002). Cowden disease or multiple hamartoma syndrome – cutaneous clue to internal malignancy. Eur J Dermatol 12: 411-421.

749. Fitzpatrick TB, Johnson RA, Wolff K, Suurmond D, Wolf K (2001). Color Atlas & Synopsis of Clinical Dermatology. In: McGraw-Hill: pp. 272-277.

750. Flanagan BP, Helwig EB (1977). Cutaneous lymphangioma. Arch Dermatol 113: 24-30.

751. Fletcher CD (1988). Giant cell fibroblastoma of soft tissue: a clinicopathological

and immunohistochemical study. Histopathology 13: 499-508.

752. Fletcher CD (1989). Solitary circumscribed neuroma of the skin (so-called palisaded, encapsulated neuroma). A clinicopathologic and immunohistochemical study. Am J Surg Pathol 13: 574-580.

753. Fletcher CD, Achu P, Van Noorden S, McKee PH (1987). Infantile myofibromatosis: a light microscopic, histochemical and immunohistochemical study suggesting true smooth muscle differentiation. Histopathology 11: 245-258.

754. Fletcher CD, Beham A, Schmid C (1991). Spindle cell haemangioendothelioma: a clinicopathological and immunohistochemical study indicative of a non-neoplastic lesion. Histopathology 18: 291-301.

755. Fletcher CD, Chan JK, McKee PH (1986). Dermal nerve sheath myxoma: a study of three cases. Histopathology 10: 135-145.

756. Fletcher CDM, Unni K, Mertens F (2002). World Health Organization Classification of Tumours. Pathology and Genetics of Tumours of Soft Tissue and Bone. IARC Press: Lyon.

757. Fletcher V, Sagebiel RW (1981). The combined naevus: Mixed patterns of benign melanocytic lesions must be differentiated from malignant melanomas. In: Pathology of Malignant Melanoma, Ackerman AB, ed., Masson Publishing: Philadelphia , pp. 273-283.

758. Flotte TJ, Bell DA, Sidhu GS, Plair CM (1981). Leiomyosarcoma of the dartos muscle. J Cutan Pathol 8: 69-74.

759. Flotte TJ, Mihm MCJr (1999). Lentigo maligna and malignant melanoma in situ, lentigo maligna type. Hum Pathol 30: 533-536.

760. Fogt F, Vortmeyer AO, Tahan SR (1995). Nucleolar organizer regions (AgNOR) and Ki-67 immunoreactivity in cutaneous melanocytic lesions. Am J Dermatopathol 17: 12-17.

761. Folpe AL, Chand EM, Goldblum JR, Weiss SW (2001). Expression of Fli-1, a nuclear transcription factor, distinguishes vascular neoplasms from potential mimics. Am J Surg Pathol 25: 1061-1066.

762. Folpe AL, Reisenauer AK, Mentzel T, Rutten A, Solomon AR (2003). Proliferating trichilemmal tumors: clinicopathologic evaluation is a guide to biologic behavior. J Cutan Pathol 30: 492-498.

763. Folpe AL, Veikkola T, Valtola R, Weiss SW (2000). Vascular endothelial growth factor receptor-3 (VEGFR-3): a marker of vascular tumors with presumed lymphatic differentiation, including Kaposi's sarcoma, kaposiform and Dabska-type hemangioendotheliomas, and a subset of angiosarcomas. Mod Pathol 13: 180-185.

764. Fontaine D, Parkhill W, Greer W, Walsh N (2003). Partial regression of primary cutaneous melanoma: is there an association with sub-clinical sentinel lymph node metastasis? Am J Dermatopathol 25: 371-376.

765. Fordyce JA (1895). Adenocarcinoma of the skin originating in the coil glands. J Cutan Dis 13: 41-50.

766. Fortier-Beaulieu M, Thomine E, Boullie MC, Le Loet X, Lauret P, Hemet J (1993). New electron microscopic findings in a case of multicentric reticulohistiocytosis. Long spacing collagen inclusions. Am J Dermatopathol 15: 587-589.

767. Fortin PT, Freiberg AA, Rees R, Sondak VK, Johnson TM (1995). Malignant

melanoma of the foot and ankle. J Bone Joint Surg Am 77: 1396-1403.

768. Foucar E, Mason WV (1986). Angiokeratoma circumscriptum following damage to underlying vasculature. Arch Dermatol 122: 245-246.

769. Fouilloux B, Perrin C, Dutoit M, Cambazard F (2001). Clear cell syringofibroadenoma (of Mascaro) of the nail. Br J Dermatol 144: 625-627.

770. Fox MF, DuToit DL, Warnich L, Retief AE (1984). Regional localization of alpha-galactosidase (GLA) to Xpter-q22, hexosaminidase B (HEXB) to 5q13-qter, and arylsulfatase B (ARSB) to 5pter-q13. Cytogenet Cell Genet 38: 45-49.

771. Fox SB, Cotton DW (1992). Tubular apocrine adenoma and papillary eccrine adenoma. Entities or unity? Am J Dermatopathol 14: 149-154.

772. Franceschi S, Levi F, Randimbison L, La Vecchia C (1996). Site distribution of different types of skin cancer: new aetiological clues. Int J Cancer 67: 24-28.

773. Franchi A, Dini M, Paglierani M, Bondi R (1995). Immunolocalization of extracellular matrix components in mixed tumors of the skin. Am J Dermatopathol 17: 36-41.

774. Franco R, Fernandez-Vazquez A, Rodriguez-Peralto JL, Bellas C, Lopez-Rios F, Saez A, Villuendas R, Navarrete M, Fernandez I, Zarco C, Piris MA (2001). Cutaneous follicular B-cell lymphoma: description of a series of 18 cases. Am J Surg Pathol 25: 875-883.

775. Franke W, Neumann NJ, Ruzicka T, Schulte KW (2000). Plantar malignant melanoma – a challenge for early recognition. Melanoma Res 10: 571-576.

776. Fraser-Andrews E, Ashton R, Russell-Jones R (1999). Pilotropic mycosis fungoides presenting with multiple cysts, comedones and alopecia. Br J Dermatol 140: 141-144.

777. Fraser-Andrews EA, Russell-Jones R, Woolford AJ, Wolstencroft RA, Dean AJ, Whittaker SJ (2001). Diagnostic and prognostic importance of T-cell receptor gene analysis in patients with Sezary syndrome. Cancer 92: 1745-1752.

778. Freedberg IM, Eisen AZ, Wolff K, Austen KF, Goldsmith LO, Katz SI, Fitzpatrick TB (1999). Fitzpatrick's Dermatology in General Medicine. 5th ed. McGraw-Hill: New York.

779. French LE (1997). Reactive eccrine syringofibroadenoma: an emerging subtype. Dermatology 195: 309-310.

780. French LE, Masgrau E, Chavaz P, Saurat JH (1997). Eccrine syringofibroadenoma in a patient with erosive palmoplantar lichen planus. Dermatology 195: 399-401.

781. Fretzin DF, Sloan JB, Beer K, Fretzin SA (1995). Eccrine syringofibroadenoma. A clear-cell variant. Am J Dermatopathol 17: 591-593.

782. Friedman RJ, Ackerman AB (1981). Difficulties in the histological diagnosis of melanocytic nevi on the vulvae of premenopausal women. In: Pathology of Malignant Melanoma, Ackerman AB, ed., Masson Publishing: New York , pp. 119-128.

783. Friedmann D, Wechsler J, Delfau MH, Esteve E, Farcet JP, de Muret A, Parneix-Spake A, Vaillant L, Revuz J, Bagot M (1995). Primary cutaneous pleomorphic small T-cell lymphoma. A review of 11 cases. The French Study Group on Cutaneous Lymphomas. Arch Dermatol 131: 1009-1015.

784. Friedrich EGJr, Burch K, Bahr JP (1979). The vulvar clinic: an eight-year appraisal. Am J Obstet Gynecol 135: 1036-1040.

785. Frigy AF, Cooper PH (1985). Benign lichenoid keratosis. Am J Clin Pathol 83: 439-443.

786. Fritz A, Percy C, Jack A, Shanmugaratnam K, Sobin LH, Parkin DM, Whelan S (2000). International Classification of Diseases for Oncology. 3rd ed. World Health Organization: Geneva.

787. Frizzera G, Moran EM, Rappaport H (1975). Angio-immunoblastic lymphadenopathy. Diagnosis and clinical course. Am J Med 59: 803-818.

788. Frost C, Williams G, Green A (2000). High incidence and regression rates of solar keratoses in a Queensland community. J Invest Dermatol 115: 273-277.

789. Frost CA, Green AC (1994). Epidemiology of solar keratoses. Br J Dermatol 131: 455-464.

790. Frost CA, Green AC, Williams GM (1998). The prevalence and determinants of solar keratoses at a subtropical latitude (Queensland, Australia). Br J Dermatol 139: 1033-1039.

791. Fu W, Cockerell CJ (2003). The actinic (solar) keratosis: a 21st-century perspective. Arch Dermatol 139: 66-70.

792. Fujiwara Y, Abe Y, Kuyama M, Arata J, Yoshino T, Akagi T, Miyoshi K (1990). CD8+ cutaneous T-cell lymphoma with pagetoid epidermotropism and angiocentric and angiodestructive infiltration. Arch Dermatol 126: 801-804.

793. Fukai K, Ishii M, Kobayashi H, Chanoki M, Furukawa M, Nakagawa K, Hamada T, Abe Y, Ooshima A (1990). Primary cutaneous adenoid cystic carcinoma: ultrastructural study and immunolocalization of types I, III, IV, V collagens and laminin. J Cutan Pathol 17: 374-380.

794. Fukamizu H, Oku T, Inoue K, Matsumoto K, Okayama H, Tagami H (1983). Atypical ("pseudosarcomatous") cutaneous histiocytoma. J Cut Pathol 10: 327-333.

795. Fukunaga M (2000). Intravenous tufted angioma. APMIS 108: 287-292.

796. Fukunaga M, Ushigome S, Nikaido T, Ishikawa E, Nakamori K (1995). Spindle cell hemangioendothelioma: an immunohistochemical and flow cytometric study of six cases. Pathol Int 45: 589-595.

797. Fullen DR, Jacobson SN, Valdez R, Novice FM, Lowe L (2003). Granuloma annulare-like infiltrates with concomitant cutaneous involvement by B-cell non-Hodgkin's lymphoma: report of a case. Am J Dermatopathol 25: 57-61.

798. Fullen DR, Lowe L, Su LD (2003). Antibody to S100a6 protein is a sensitive immunohistochemical marker for neurothekeoma. J Cutan Pathol 30: 118-122.

799. Fung DC, Holland EA, Becker TM, Hayward NK, Bressac de Paillerets B, Mann GJ (2003). eMelanoBase: an online locus-specific variant database for familial melanoma. Hum Mutat 21: 2-7.

800. Furue M, Hori Y, Nakabayashi Y (1984). Clear-cell syringoma. Association with diabetes mellitus. Am J Dermatopathol 6: 131-138.

801. Gaasterland DE, Rodrigues MM, Moshell AN (1982). Ocular involvement in xeroderma pigmentosum. Ophthalmology 89: 980-986.

802. Gailani MR, Stahle-Backdahl M, Leffell DJ, Glynn M, Zaphiropoulos PG, Pressman C, Unden AB, Dean M, Brash DE,

Bale AE, Toftgard R (1996). The role of the human homologue of Drosophila patched in sporadic basal cell carcinomas. Nat Genet 14: 78-81.
803. Gallager MS, Miller GV, Grampa G (1959). Primary mucoepidermoid carcinoma of the skin. Report of a case. Cancer 12: 286-288.
804. Galvez-Aranda MV, Herrera-Ceballos E, Sanchez-Sanchez P, Bosch-Garcia RJ, Matilla-Vicente A (2002). Pilomatrix carcinoma with lymph node and pulmonary metastasis: report of a case arising on the knee. Am J Dermatopathol 24: 139-143.
805. Gambichler T, Herde M, Hoffmann K, Altmeyer P, Jansen T (2002). Poor prognosis of acute myeloid leukaemia associated with leukaemia cutis. J Eur Acad Dermatol Venereol 16: 177-178.
806. Gambini C, Rongioletti F, Semino MT, Rebora A (1996). Solitary eccrine syringofibroadenoma (or eccrine syringofibroadenomatous hyperplasia?) and diabetic polyneuropathy. Dermatology 193: 68-69.
807. Garbe C, Stein H, Dienemann D, Orfanos CE (1991). Borrelia burgdorferi-associated cutaneous B cell lymphoma: clinical and immunohistologic characterization of four cases. J Am Acad Dermatol 24: 584-590.
808. Garcia-Doval I, Casas L, Toribio J (1998). Pleomorphic fibroma of the skin, a form of sclerotic fibroma: an immunohistochemical study. Clin Exp Dermatol 23: 22-24.
809. Gascoyne RD, Aoun P, Wu D, Chhanabhai M, Skinnider BF, Greiner TC, Morris SW, Connors JM, Vose JM, Viswanatha DS, Coldman A, Weisenburger DD (1999). Prognostic significance of anaplastic lymphoma kinase (ALK) protein expression in adults with anaplastic large cell lymphoma. Blood 93: 3913-3921.
810. Gasior-Chrzan B (2001). Cellular blue nevus in association with phototherapy. Dermatology 202: 140.
811. Gatta G, Capocaccia R, Stiller C, Kaatsch P, Berrino F, Terenziani M (2005). Childhood cancer survival trends in Europe: a EUROCARE Working Group study. J Clin Oncol 23: 3742-3751.
812. Gauthier Y, Surleve-Bazeille JE, Texier L (1978). Halo nevi without dermal infiltrate. Arch Dermatol 114: 1718.
813. Gayraud A, Lorenzato M, Sartelet H, Grosshans E, Hopfner C, Mehaut S, Bernard P, Durlach A (2002). [Malignant blue nevus: clinicopathologic study with AgNOR measurement. Seven cases]. Ann Dermatol Venereol 129: 1359-1364.
814. Geelen FA, Vermeer MH, Meijer CJ, Van der Putte SC, Kerkhof E, Kluin PM, Willemze R (1998). bcl-2 protein expression in primary cutaneous large B-cell lymphoma is site-related. J Clin Oncol 16: 2080-2085.
815. Gellis SS, Feingold M (1971). Mucosal neuroma syndrome. Syndrome of bilateral pheochromocytoma, medullary thyroid carcinoma, and multiple neuromas. Am J Dis Child 121: 235-236.
816. Gellrich S, Rutz S, Golembowski S, Jacobs C, von Zimmermann M, Lorenz P, Audring H, Muche M, Sterry W, Jahn S (2001). Primary cutaneous follicle center cell lymphomas and large B cell lymphomas of the leg descend from germinal center cells. A single cell polymerase chain reaction analysis. J Invest Dermatol 117: 1512-1520.
817. George E, Swanson PE, Wick MR (1989). Neuroendocrine differentiation in basal cell carcinoma. An immunohistochemical study. Am J Dermatopathol 11: 131-135.
818. Gerbig AW, Zala L, Hunziker T (2000). Tumorlike eosinophilic granuloma of the skin. Am J Dermatopathol 22: 75-78.
819. Gerdsen R, Lagarde C, Steen A, Steen KH, Uerlich M, Bieber T (1999). Congenital smooth muscle hamartoma of the skin: clinical classification. Acta Derm Venereol 79: 408-409.
820. Gerdsen R, Stockfleth E, Uerlich M, Fartasch M, Steen KH, Bieber T (2000). Papular palmoplantar hyperkeratosis following chronic medical exposure to arsenic: human papillomavirus as a co-factor in the pathogenesis of arsenical keratosis? Acta Derm Venereol 80: 292-293.
821. Germain DP (2001). Co-occurrence and contribution of Fabry disease and Klippel-Trenaunay-Weber syndrome to a patient with atypical skin lesions. Clin Genet 60: 63-67.
822. Ghiorzo P, Ciotti P, Mantelli M, Heouaine A, Queirolo P, Rainero ML, Ferrari C, Santi PL, De Marchi R, Farris A, Ajmar F, Bruzzi P, Bianchi-Scarra G (1999). Characterization of ligurian melanoma families and risk of occurrence of other neoplasia. Int J Cancer 83: 441-448.
823. Giannotti B, Santucci M (1993). Skin-associated lymphoid tissue (SALT)-related B-cell lymphoma (primary cutaneous B-cell lymphoma). A concept and a clinicopathologic entity. Arch Dermatol 129: 353-355.
824. Gianotti F, Caputo R (1985). Histiocytic syndromes: a review. J Am Acad Dermatol 13: 383-404.
825. Gianotti R, Alessi E (1997). Clear cell hidradenoma associated with the folliculo-sebaceous-apocrine unit. Histologic study of five cases. Am J Dermatopathol 19: 351-357.
826. Giles FJ, O'Brien SM, Keating MJ (1998). Chronic lymphocytic leukemia in (Richter's) transformation. Semin Oncol 25: 117-125.
827. Giles GG, Armstrong BK, Burton RC, Staples MP, Thursfield VJ (1996). Has mortality from melanoma stopped rising in Australia? Analysis of trends between 1931 and 1994. BMJ 312: 1121-1125.
828. Giles GG, Marks R, Foley P (1988). Incidence of non-melanocytic skin cancer treated in Australia. Br Med J (Clin Res Ed) 296: 13-17.
829. Gilliam AC, Lessin SR, Wilson DM, Salhany KE (1997). Folliculotropic mycosis fungoides with large-cell transformation presenting as dissecting cellulitis of the scalp. J Cutan Pathol 24: 169-175.
830. Gimotty PA, Botbyl JD, Soong SJ, Guerry DIV (2005). A population-based validation of the AJCC melanoma staging system. J Clin Oncol in press.
831. Gimotty PA, Guerry D, Ming ME, Elenitsas R, Xu X, Czerniecki B, Spitz F, Schuchter L, Elder D (2004). Thin primary cutaneous malignant melanoma: a prognostic tree for 10-year metastasis is more accurate than American Joint Committee on Cancer staging. J Clin Oncol 22: 3668-3676.
832. Gimotty PA, Van Belle P, Elder DE, Murry T, Montone KT, Xu X, Hotz S, Raines S, Ming ME, Wahl PM, Guerry DIV (2005). The biologic and prognostic signifi^cance of dermal Ki-67 expression , mitoses and tumorigenicity in thin invasive cutaneous melanoma. J Clin Oncol (in press).
833. Gioglio L, Porta C, Moroni M, Nastasi G, Gangarossa I (1992). Scrotal angiokeratoma (Fordyce): histopathological and ultrastructural findings. Histol Histopathol 7: 47-55.
834. Girard C, Graham JH, Johnson WC (1974). Arteriovenous hemangioma (arteriovenous shunt). A clinicopathological and histochemical study. J Cutan Pathol 1: 73-87.
835. Giroux L, Delorme F, Bettez P (1975). [Multiple mucosal neuroma syndrome]. Union Med Can 104: 605-610.
836. Gisselbrecht C, Gaulard P, Lepage E, Coiffier B, Briere J, Haioun C, Cazals-Hatem D, Bosly A, Xerri L, Tilly H, Berger F, Bouhabdallah R, Diebold J (1998). Prognostic significance of T-cell phenotype in aggressive non-Hodgkin's lymphomas. Groupe d'Etudes des Lymphomes de l'Adulte (GELA). Blood 92: 76-82.
837. Glass J, Hochberg FH, Miller DC (1993). Intravascular lymphomatosis. A systemic disease with neurologic manifestations. Cancer 71: 3156-3164.
838. Glogau RG (2000). The risk of progression to invasive disease. J Am Acad Dermatol 42: 23-24.
839. Gloor P, Ansari I, Sinard J (1999). Sebaceous carcinoma presenting as a unilateral papillary conjunctivitis. Am J Ophthalmol 127: 458-459.
840. Glusac EJ, McNiff JM (1999). Epithelioid cell histiocytoma: a simulant of vascular and melanocytic neoplasms. Am J Dermatopathol 21: 1-7.
841. Goble RR, Frangoulis MA (1990). Lymphangioma circumscriptum of the eyelids and conjunctiva. Br J Ophthalmol 74: 574-575.
842. Godbolt AM, Sullivan JJ, Weedon D (2001). Keratoacanthoma with perineural invasion: a report of 40 cases. Australas J Dermatol 42: 168-171.
843. Goessling W, McKee PH, Mayer RJ (2002). Merkel cell carcinoma. J Clin Oncol 20: 588-598.
844. Goette DK (1980). Benign lichenoid keratosis. Arch Dermatol 116: 780-782.
845. Goette DK (1988). Hidradenoma papilliferum. J Am Acad Dermatol 19: 133-135.
846. Goette DK, McConnell MA, Fowler VR (1982). Cylindroma and eccrine spiradenoma coexistent in the same lesion. Arch Dermatol 118: 274.
847. Goette DK, Odom RB, Fitzwater JEJr (1982). Diffuse cutaneous reticulohistiocytosis. Arch Dermatol 118: 173-176.
848. Gogusev J, Telvi L, Murakami I, Lepelletier Y, Nezelof C, Stojkoski A, Glorion C, Jaubert F (2005). DOR-1, A novel CD10+ stromal cell line derived from progressive Langerhans cell histiocytosis of bone. Pediatr Blood Cancer 44: 128-137.
849. Goldberg NS, Bauer BS, Kraus H, Crussi FG, Esterly NB (1988). Infantile myofibromatosis: a review of clinicopathology with perspectives on new treatment choices. Pediatr Dermatol 5: 37-46.
850. Goldberg NS, Hebert AA, Esterly NB (1986). Sacral hemangiomas and multiple congenital abnormalities. Arch Dermatol 122: 684-687.
851. Goldblum JR, Hart WR (1997). Vulvar Paget's disease: a clinicopathologic and immunohistochemical study of 19 cases. Am J Surg Pathol 21: 1178-1187.
852. Goldblum JR, Hart WR (1998). Perianal Paget's disease: a histologic and immunohistochemical study of 11 cases with and without associated rectal adenocarcinoma. Am J Surg Pathol 22: 170-179.
853. Goldblum JR, Reith JD, Weiss SW (2000). Sarcomas arising in dermatofibrosarcoma protuberans: a reappraisal of biologic behavior in eighteen cases treated by wide local excision with extended clinical follow up. Am J Surg Pathol 24: 1125-1130.
854. Golden N, Maliawan S, Mulyadi K (2000). Cellular blue naevus of the scalp with brain invasion. J Clin Neurosci 7: 453-454.
855. Goldenberger D, Zbinden R, Perschil I, Altwegg M (1996). [Detection of Bartonella (Rochalimaea) henselae/B. quintana by polymerase chain reaction (PCR)]. Schweiz Med Wochenschr 126: 207-213.
856. Goldenhersh MA, Savin RC, Barnhill RL, Stenn KS (1988). Malignant blue nevus. Case report and literature review. J Am Acad Dermatol 19: 712-722.
857. Goldman L, Gibson SH, Richfield DF (1981). Thrombotic angiokeratoma circumscriptum simulating melanoma. Arch Dermatol 117: 138-139.
858. Goldman RL (1981). Blue naevus of lymph node capsule: report of a unique case. Histopathology 5: 445-450.
859. Goldstein AM, Fraser MC, Struewing JP, Hussussian CJ, Ranade K, Zametkin DP, Fontaine LS, Organic SM, Dracopoli NC, Clark WHJr, Tucker MA (1995). Increased risk of pancreatic cancer in melanoma-prone kindreds with p16INK4 mutations. N Engl J Med 333: 970-974.
859A. Goldstein AM, Liu L, Shennan MG, Hogg D, Tucker MA, Struewing JP (2001). A common founder for the V126D CDKN2A mutation in seven North American melanoma-prone families. Br J Cancer 85: 527-530.
860. Goldstein AM, Martinez M, Tucker MA, Demenais F (2000). Gene-covariate interaction between dysplastic nevi and the CDKN2A gene in American melanoma-prone families. Cancer Epidemiol Biomarkers Prev 9: 889-894.
861. Goldstein DJ, Barr RJ, Santa Cruz DJ (1982). Microcystic adnexal carcinoma: a distinct clinicopathologic entity. Cancer 50: 566-572.
862. Gomez CS, Calonje E, Ferrar DW, Browse NL, Fletcher CD (1995). Lymphangiomatosis of the limbs. Clinicopathologic analysis of a series with a good prognosis. Am J Surg Pathol 19: 125-133.
863. Gonzalez CL, Medeiros LJ, Braziel RM, Jaffe ES (1991). T-cell lymphoma involving subcutaneous tissue. A clinicopathologic entity commonly associated with hemophagocytic syndrome. Am J Surg Pathol 15: 17-27.
864. Goodlad JR, Krajewski AS, Batstone PJ, McKay P, White JM, Benton EC, Kavanagh GM, Lucraft HH (2002). Primary cutaneous follicular lymphoma: a clinicopathologic and molecular study of 16 cases in support of a distinct entity. Am J Surg Pathol 26: 733-741.
865. Goovaerts G, Buyssens N (1988). Nevus cell maturation or atrophy? Am J Dermatopathol 10: 20-27.
866. Gordon CJ (1991). Proliferating trichilemmal cyst in an organoid nevus. Cutis 48: 49-52.
867. Gorlin RJ (1987). Nevoid basal-cell carcinoma syndrome. Medicine (Baltimore) 66: 98-113.
868. Gorlin RJ (1995). Nevoid basal cell carcinoma syndrome. Dermatol Clin 13:

1137. Jemal A, Devesa SS, Hartge P, Tucker MA (2001). Recent trends in cutaneous melanoma incidence among whites in the United States. J Natl Cancer Inst 93: 678-683.

1138. Jensen K, Kohler S, Rouse RV (2000). Cytokeratin staining in Merkel cell carcinoma: an immunohistochemical study of cytokeratins 5/6, 7, 17, and 20. Appl Immunohistochem Mol Morphol 8: 310-315.

1139. Jensen ML, Jensen OM, Michalski W, Nielsen OS, Keller J (1996). Intradermal and subcutaneous leiomyosarcoma: a clinicopathological and immunohistochemical study of 41 cases. J Cutan Pathol 23: 458-463.

1140. Jensen NE, Sabharwal S, Walker AE (1971). Naevoxanthoendothelioma and neurofibromatosis. Br J Dermatol 85: 326-330.

1141. Jessner M, Kanoff NB (1953). Lymphocytic infiltration of the skin. Arch Dermatol 68: 447-449.

1142. Jin F, Devesa SS, Chow WH, Zheng W, Ji BT, Fraumeni JF, Jr., Gao YT (1999). Cancer incidence trends in urban shanghai, 1972-1994: an update. Int J Cancer 83: 435-440.

1143. Jin Y, Jin C, Salemark L, Wennerberg J, Persson B, Jonsson N (2002). Clonal chromosome abnormalities in premalignant lesions of the skin. Cancer Genet Cytogenet 136: 48-52.

1144. Johno M, Ohishi M, Kojo Y, Yamamoto S, Ono T (1992). Cutaneous manifestations of adult T-cell leukemia/lymphoma. Gann Monograph Cancer Res 39: 33-41.

1145. Johnson MD, Jacobs AH (1989). Congenital smooth muscle hamartoma. A report of six cases and a review of the literature. Arch Dermatol 125: 820-822.

1146. Johnson RL, Rothman AL, Xie J, Goodrich LV, Bare JW, Bonifas JM, Quinn AG, Myers RM, Cox DR, Epstein EHJr, Scott MP (1996). Human homolog of patched, a candidate gene for the basal cell nevus syndrome. Science 272: 1668-1671.

1147. Johnson TM, Saluja A, Fader D, Blum D, Cotton J, Wang TS, Lowe L (1999). Isolated extragenital bowenoid papulosis of the neck. J Am Acad Dermatol 41: 867-870.

1148. Johnson WC, Graham JH, Helwig EB (1965). Cutaneous myxoid cysts-A clinicopathological and histochemical study. JAMA 191: 15-20.

1149. Johnson WC, Helwig EB (1966). Adenoid squamous cell carcinoma (adenoacanthoma). A clinicopathologic study of 155 patients. Cancer 19: 1639-1650.

1150. Jonason AS, Kunala S, Price GJ, Restifo RJ, Spinelli HM, Persing JA, Leffell DJ, Tarone RE, Brash DE (1996). Frequent clones of p53-mutated keratinocytes in normal human skin. Proc Natl Acad Sci U S A 93: 14025-14029.

1151. Jones D, Vega F, Sarris AH, Medeiros LJ (2002). CD4-CD8-"Double-negative" cutaneous T-cell lymphomas share common histologic features and an aggressive clinical course. Am J Surg Pathol 26: 225-231.

1152. Jones EW (1966). Proliferating epidermoid cysts. Arch Dermatol 94: 11-19.

1153. Jones EW (1976). Dowling oration 1976. Malignant vascular tumours. Clin Exp Dermatol 1: 287-312.

1154. Jones EW, Bleehen SS (1969). Inflammatory angiomatous nodules with abnormal blood vessels occurring about the ears and scalp (pseudo or atypical pyogenic granuloma). Br J Dermatol 81: 804-816.

1155. Jones EW, Cerio R, Smith NP (1989). Epithelioid cell histiocytoma: a new entity. Br J Dermatol 120: 185-195.

1156. Jones EW, Orkin M (1989). Tufted angioma (angioblastoma). A benign progressive angioma, not to be confused with Kaposi's sarcoma or low-grade angiosarcoma. J Am Acad Dermatol 20: 214-225.

1157. Jones EW, Winkelmann RK, Zachary CB, Reda AM (1990). Benign lymphangioendothelioma. J Am Acad Dermatol 23: 229-235.

1158. Jones REJr (1984). What is the boundary that separates a thick solar keratosis and a thin squamous cell carcinoma? Am J Dermatopathol 6: 301-306.

1159. Jones REJr (1985). Mammary Paget's disease without underlying carcinoma. Am J Dermatopathol 7: 361-365.

1160. Jonjic N, Zamolo G, Stifter S, Fuckar D, Gruber F, Sasso F, Rizzardi C, Melato M (2003). Cytomorphological variations, proliferation and angiogenesis in the prognosis of cutaneous melanoma. Clin Exp Dermatol 28: 310-314.

1161. Joshi PC (1998). Copper(II) as an efficient scavenger of singlet molecular oxygen. Indian J Biochem Biophys 35: 208-215.

1162. Junkins-Hopkins JM (2000). Polypoid malignant acrospiroma: a clinical variant with aggressive behaviour. J Cutan Pathol 27: 561.

1163. Kaddu S, Beham-Schmid C, Zenahlik P, Kerl H, Cerroni L (1999). CD56+ blastic transformation of chronic myeloid leukemia involving the skin. J Cutan Pathol 26: 497-503.

1164. Kaddu S, Beham A, Cerroni L, Humer-Fuchs U, Salmhofer W, Kerl H, Soyer HP (1997). Cutaneous leiomyosarcoma. Am J Surg Pathol 21: 979-987.

1165. Kaddu S, Cerroni L, Pilatti A, Soyer HP, Kerl H (1994). Acral pseudolymphomatous angiokeratoma. A variant of the cutaneous pseudolymphomas. Am J Dermatopathol 16: 130-133.

1166. Kaddu S, Dong H, Mayer G, Kerl H, Cerroni L (2002). Warty dyskeratoma – "follicular dyskeratoma": analysis of clinicopathologic features of a distinctive follicular adnexal neoplasm. J Am Acad Dermatol 47: 423-428.

1167. Kaddu S, Smolle J, Cerroni L, Kerl H (1996). Prognostic evaluation of specific cutaneous infiltrates in B-chronic lymphocytic leukemia. J Cutan Pathol 23: 487-494.

1168. Kaddu S, Smolle J, Zenahlik P, Hofmann-Wellenhof R, Kerl H (2002). Melanoma with benign melanocytic naevus components: reappraisal of clinicopathological features and prognosis. Melanoma Res 12: 271-278.

1169. Kaddu S, Soyer HP, Hodl S, Kerl H (1996). Morphological stages of pilomatricoma. Am J Dermatopathol 18: 333-338.

1170. Kaddu S, Soyer HP, Wolf IH, Kerl H (1997). Proliferating pilomatricoma. A histopathologic simulator of matrical carcinoma. J Cutan Pathol 24: 228-234.

1171. Kaddu S, Soyer HP, Wolf IH, Rieger E, Kerl H (1997). [Reticular lentigo]. Hautarzt 48: 181-185.

1172. Kaddu S, Zenahlik P, Beham-Schmid C, Kerl H, Cerroni L (1999). Specific cutaneous infiltrates in patients with myelogenous leukemia: a clinicopathologic study of 26 patients with assessment of diagnostic criteria. J Am Acad Dermatol 40: 966-978.

1173. Kadin ME (1985). Common activated helper-T-cell origin for lymphomatoid papulosis, mycosis fungoides, and some types of Hodgkin's disease. Lancet 2: 864-865.

1174. Kadin ME (1990). The spectrum of Ki-1+ cutaneous lymphomas. Curr Probl Dermatol 19: 132-143.

1175. Kadin ME (1993). Lymphomatoid papulosis and associated lymphomas. How are they related? Arch Dermatol 129: 351-353.

1176. Kadin ME, Drews R, Samel A, Gilchrist A, Kocher O (2001). Hodgkin's lymphoma of T-cell type: clonal association with a CD30+ cutaneous lymphoma. Hum Pathol 32: 1269-1272.

1177. Kadin ME, Levi E, Kempf W (2001). Progression of lymphomatoid papulosis to systemic lymphoma is associated with escape from growth inhibition by transforming growth factor-beta and CD30 ligand. Ann N Y Acad Sci 941: 59-68.

1178. Kagen MH, Hirsch RJ, Chu P, McCormack PC, Weinberg JM (2000). Multiple infundibulocystic basal cell carcinomas in association with human immunodeficiency virus. J Cutan Pathol 27: 316-319.

1179. Kahn HJ, Bailey D, Marks A (2002). Monoclonal antibody D2-40, a new marker of lymphatic endothelium, reacts with Kaposi's sarcoma and a subset of angiosarcomas. Mod Pathol 15: 434-440.

1180. Kahn HJ, Fekete E, From L (2001). Tenascin differentiates dermatofibroma from dermatofibrosarcoma protuberans: comparison with CD34 and factor XIIIa. Hum Pathol 32: 50-56.

1181. Kakurai M, Yamada T, Kiyosawa T, Ohtsuki M, Nakagawa H (2003). Giant acquired digital fibrokeratoma. J Am Acad Dermatol 48: S67-S68.

1182. Kakuta M, Tsuboi R, Yamazaki M, Sakuma M, Yoshikata R, Ogawa H (1996). Giant mixed tumor of the face. J Dermatol 23: 369-371.

1183. Kalidas M, Kantarjian H, Talpaz M (2001). Chronic myelogenous leukemia. JAMA 286: 895-898.

1184. Kamb A, Shattuck-Eidens D, Eeles R, Liu Q, Gruis NA, Ding W, Hussey C, Tran T, Miki Y, Weaver-Feldhaus J, McClure M, Aitken JF, Anderson DE, Bergman W, Frants R, Goldgar DE, Green A, MacLennan R, Martin NG, Meyer LJ, Youl P, Zone JJ, Skolnick MH, Cannon-Albright LA (1994). Analysis of the p16 gene (CDKN2) as a candidate for the chromosome 9p melanoma susceptibility locus. Nat Genet 8: 23-26.

1185. Kambic V, Gale N, Radsel Z (1982). Warty dyskeratosis of the vocal cord. First reported case. Arch Otolaryngol 108: 385-387.

1186. Kamino H, Flotte TJ, Misheloff E, Greco MA, Ackerman AB (1979). Eosinophilic globules in Spitz's nevi. New findings and a diagnostic sign. Am J Dermatopathol 1: 319-324.

1187. Kamino H, Jacobson M (1990). Dermatofibroma extending into the subcutaneous tissue. Differential diagnosis from dermatofibrosarcoma protuberans. Am J Surg Pathol 14: 1156-1164.

1188. Kamino H, Lee JY, Berke A (1989). Pleomorphic fibroma of the skin: a benign neoplasm with cytologic atypia. A clinicopathologic study of eight cases. Am J Surg Pathol 13: 107-113.

1189. Kamino H, Reddy VB, Gero M, Greco MA (1992). Dermatomyofibroma. A benign cutaneous, plaque-like proliferation of fibroblasts and myofibroblasts in young adults. J Cutan Pathol 19: 85-93.

1190. Kamino H, Tam ST (1990). Compound blue nevus: a variant of blue nevus with an additional junctional dendritic component. A clinical, histopathologic, and immunohistochemical study of six cases. Arch Dermatol 126: 1330-1333.

1191. Kanavaros P, De Bruin PC, Briere J, Meijer CJ, Gaulard P (1995). Epstein-Barr virus (EBV) in extranodal T-cell non-Hodgkin's lymphomas (T-NHL). Identification of nasal T-NHL as a distinct clinicopathological entity associated with EBV. Leuk Lymphoma 18: 27-34.

1192. Kanavaros P, Ioannidou D, Tzardi M, Datseris G, Katsantonis J, Delidis G, Tosca A (1994). Mycosis fungoides: expression of C-myc p62 p53, bcl-2 and PCNA proteins and absence of association with Epstein-Barr virus. Pathol Res Pract 190: 767-774.

1193. Kanda M, Suzumiya J, Ohshima K, Haraoka S, Nakamura N, Abe M, Tamura K, Kikuchi M (2001). Analysis of the immunoglobulin heavy chain gene variable region of intravascular large B-cell lymphoma. Virchows Arch 439: 540-546.

1194. Kaneishi NK, Cockerell CJ (1998). Histologic differentiation of desmoplastic melanoma from cicatrices. Am J Dermatopathol 20: 128-134.

1195. Kang DS, Chung KY (1999). Common blue naevus with satellite lesions: possible perivascular dissemination resulting in a clinical resemblance to malignant melanoma. Br J Dermatol 141: 922-925.

1196. Kang S, Barnhill RL, Mihm MC, Jr., Sober AJ (1992). Multiple primary cutaneous melanomas. Cancer 70: 1911-1916.

1197. Kang S, Milton GW, Sober AJ (1992). Childhood melanoma. In: Cutaneous Melanoma, Balch CM, Houghton AN, Milton GW, eds., 2nd ed. JB Lippincott: Philadelphia , p. 312.

1198. Kang WH, Chun SI, Lee S (1987). Generalized anhidrosis associated with Fabry's disease. J Am Acad Dermatol 17: 883-887.

1199. Kanitakis J, Brutzkus A, Butnaru AC, Claudy A (2002). Melanotrichoblastoma: immunohistochemical study of a variant of pigmented trichoblastoma. Am J Dermatopathol 24: 498-501.

1199A. Kannengiesser C, Avril MF, Spatz A, Laud K, Lenoir GM, Bressac-de-Paillerets B (2003) CDKN2A as a uveal and cutaneous melanoma susceptibility gene. Genes Chromosomes Cancer 38: 265-268

1200. Kanold J, Vannier JP, Fusade T, Drouin V, Thomine E, Prudent M, Tron P (1994). [Langerhans-cell histiocytosis in twin sisters]. Arch Pediatr 1: 49-53.

1201. Kanter L, Blegen H, Wejde J, Lagerlof B, Larsson O (1995). Utility of a proliferation marker in distinguishing between benign naevocellular naevi and naevocellular naevus-like lesions with malignant properties. Melanoma Res 5: 345-350.

1202. Kanzler MH, Mraz-Gernhard S (2001). Primary cutaneous malignant melanoma and its precursor lesions: diagnostic and therapeutic overview. J Am Acad Dermatol 45: 260-276.

1203. Kao GF (1986). Carcinoma arising in Bowen's disease. Arch Dermatol 122: 1124-1126.

1204. Kao GF, Farmer EV (1999). Benign tumors and carcinoma in situ of the skin. In: Pathology of the Skin, Farmer ER, Hood AF, eds., 2nd ed. McGraw Hill Professional: New York , pp. 931-968.

1205. Kao GF, Helwig EB, Graham JH (1987). Aggressive digital papillary adeno-

ma and adenocarcinoma. A clinicopathological study of 57 patients, with histochemical, immunopathological, and ultrastructural observations. J Cutan Pathol 14: 129-146.
1206. Kao GF, Laskin WB, Weiss SW (1990). Eccrine spiradenoma occurring in infancy mimicking mesenchymal tumor. J Cutan Pathol 17: 214-219.
1207. Kaplan EN (1974). The risk of malignancy in large congenital nevi. Plast Reconstr Surg 53: 421-428.
1208. Karagas MR (1994). Occurrence of cutaneous basal cell and squamous cell malignancies among those with a prior history of skin cancer. The Skin Cancer Prevention Study Group. J Invest Dermatol 102: 10S-13S.
1209. Karenko L, Hyytinen E, Sarna S, Ranki A (1997). Chromosomal abnormalities in cutaneous T-cell lymphoma and in its premalignant conditions as detected by G-banding and interphase cytogenetic methods. J Invest Dermatol 108: 22-29.
1210. Karenko L, Kahkonen M, Hyytinen ER, Lindlof M, Ranki A (1999). Notable losses at specific regions of chromosomes 10q and 13q in the Sezary syndrome detected by comparative genomic hybridization. J Invest Dermatol 112: 392-395.
1211. Kari L, Loboda A, Nebozhyn M, Rook AH, Vonderheid EC, Nichols C, Virok D, Chang C, Horng WH, Johnston J, Wysocka M, Showe MK, Showe LC (2003). Classification and prediction of survival in patients with the leukemic phase of cutaneous T cell lymphoma. J Exp Med 197: 1477-1488.
1212. Karimipour DJ, Johnson TM, Kang S, Wang TS, Lowe L (1997). Mucinous carcinoma of the skin. J Am Acad Dermatol 36: 323-326.
1213. Kashani-Sabet M, Sagebiel RW, Ferreira CM, Nosrati M, Miller JR, III (2001). Vascular involvement in the prognosis of primary cutaneous melanoma. Arch Dermatol 137: 1169-1173.
1214. Kashima M, Adachi M, Honda M, Niimura M, Nakabayashi Y (1994). A case of peculiar plantar warts. Human papillomavirus type 60 infection. Arch Dermatol 130: 1418-1420.
1215. Katane M, Akiyama M, Ohnishi T, Watanabe S, Matsuo I (2003). Carcinomatous transformation of eccrine syringofibroadenoma. J Cutan Pathol 30: 211-214.
1216. Kato N, Onozuka T, Yasukawa K, Kimura K, Sasaki K (2000). Penile hybrid verrucous-squamous carcinoma associated with a superficial inguinal lymph node metastasis. Am J Dermatopathol 22: 339-343.
1217. Kato N, Ueno H (1992). Eccrine hidrocystoma: two cases of Robinson and Smith types. J Dermatol 19: 493-497.
1218. Kato N, Ueno H (1993). Infundibulocystic basal cell carcinoma. Am J Dermatopathol 15: 265-267.
1219. Kato N, Yasukawa K, Onozuka T (1998). Primary cutaneous adenoid cystic carcinoma with lymph node metastasis. Am J Dermatopathol 20: 571-577.
1220. Kato T, Kumasaka N, Suetake T, Tabata N, Tagami H (1996). Clinicopathological study of acral melanoma in situ in 44 Japanese patients. Dermatology 193: 192-197.
1221. Kato T, Suetake T, Sugiyama Y, Tabata N, Tagami H (1996). Epidemiology and prognosis of subungual melanoma in 34 Japanese patients. Br J Dermatol 134: 383-387.
1222. Katsourakis M, Kapranos N, Papanicolaou SI, Patrikiou A (1996). Nerve-sheath myxoma (neurothekeoma) of the oral cavity: a case report and review of the literature. J Oral Maxillofac Surg 54: 904-906.
1223. Katzenstein AL, Carrington CB, Liebow AA (1979). Lymphomatoid granulomatosis: a clinicopathologic study of 152 cases. Cancer 43: 360-373.
1224. Katzenstein AL, Peiper SC (1990). Detection of Epstein-Barr virus genomes in lymphomatoid granulomatosis: analysis of 29 cases by the polymerase chain reaction technique. Mod Pathol 3: 435-441.
1225. Kaudewitz P, Burg G (1991). Lymphomatoid papulosis and Ki-1 (CD30)-positive cutaneous large cell lymphomas. Semin Diagn Pathol 8: 117-124.
1226. Kaudewitz P, Burg G, Stein H (1990). Ki-1 (CD30) positive cutaneous anaplastic large cell lymphomas. Curr Probl Dermatol 19: 150-156.
1227. Kaudewitz P, Burg G, Stein H, Klepzig K, Mason DY, Braun-Falco O (1985). Monoclonal antibody patterns in lymphomatoid papulosis. Dermatol Clin 3: 749-757.
1228. Kaudewitz P, Stein H, Dallenbach F, Eckert F, Bieber K, Burg G, Braun-Falco O (1989). Primary and secondary cutaneous Ki-1+ (CD30+) anaplastic large cell lymphomas. Morphologic, immunohistologic, and clinical-characteristics. Am J Pathol 135: 359-367.
1229. KAUFFMAN SL, Stout AP (1965). CONGENITAL MESENCHYMAL TUMORS. Cancer 18: 460-476.
1230. Kaufman DK, Kimmel DW, Parisi JE, Michels VV (1993). A familial syndrome with cutaneous malignant melanoma and cerebral astrocytoma. Neurology 43: 1728-1731.
1231. Kavanagh GM, Rigby HS, Archer CB (1993). Giant primary mucinous sweat gland carcinoma of the scalp. Clin Exp Dermatol 18: 375-377.
1232. Kawabata Y, Tamaki K (1998). Distinctive dermatoscopic features of acral lentiginous melanoma in situ from plantar melanocytic nevi and their histopathologic correlation. J Cutan Med Surg 2: 199-204.
1233. Kayaselcuk F, Ceken I, Bircan S, Tuncer I (2002). Bacillary angiomatosis of the scalp in a human immunodeficiency virus-negative patient. J Eur Acad Dermatol Venereol 16: 612-614.
1234. Kazakov DV, Burg G, Kempf W (2004). Clinicopathological spectrum of mycosis fungoides. J Eur Acad Dermatol Venereol 18: 397-415.
1235. Kazakov DV, Kutzner H, Rutten A, Mukensnabl P, Michal M (2005). Carcinoid-like pattern in sebaceous neoplasms: another distinctive, previously unrecognized pattern in extraocular sebaceous carcinoma and sebaceoma. Am J Dermatopathol 27: 195-203.
1236. Kazakov DV, Mentzel T, Burg G, Dummer R, Kempf W (2003). Blastic natural killer-cell lymphoma of the skin associated with myelodysplastic syndrome or myelogenous leukaemia: a coincidence or more? Br J Dermatol 149: 869-876.
1237. Keasbey LE, Hadley CG (1954). Clear-cell hidradenoma. Report of three cases with widespread metastases. Cancer 7: 934-952.
1238. Kefford R, Bishop JN, Tucker M, Bressac de Paillerets B, Bianchi-Scarra G, Bergman W, Goldstein A, Puig S, Mackie R, Elder D, Hansson J, Hayward N, Hogg D, Olsson H (2002). Genetic testing for melanoma. Lancet Oncol 3: 653-654.
1239. Kefford RF, Newton Bishop JA, Bergman W, Tucker MA (1999). Counseling and DNA testing for individuals perceived to be genetically predisposed to melanoma: A consensus statement of the Melanoma Genetics Consortium. J Clin Oncol 17: 3245-3251.
1240. Kelfkens G, Bregman A, de Gruijl FR, van der Leun JC, Piquet A, van Oijen T, Gieskes WWC, van Loveren H, Velders GJM, Martens P, Slaper H (2002). Ozone layer - climate change interactions: Influence on UV levels and UV related effects. RIVM: Bilthoven.
1241. Kempf W, Haeffner AC, Zepter K, Sander CA, Flaig MJ, Mueller B, Panizzon RG, Hardmeier T, Adams V, Burg G (2002). Angiolymphoid hyperplasia with eosinophilia: evidence for a T-cell lymphoproliferative origin. Hum Pathol 33: 1023-1029.
1242. Kempf W, Kadin ME, Dvorak AM, Lord CC, Burg G, Letvin NL, Koralnik IJ (2003). Endogenous retroviral elements, but not exogenous retroviruses, are detected in CD30-positive lymphoproliferative disorders of the skin. Carcinogenesis 24: 301-306.
1243. Kempf W, Levi E, Kamarashev J, Kutzner H, Pfeifer W, Petrogiannis-Haliotis T, Burg G, Kadin ME (2002). Fascin expression in CD30-positive cutaneous lymphoproliferative disorders. J Cutan Pathol 29: 295-300.
1244. Kennedy RH, Waller RR, Carney JA (1987). Ocular pigmented spots and eyelid myxomas. Am J Ophthalmol 104: 533-538.
1245. Kerl H, Smolle J, Hodl S, Soyer HP (1989). [Congenital pseudomelanoma]. Z Hautkr 64: 564, 567-564, 568.
1246. Kerl H, Trau H, Ackerman AB (1984). Differentiation of melanocytic nevi from malignant melanomas in palms, soles, and nail beds solely by signs in the cornified layer of the epidermis. Am J Dermatopathol 6 Suppl: 159-160.
1247. Kerr DA (21951). Granuloma pyogenicum. Oral Surg Oral Med Oral Pathol 4: 158-176.
1248. Kerschmann RL, Berger TG, Weiss LM, Herndier BG, Abrahms KM, Heon V, Schulze K, Kaplan LD, Resnik SD, LeBoit PE (1995). Cutaneous presentations of lymphoma in human immunodeficiency virus disease. Predominance of T cell lineage. Arch Dermatol 131: 1281-1288.
1249. Kersting DW (2003). Clear cell hidradenoma and hidradenoarcinoma. Arch Dermatol 87: 323-333.
1250. Kersting DW, Helwig EB (1956). Eccrine spiradenoma. Arch Dermatol 73: 199-227.
1251. Kesmodel SB, Karakousis GC, Botbyl JD, Canter RJ, Lewis RT, Wahl PM, Terhune KP, Alavi A, Elder DE, Ming ME, Guerry D, Gimotty PA, Fraker DL, Czerniecki BJ, Spitz FR (2005). Mitotic rate as a predictor of sentinel lymph node positivity in patients with thin melanomas. Ann Surg Oncol 12: 449-458.
1252. Ketron LW, Goodman MH (1931). Multiple lesions of the skin apparently of epithelial origin resembling clinically mycosis fungoides. Arch Dermatol 24: 758-777.
1253. Khalidi HS, Brynes RK, Browne P, Koo CH, Battifora H, Medeiros LJ (1998). Intravascular large B-cell lymphoma: the CD5 antigen is expressed by a subset of cases. Mod Pathol 11: 983-988.
1254. Khanna M, Fortier-Riberdy G, Smoller B, Dinehart S (2002). Reporting tumor thickness for cutaneous squamous cell carcinoma. J Cutan Pathol 29: 321-323.
1255. Khlat M, Vail A, Parkin M, Green A (1992). Mortality from melanoma in migrants to Australia: variation by age at arrival and duration of stay. Am J Epidemiol 135: 1103-1113.
1256. Khoo SK, Bradley M, Wong FK, Hedblad MA, Nordenskjold M, Teh BT (2001). Birt-Hogg-Dube syndrome: mapping of a novel hereditary neoplasia gene to chromosome 17p12-q11.2. Oncogene 20: 5239-5242.
1257. Khoury H, Lestou VS, Gascoyne RD, Bruyere H, Li CH, Nantel SH, Dalal BI, Naiman SC, Horsman DE (2003). Multicolor karyotyping and clinicopathological analysis of three intravascular lymphoma cases. Mod Pathol 16: 716-724.
1258. Khoury JD, Medeiros LJ, Manning JT, Sulak LE, Bueso-Ramos C, Jones D (2002). CD56(+) TdT(+) blastic natural killer cell tumor of the skin: a primitive systemic malignancy related to myelomonocytic leukemia. Cancer 94: 2401-2408.
1259. Kibar Z, Der Kaloustian V, Brais B, Hani V, Fraser FC, Rouleau GA (1996). The gene responsible for Clouston hidrotic ectodermal dysplasia maps to the pericentromeric region of chromosome 13q. Hum Mol Genet 5: 543-547.
1260. Kikuchi I (1980). Mongolian spots remaining in schoolchildren a statistical survey in Central Okinawa. J Dermatol 7: 213-216.
1261. Kikuchi I, Inoue S (1980). Natural history of the Mongolian spot. J Dermatol 7: 449-450.
1262. Kilkenny M, Merlin K, Young R, Marks R (1998). The prevalence of common skin conditions in Australian school students: 1. Common, plane and plantar viral warts. Br J Dermatol 138: 840-845.
1263. Kim BK, Surti U, Pandya AG, Swerdlow SH (2003). Primary and secondary cutaneous diffuse large B-cell lymphomas: a multiparameter analysis of 25 cases including fluorescence in situ hybridization for t(14;18) translocation. Am J Surg Pathol 27: 356-364.
1264. Kim KJ, Lee MW, Choi JH, Sung KJ, Moon KC, Koh JK (2001). A case of congenital tufted angioma mimicking cavernous hemangioma. J Dermatol 28: 514-515.
1265. Kim MY, Park HJ, Baek SC, Byun DG, Houh D (2002). Mutations of the p53 and PTCH gene in basal cell carcinomas: UV mutation signature and strand bias. J Dermatol Sci 29: 1-9.
1266. Kim S, Elenitsas R, James WD (2002). Diffuse dermal angiomatosis: a variant of reactive angioendotheliomatosis associated with peripheral vascular atherosclerosis. Arch Dermatol 138: 456-458.
1267. Kim TH, Choi EH, Ahn SK, Lee SH (1999). Vascular tumors arising in port-wine stains: two cases of pyogenic granuloma and a case of acquired tufted angioma. J Dermatol 26: 813-816.
1268. Kim YC, Lee MG, Choe SW, Lee MC, Chung HG, Cho SH (2003). Acral lentiginous melanoma: an immunohistochemical study of 20 cases. Int J Dermatol 42: 123-129.
1269. Kim YC, Vandersteen DP, Chung YJ, Myong NH (2001). Signet ring cell basal cell carcinoma: a basal cell carcinoma with myoepithelial differentiation. Am J Dermatopathol 23: 525-529.
1270. Kim YD, Lee EJ, Song MH, Suhr KB, Lee JH, Park JK (2002). Multiple eccrine hidrocystomas associated with Graves'

disease. Int J Dermatol 41: 295-297.

1271. Kim YH, Chow S, Varghese A, Hoppe RT (1999). Clinical characteristics and long-term outcome of patients with generalized patch and/or plaque (T2) mycosis fungoides. Arch Dermatol 135: 26-32.

1272. Kim YK, Kim HJ, Lee KG (1992). Acquired tufted angioma associated with pregnancy. Clin Exp Dermatol 17: 458-459.

1273. Kimonis VE, Goldstein AM, Pastakia B, Yang ML, Kase R, DiGiovanna JJ, Bale AE, Bale SJ (1997). Clinical manifestations in 105 persons with nevoid basal cell carcinoma syndrome. Am J Med Genet 69: 299-308.

1274. Kimura S, Hirai A, Harada R, Nagashima M (1978). So-called multicentric pigmented Bowen's disease. Report of a case and a possible etiologic role of human papilloma virus. Dermatologica 157: 229-237.

1275. Kimura T, Miyazawa H, Aoyagi T, Ackerman AB (1991). Folliculosebaceous cystic hamartoma. A distinctive malformation of the skin. Am J Dermatopathol 13: 213-220.

1276. Kimyai-Asadi A, Nousari HC, Ketabchi N, Henneberry JM, Costarangos C (1999). Diffuse dermal angiomatosis: a variant of reactive angioendotheliomatosis associated with atherosclerosis. J Am Acad Dermatol 40: 257-259.

1277. Kindblom LG, Stenman G, Angervall L (1991). Morphological and cytogenetic studies of angiosarcoma in Stewart-Treves syndrome. Virchows Arch A Pathol Anat Histopathol 419: 439-445.

1278. Kingdon EJ, Phillips BB, Jarmulowicz M, Powis SH, Vanderpump MP (2001). Glomeruloid haemangioma and POEMS syndrome. Nephrol Dial Transplant 16: 2105-2107.

1279. Kint A, Baran R (1988). Histopathologic study of Koenen tumors. Are they different from acquired digital fibrokeratoma? J Am Acad Dermatol 18: 369-372.

1280. Kint A, Baran R, De Keyser H (1985). Acquired (digital) fibrokeratoma. J Am Acad Dermatol 12: 816-821.

1281. Kirkham N (2000). Optimal handling and criteria for melanoma diagnosis. Histopathology 37: 467-469.

1282. Kirnbauer R, Lenz P, Okun MM (2003). Human papillomaviruses. In: Dermatology, Bolognia JL, Jorizzo JL, eds., Mosby Publishers: pp. 1217-1233.

1283. Kirova YM, Piedbois Y, Le Bourgeois JP (1999). Radiotherapy in the management of cutaneous B-cell lymphoma. Our experience in 25 cases. Radiother Oncol 52: 15-18.

1284. Kirschner LS, Sandrini F, Monbo J, Lin JP, Carney JA, Stratakis CA (2000). Genetic heterogeneity and spectrum of mutations of the PRKAR1A gene in patients with the carney complex. Hum Mol Genet 9: 3037-3046.

1285. Kishimoto S, Takenaka H, Shibagaki R, Noda Y, Yamamoto M, Yasuno H (2000). Glomeruloid hemangioma in POEMS syndrome shows two different immunophenotypic endothelial cells. J Cutan Pathol 27: 87-92.

1286. Kittler H, Binder M (2001). Risks and benefits of sequential imaging of melanocytic skin lesions in patients with multiple atypical nevi. Arch Dermatol 137: 1590-1595.

1287. Kleihues P, Cavenee WK (2000). World Health Organization Classification of Tumours. Pathology and Genetics of Tumours of the Nervous System. IARC Press: Lyon.

1288. Klein U, Tu Y, Stolovitzky GA, Mattioli M, Cattoretti G, Husson H, Freedman A, Inghirami G, Cro L, Baldini L, Neri A, Califano A, Dalla-Favera R (2001). Gene expression profiling of B cell chronic lymphocytic leukemia reveals a homogeneous phenotype related to memory B cells. J Exp Med 194: 1625-1638.

1289. Kleinegger CL, Hammond HL, Vincent SD, Finkelstein MW (2000). Acquired tufted angioma: a unique vascular lesion not previously reported in the oral mucosa. Br J Dermatol 142: 794-799.

1290. Knable A, Treadwell P (1996). Pigmented plaque with hypertrichosis on the scalp of an infant. Pediatr Dermatol 13: 431-433.

1291. Knipper JE, Hud JA, Cockerell CJ (1993). Disseminated epidermolytic acanthoma. Am J Dermatopathol 15: 70-72.

1292. Knoell KA, Nelson KC, Patterson JW (1998). Familial multiple blue nevi. J Am Acad Dermatol 39: 322-325.

1293. Knudsen H, Gronbaek K, thor SP, Gisselo C, Johansen P, Timshel S, Bergmann OJ, Hansen NE, Ralfkiaer E (2002). A case of lymphoblastoid natural killer (NK)-cell lymphoma: association with the NK-cell receptor complex CD94/NKG2 and TP53 intragenic deletion. Br J Dermatol 146: 148-153.

1294. Koch MB, Shih IM, Weiss SW, Folpe AL (2001). Microphthalmia transcription factor and melanoma cell adhesion molecule expression distinguish desmoplastic/spindle cell melanoma from morphologic mimics. Am J Surg Pathol 25: 58-64.

1295. Koh D, Wang H, Lee J, Chia KS, Lee HP, Goh CL (2003). Basal cell carcinoma, squamous cell carcinoma and melanoma of the skin: analysis of the Singapore Cancer Registry data 1968-97. Br J Dermatol 148: 1161-1166.

1296. Koh HK, Michalik E, Sober AJ, Lew RA, Day CL, Clark W, Mihm MC, Kopf AW, Blois MS, Fitzpatrick TB (1984). Lentigo maligna melanoma has no better prognosis than other types of melanoma. J Clin Oncol 2: 994-1001.

1297. Kohler S, Rouse RV, Smoller BR (1998). The differential diagnosis of pagetoid cells in the epidermis. Mod Pathol 11: 79-92.

1298. Kohler S, Smoller BR (1996). Gross cystic disease fluid protein-15 reactivity in extramammary Paget's disease with and without associated internal malignancy. Am J Dermatopathol 18: 118-123.

1299. Koizumi H, Kodama K, Tsuji Y, Matsumura T, Nabeshima M, Ohkawara A (1999). CD34-positive dendritic cells are an intrinsic part of smooth muscle hamartoma. Br J Dermatol 140: 172-174.

1300. Koizumi K, Sawada K, Nishio M, Katagiri E, Fukae J, Fukada Y, Tarumi T, Notoya A, Shimizu T, Abe R, Kobayashi H, Koike T (1997). Effective high-dose chemotherapy followed by autologous peripheral blood stem cell transplantation in a patient with the aggressive form of cytophagic histiocytic panniculitis. Bone Marrow Transplant 20: 171-173.

1301. Kojima M, Sakuma H, Mori N (1983). Histopathological features of plasma cell dyscrasia with polyneuropathy and endocrine disturbances, with special reference to germinal center lesions. Jpn J Clin Oncol 13: 557-575.

1302. Kolde G, Brocker EB (1986). Multiple skin tumors of indeterminate cells in an adult. J Am Acad Dermatol 15: 591-597.

1303. Kolmel KF, Grange JM, Krone B, Mastrangelo G, Rossi CR, Henz BM, Seebacher C, Botev IN, Niin M, Lambert D, Shafir R, Kokoschka EM, Kleeberg UR, Gefeller O, Pfahlberg A (2005). Prior immunisation of patients with malignant melanoma with vaccinia or BCG is associated with better survival. An European Organization for Research and Treatment of Cancer cohort study on 542 patients. Eur J Cancer 41: 118-125.

1304. Komine M, Hattori N, Tamaki K (2000). Eccrine syringofibroadenoma (Mascaro): an immunohistochemical study. Am J Dermatopathol 22: 171-175.

1305. Kopf AW, Bart RS (1977). Tumor conference No. 11: multiple bowenoid papules of the penis: a new entity? J Dermatol Surg Oncol 3: 265-269.

1306. Kopf AW, Bart RS, Hennessey P (1979). Congenital nevocytic nevi and malignant melanomas. J Am Acad Dermatol 1: 123-130.

1307. Kopf AW, Weidman AI (1962). Nevus of Ota. Arch Dermatol 85: 195-208.

1308. Korabiowska M, Brinck U, Middel P, Brinkmann U, Berger H, Radzun HJ, Ruschenburg I, Droese M (2000). Proliferative activity in the progression of pigmented skin lesions, diagnostic and prognostic significance. Anticancer Res 20: 1781-1785.

1309. Kore-eda S, Tanaka T, Moriwaki S, Nishigori C, Imamura S (1992). A case of xeroderma pigmentosum group A diagnosed with a polymerase chain reaction (PCR) technique. Usefulness of PCR in the detection of point mutation in a patient with a hereditary disease. Arch Dermatol 128: 971-974.

1310. Kornberg R, Ackerman AB (1975). Pseudomelanoma: recurrent melanocytic nevus following partial surgical removal. Arch Dermatol 111: 1588-1590.

1311. Korsmeyer SJ, Arnold A, Bakhshi A, Ravetch JV, Siebenlist U, Hieter PA, Sharrow SO, LeBien TW, Kersey JH, Poplack DG, Leder P, Waldmann TA (1983). Immunoglobulin gene rearrangement and cell surface antigen expression in acute lymphocytic leukemias of T cell and B cell precursor origins. J Clin Invest 71: 301-313.

1312. Kort R, Fazaa B, Bouden S, Nikkels AF, Pierard GE, Kamoun MR (1995). Perianal basal cell carcinoma. Int J Dermatol 34: 427-428.

1313. Kossard S (2002). Atypical lentiginous junctional naevi of the elderly and melanoma. Australas J Dermatol 43: 93-101.

1314. Kossard S, Kumar A, Wilkinson B (1999). Neural spectrum: palisaded encapsulated neuroma and verocay body poor dermal schwannoma. J Cutan Pathol 26: 31-36.

1315. Kossard S, Rosen R (1992). Cutaneous Bowen's disease. An analysis of 1001 cases according to age, sex, and site. J Am Acad Dermatol 27: 406-410.

1316. Kossard S, Wilkinson B (1995). Nucleolar organizer regions and image analysis nuclear morphometry of small cell (nevoid) melanoma. J Cutan Pathol 22: 132-136.

1317. Kossard S, Wilkinson B (1997). Small cell (naevoid) melanoma: a clinicopathologic study of 131 cases. Australas J Dermatol 38 Suppl 1: S54-S58.

1318. Koutlas IG, Jessurun J (1994). Arteriovenous hemangioma: a clinicopathological and immunohistochemical study. J Cutan Pathol 21: 343-349.

1319. Kraemer KH (1977). Progressive degenerative diseases associated with defective DNA repair: xeroderma pigmentosum and ataxia telangiesctasia. 37-71.

1320. Kraemer KH, Greene MH, Tarone R, Elder DE, Clark WHJr, Guerry D (1983). Dysplastic naevi and cutaneous melanoma risk. Lancet 2: 1076-1077.

1321. Kraemer KH, Lee MM, Andrews AD, Lambert WC (1994). The role of sunlight and DNA repair in melanoma and non-melanoma skin cancer. The xeroderma pigmentosum paradigm. Arch Dermatol 130: 1018-1021.

1322. Kraemer KH, Lee MM, Scotto J (1987). Xeroderma pigmentosum. Cutaneous, ocular, and neurologic abnormalities in 830 published cases. Arch Dermatol 123: 241-250.

1323. Kraus MD, Lind AC, Alder SL, Dehner LP (1999). Angiomatosis with angiokeratoma-like features in children: a light microscopic and immunophenotypic examination of four cases. Am J Dermatopathol 21: 350-355.

1324. Kremer M, Sandherr M, Geist B, Cabras AD, Hofler H, Fend F (2001). Epstein-Barr virus-negative Hodgkin's lymphoma after mycosis fungoides: molecular evidence for distinct clonal origin. Mod Pathol 14: 91-97.

1325. Krenacs L, Smyth MJ, Bagdi E, Krenacs T, Kopper L, Rudiger T, Zettl A, Muller-Hermelink HK, Jaffe ES, Raffeld M (2003). The serine protease granzyme M is preferentially expressed in NK-cell, gamma delta T-cell, and intestinal T-cell lymphomas: evidence of origin from lymphocytes involved in innate immunity. Blood 101: 3590-3593.

1326. Krenek G, Orengo IF, Baer S, Byrd D (1998). Desmoplastic malignant melanoma presenting as an erythematous nodule tumor. Cutis 61: 275-276.

1327. Krige JE, Isaacs S, Hudson DA, King HS, Strover RM, Johnson CA (1991). Delay in the diagnosis of cutaneous malignant melanoma. A prospective study in 250 patients. Cancer 68: 2064-2068.

1328. Krischer J, Pechere M, Salomon D, Harms M, Chavaz P, Saurat JH (1999). Interferon alfa-2b-induced Meyerson's nevi in a patient with dysplastic nevus syndrome. J Am Acad Dermatol 40: 105-106.

1329. Krivanek JF, Cains GD, Paver K (1977). Halo eczema and junctional naevi: a case report. Australas J Dermatol 18: 81-83.

1330. Krone B, Kolmel KF, Grange JM, Mastrangelo G, Henz BM, Botev IN, Niin M, Seebacher C, Lambert D, Shafir R, Kokoschka EM, Kleeberg UR, Gefeller O, Pfahlberg A (2003). Impact of vaccinations and infectious diseases on the risk of melanoma – evaluation of an EORTC case-control study. Eur J Cancer 39: 2372-2378.

1331. Krone B, Kolmel KF, Henz BM, Grange JM (2005). Protection against melanoma by vaccination with Bacille Calmette-Guerin (BCG) and/or vaccinia: an epidemiology-based hypothesis on the nature of a melanoma risk factor and its immunological control. Eur J Cancer 41: 104-117.

1332. Kruse R, Rutten A, Lamberti C, Hosseiny-Malayeri HR, Wang Y, Ruelfs C, Jungck M, Mathiak M, Ruzicka T, Hartschuh W, Bisceglia M, Friedl W, Propping P (1998). Muir-Torre phenotype has a frequency of DNA mismatch-repair-gene mutations similar to that in hereditary nonpolyposis colorectal cancer families

defined by the Amsterdam criteria. Am J Hum Genet 63: 63-70.
1333. Kruse R, Rutten A, Malayeri HR, Gunzl HJ, Friedl W, Propping P (1999). A novel germline mutation in the hMLH1 DNA mismatch repair gene in a patient with an isolated cystic sebaceous tumor. J Invest Dermatol 112: 117-118.
1334. Kruse R, Rutten A, Schweiger N, Jakob E, Mathiak M, Propping P, Mangold E, Bisceglia M, Ruzicka T (2003). Frequency of microsatellite instability in unselected sebaceous gland neoplasias and hyperplasias. J Invest Dermatol 120: 858-864.
1335. Kubo M, Kikuchi K, Nashiro K, Kakinuma T, Hayashi N, Nanko H, Tamaki K (1998). Expression of fibrogenic cytokines in desmoplastic malignant melanoma. Br J Dermatol 139: 192-197.
1336. Kubo Y, Murao K, Matsumoto K, Arase S (2002). Molecular carcinogenesis of squamous cell carcinomas of the skin. J Med Invest 49: 111-117.
1337. Kuchelmeister C, Schaumburg-Lever G, Garbe C (2000). Acral cutaneous melanoma in caucasians: clinical features, histopathology and prognosis in 112 patients. Br J Dermatol 143: 275-280.
1338. Kukita A, Ishihara K (1989). Clinical features and distribution of malignant melanoma and pigmented nevi on the soles of the feet in Japan. J Invest Dermatol 92: 210S-213S.
1339. Kulow BF, Cualing H, Steele P, VanHorn J, Breneman JC, Mutasim DF, Breneman DL (2002). Progression of cutaneous B-cell pseudolymphoma to cutaneous B-cell lymphoma. J Cutan Med Surg 6: 519-528.
1340. Kumar S, Kingma DW, Weiss WB, Raffeld M, Jaffe ES (1996). Primary cutaneous Hodgkin's disease with evolution to systemic disease. Association with the Epstein-Barr virus. Am J Surg Pathol 20: 754-759.
1341. Kumar S, Krenacs L, Medeiros J, Elenitoba-Johnson KS, Greiner TC, Sorbara L, Kingma DW, Raffeld M, Jaffe ES (1998). Subcutaneous panniculitic T-cell lymphoma is a tumor of cytotoxic T lymphocytes. Hum Pathol 29: 397-403.
1342. Kummer JA, Vermeer MH, Dukers D, Meijer CJ, Willemze R (1997). Most primary cutaneous CD30-positive lymphoproliferative disorders have a CD4-positive cytotoxic T-cell phenotype. J Invest Dermatol 109: 636-640.
1343. Kuno Y, Tsuji T, Yamamoto K (1999). Adenocarcinoma with signet ring cells of the axilla: two case reports and review of the literature. J Dermatol 26: 390-395.
1344. Kuo T (1980). Clear cell carcinoma of the skin. A variant of the squamous cell carcinoma that simulates sebaceous carcinoma. Am J Surg Pathol 4: 573-583.
1345. Kuo TT, Chan HL (1994). Ossifying dermatofibroma with osteoclast-like giant cells. Am J Dermatopathol 16: 193-195.
1346. Kuo TT, Hu S, Chan HL (1998). Keloidal dermatofibroma: report of 10 cases of a new variant. Am J Surg Pathol 22: 564-568.
1347. Kurman RJ (2002). Blaustein's Pathology of the Female Genital Tract. 5th ed. Springer: New York Berlin.
1348. Kurokawa M, Amano M, Miyaguni H, Tateyama S, Ogata K, Idemori M, Setoyama M (2001). Eccrine poromas in a patient with mycosis fungoides treated with electron beam therapy. Br J Dermatol 145: 830-833.
1349. Kurzen H, Esposito L, Langbein L, Hartschuh W (2001). Cytokeratins as markers of follicular differentiation: an immunohistochemical study of trichoblastoma and basal cell carcinoma. Am J Dermatopathol 23: 501-509.
1350. Kushida Y, Miki H, Ohmori M (1999). Loss of heterozygosity in actinic keratosis, squamous cell carcinoma and sun-exposed normal-appearing skin in Japanese: difference between Japanese and Caucasians. Cancer Lett 140: 169-175.
1351. Kutzner H, Winzer M, Mentzel T (2000). [Symplastic hemangioma]. Hautarzt 51: 327-331.
1352. Kwittken J, Negri L (1966). Malignant blue nevus. Case report of a Negro woman. Arch Dermatol 94: 64-69.
1353. La Vecchia C, Lucchini F, Negri E, Levi F (1999). Recent declines in worldwide mortality from cutaneous melanoma in youth and middle age. Int J Cancer 81: 62-66.
1354. Lack EE, Worsham GF, Callihan MD, Crawford BE, Klappenbach S, Rowden G, Chun B (1980). Granular cell tumor: a clinicopathologic study of 110 patients. J Surg Oncol 13: 301-316.
1355. Lakhani SR, Hulman G, Hall JM, Slack DN, Sloane JP (1994). Intravascular malignant lymphomatosis (angiotropic large-cell lymphoma). A case report with evidence for T-cell lineage with polymerase chain reaction analysis. Histopathology 25: 283-286.
1356. Lamberg SI, Bunn PAJr (1979). Cutaneous T-cell lymphomas. Summary of the Mycosis Fungoides Cooperative Group-National Cancer Institute Workshop. Arch Dermatol 115: 1103-1105.
1357. Lambert WC, Brodkin RH (1984). Nodal and subcutaneous cellular blue nevi. A pseudometastasizing pseudomelanoma. Arch Dermatol 120: 367-370.
1358. Lamovec J (1984). Blue nevus of the lymph node capsule. Report of a new case with review of the literature. Am J Clin Pathol 81: 367-372.
1359. Landa NG, Winkelmann RK (1991). Epidermotropic eccrine porocarcinoma. J Am Acad Dermatol 24: 27-31.
1360. Landi MT, Baccarelli A, Tarone RE, Pesatori A, Tucker MA, Hedayati M, Grossman L (2002). DNA repair, dysplastic nevi, and sunlight sensitivity in the development of cutaneous malignant melanoma. J Natl Cancer Inst 94: 94-101.
1361. Landry M, Winkelmann RK (1972). An unusual tubular apocrine adenoma. Arch Dermatol 105: 869-879.
1362. Langard S, Rosenberg J, Andersen A, Heldaas SS (2000). Incidence of cancer among workers exposed to vinyl chloride in polyvinyl chloride manufacture. Occup Environ Med 57: 65-68.
1363. Langer K, Rappersberger K, Steiner A, Konrad K, Wolff K (1990). The ultrastructure of dysplastic naevi: comparison with superficial spreading melanoma and common naevocellular naevi. Arch Dermatol Res 282: 353-362.
1364. Langholz B, Richardson J, Rappaport E, Waisman J, Cockburn M, Mack T (2000). Skin characteristics and risk of superficial spreading and nodular melanoma (United States). Cancer Causes Control 11: 741-750.
1365. Lao LM, Kumakiri M, Kiyohara T, Kuwahara H, Ueda K (2001). Sub-populations of melanocytes in pigmented basal cell carcinoma: a quantitative, ultrastructural investigation. J Cutan Pathol 28: 34-43.
1366. Lao LM, Kumakiri M, Mima H, Kuwahara H, Ishida H, Ishiguro K, Fujita T, Ueda K (1998). The ultrastructural characteristics of eccrine sweat glands in a Fabry disease patient with hypohidrosis. J Dermatol Sci 18: 109-117.
1367. Lapid O, Shaco-Levy R, Krieger Y, Kachko L, Sagi A (2001). Congenital epulis. Pediatrics 107: E22.
1368. Laroche L, Bach JF (1981). T cell imbalance in nonleukemic and leukemic cutaneous lymphoma defined by monoclonal antibodies. Clin Immunol Immunopathol 20: 278-284.
1369. Larralde M, Rositto A, Giardelli M, Gatti CF, Santos MA (1999). Congenital self-healing histiocytosis (Hashimoto-Pritzker). Int J Dermatol 38: 693-696.
1370. Laskin WB, Fetsch JF, Miettinen M (2000). The "neurothekeoma": immunohistochemical analysis distinguishes the true nerve sheath myxoma from its mimics. Hum Pathol 31: 1230-1241.
1371. Lasota J, Miettinen M (1999). Absence of Kaposi's sarcoma-associated virus (human herpesvirus-8) sequences in angiosarcoma. Virchows Arch 434: 51-56.
1372. Laugier P, Hunziker N, Laut J, Orusco M, Osmos L (1975). [Reticulohistiocytosis of benign evolution (Hashimoto-Pritzker type). Electron microscopy study]. Ann Dermatol Syphiligr (Paris) 102: 21-31.
1373. Laur WE, Posey RE, Waller JD (1981). Lichen planus-like keratosis. A clinicohistopathologic correlation. J Am Acad Dermatol 4: 329-336.
1374. Laws RA, English JCI, Elston DM (1996). Acrospiroma: a case report and review. Cutis 58: 349-351.
1375. Lazar AP, Caro WA, Roenigk HHJr, Pinski KS (1989). Parapsoriasis and mycosis fungoides: the Northwestern University experience, 1970 to 1985. J Am Acad Dermatol 21: 919-923.
1376. Lazarou G, Goldberg MI (2000). Vulvar arteriovenous hemangioma. A case report. J Reprod Med 45: 439-441.
1377. Leake JF, Buscema J, Cho KR, Currie JL (1991). Dermatofibrosarcoma protuberans of the vulva. Gynecol Oncol 41: 245-249.
1378. Lear JT, Smith AG, Heagerty AH, Bowers B, Jones PW, Gilford J, Alldersea J, Strange RC, Fryer AA (1997). Truncal site and detoxifying enzyme polymorphisms significantly reduce time to presentation of further primary cutaneous basal cell carcinoma. Carcinogenesis 18: 1499-1503.
1379. LeBoit PE (1994). Granulomatous slack skin. Dermatol Clin 12: 375-389.
1380. LeBoit PE (2003). Pictures of a unicorn? Am J Dermatopathol 25: 88-91.
1381. LeBoit PE, Barr RJ (1994). Smooth-muscle proliferation in dermatofibromas. Am J Dermatopathol 16: 155-160.
1382. LeBoit PE, Beckstead JH, Bond B, Epstein WL, Frieden IJ, Parslow TG (1987). Granulomatous slack skin: clonal rearrangement of the T-cell receptor beta gene is evidence for the lymphoproliferative nature of a cutaneous elastolytic disorder. J Invest Dermatol 89: 183-186.
1383. LeBoit PE, Berger TG, Egbert BM, Beckstead JH, Yen TS, Stoler MH (1989). Bacillary angiomatosis. The histopathology and differential diagnosis of a pseudoneoplastic infection in patients with human immunodeficiency virus disease. Am J Surg Pathol 13: 909-920.
1384. LeBoit PE, Crutcher WA, Shapiro PE (1992). Pagetoid intraepidermal spread in Merkel cell (primary neuroendocrine) carcinoma of the skin. Am J Surg Pathol 16: 584-592.
1385. LeBoit PE, Solomon AR, Santa Cruz DJ, Wick MR (1992). Angiomatosis with luminal cryoprotein deposition. J Am Acad Dermatol 27: 969-973.
1386. LeBoit PE, Van Fletcher H (1987). A comparative study of Spitz nevus and nodular malignant melanoma using image analysis cytometry. J Invest Dermatol 88: 753-757.
1387. LeBoit PE, Zackheim HS, White CRJr (1988). Granulomatous variants of cutaneous T-cell lymphoma. The histopathology of granulomatous mycosis fungoides and granulomatous slack skin. Am J Surg Pathol 12: 83-95.
1388. Lee AY, Kawashima M, Nakagawa H, Ishibashi Y (1991). Generalized eruptive syringoma. J Am Acad Dermatol 25: 570-571.
1389. Lee CS, Southey MC, Slater H, Auldist AW, Chow CW, Venter DJ (1995). Primary cutaneous Ewing's sarcoma/ peripheral primitive neuroectodermal tumors in childhood. A molecular, cytogenetic, and immunohistochemical study. Diagn Mol Pathol 4: 174-181.
1390. Lee ES, Locker J, Nalesnik M, Reyes J, Jaffe R, Alashari M, Nour B, Tzakis A, Dickman PS (1995). The association of Epstein-Barr virus with smooth-muscle tumors occurring after organ transplantation. N Engl J Med 332: 19-25.
1391. Lee HH, Lee KG (1998). Malignant eccrine spiradenoma with florid squamous differentiation. J Korean Med Sci 13: 191-195.
1392. Lee J, Bhawan J, Wax F, Farber J (1994). Plexiform granular cell tumor. A report of two cases. Am J Dermatopathol 16: 537-541.
1393. Lee JA, Carter AP (1970). Secular trends in mortality from malignant melanoma. J Natl Cancer Inst 45: 91-97.
1394. Lee JB, Kim M, Lee SC, Won YH (2000). Granuloma pyogenicum arising in an arteriovenous haemangioma associated with a port-wine stain. Br J Dermatol 143: 669-671.
1395. Lee PK, Olbricht SM, Gonzalez-Serva A, Harrist TH (1997). rative squamous cell carcinoma: histopathologic and clinical characterizatoin of a newly described skin cancer. J Cutan Pathol 24: 108.
1396. Leffell DJ (2000). The scientific basis of skin cancer. J Am Acad Dermatol 42: 18-22.
1397. Leinweber B, Colli C, Chott A, Kerl H, Cerroni L (2004). Differential diagnosis of cutaneous infiltrates of B lymphocytes with follicular growth pattern. Am J Dermatopathol 26: 4-13.
1398. Leitinger G, Cerroni L, Soyer HP, Smolle J, Kerl H (1990). Morphometric diagnosis of melanocytic skin tumors. Am J Dermatopathol 12: 441-445.
1399. Lele SM, Gloster ES, Heilman ER, Chen PC, Chen CK, Anzil AP, Pozner JN, Reardon MJ (1997). Eccrine syringofibroadenoma surrounding a squamous cell carcinoma: a case report. J Cutan Pathol 24: 193-196.
1400. Lenane P, Keane CO, Connell BO, Loughlin SO, Powell FC (2000). Genital melanotic macules: clinical, histologic, immunohistochemical, and ultrastructural features. J Am Acad Dermatol 42: 640-644.
1401. Lennert K, Parwaresch MR (1979). Mast cells and mast cell neoplasia: a review. Histopathology 3: 349-365.
1402. Leopold JG, Richards DB (1968). The interrelationship of blue and common naevi. J Pathol Bacteriol 95: 37-46.
1403. Lerchin E, Rahbari H (1975). Adamantinoid basal cell epithelioma. A histological variant. Arch Dermatol 111: 586-

588.

1404. Lerner AB, Nordlund JJ, Kirkwood JM (1979). Effects of oral contraceptives and pregnancy on melanomas. N Engl J Med 301: 47.

1405. Lesher JLJr, Allen BS (1984). Multicentric reticulohistiocytosis. J Am Acad Dermatol 11: 713-723.

1406. Leshin B, Whitaker DC, Foucar E (1986). Lymphangioma circumscriptum following mastectomy and radiation therapy. J Am Acad Dermatol 15: 1117-1119.

1407. Levanat S, Gorlin RJ, Fallet S, Johnson DR, Fantasia JE, Bale AE (1996). A two-hit model for developmental defects in Gorlin syndrome. Nat Genet 12: 85-87.

1408. Levanat S, Pavelic B, Crnic I, Oreskovic S, Manojlovic S (2000). Involvement of PTCH gene in various noninflammatory cysts. J Mol Med 78: 140-146.

1409. Lever L, Marks R (1989). The significance of the Darier-like solar keratosis and acantholytic change in preneoplastic lesions of the epidermis. Br J Dermatol 120: 383-389.

1410. Lever LR, Farr PM (1994). Skin cancers or premalignant lesions occur in half of high-dose PUVA patients. Br J Dermatol 131: 215-219.

1411. Levi F, Erler G, Te VC, Randimbison L, La Vecchia C (2001). Trends in skin cancer incidence in Neuchatel, 1976-98. Tumori 87: 288-289.

1412. Levi F, Te VC, Randimbison L, Erler G, La Vecchia C (2001). Trends in skin cancer incidence in Vaud: an update, 1976-1998. Eur J Cancer Prev 10: 371-373.

1413. Levisohn D, Seidel D, Phelps A, Burgdorf W (1993). Solitary congenital indeterminate cell histiocytoma. Arch Dermatol 129: 81-85.

1414. Lew S, Richter S, Jelin N, Siegal A (1991). A blue naevus of the prostate: a light microscopic study including an investigation of S-100 protein positive cells in the normal and in the diseased gland. Histopathology 18: 443-448.

1415. Lewis MG (1967). Malignant melanoma in Uganda. (The relationship between pigmentation and malignant melanoma on the soles of the feet). Br J Cancer 21: 483-495.

1416. Lewis MG, Johnson K (1968). The incidence and distribution of pigmented naevi in Ugandan Africans. Br J Dermatol 80: 362-366.

1417. Lewis MG, Kiryabwire JW (1968). Aspects of behavior and natural history of malignant melanoma in Uganda. Cancer 21: 876-887.

1418. Li C, Inagaki H, Kuo TT, Hu S, Okabe M, Eimoto T (2003). Primary cutaneous marginal zone B-cell lymphoma: a molecular and clinicopathologic study of 24 asian cases. Am J Surg Pathol 27: 1061-1069.

1419. Li DM, Sun H (1997). TEP1, encoded by a candidate tumor suppressor locus, is a novel protein tyrosine phosphatase regulated by transforming growth factor beta. Cancer Res 57: 2124-2129.

1420. Li G, Salhany KE, Rook AH, Lessin SR (1997). The pathogenesis of large cell transformation in cutaneous T-cell lymphoma is not associated with t(2;5)(p23;q35) chromosomal translocation. J Cutan Pathol 24: 403-408.

1421. Li J, Yen C, Liaw D, Podsypanina K, Bose S, Wang SI, Puc J, Miliaresis C, Rodgers L, McCombie R, Bigner SH, Giovanella BC, Ittmann M, Tycko B, Hibshoosh H, Wigler MH, Parsons R (1997). PTEN, a putative protein tyrosine phosphatase gene mutated in human brain, breast, and prostate cancer. Science 275: 1943-1947.

1422. Li JY, Gaillard F, Moreau A, Harousseau JL, Laboisse C, Milpied N, Bataille R, Avet-Loiseau H (1999). Detection of translocation t(11;14)(q13;q32) in mantle cell lymphoma by fluorescence in situ hybridization. Am J Pathol 154: 1449-1452.

1423. Li S, Griffin CA, Mann RB, Borowitz MJ (2001). Primary cutaneous T-cell-rich B-cell lymphoma: clinically distinct from its nodal counterpart? Mod Pathol 14: 10-13.

1424. Liaw D, Marsh DJ, Li J, Dahia PL, Wang SI, Zheng Z, Bose S, Call KM, Tsou HC, Peacocke M, Eng C, Parsons R (1997). Germline mutations of the PTEN gene in Cowden disease, an inherited breast and thyroid cancer syndrome. Nat Genet 16: 64-67.

1425. Lieberman PH, Jones CR, Steinman RM, Erlandson RA, Smith J, Gee T, Huvos A, Garin-Chesa P, Filippa DA, Urmacher C, Gangi MD, Sperber M (1996). Langerhans cell (eosinophilic) granulomatosis. A clinicopathologic study encompassing 50 years. Am J Surg Pathol 20: 519-552.

1426. Liebow AA, Carrington CR, Friedman PJ (1972). Lymphomatoid granulomatosis. Hum Pathol 3: 457-558.

1427. Lim SC, Lee MJ, Lee MS, Kee KH, Suh CH (1998). Giant hidradenocarcinoma: a report of malignant transformation from nodular hidradenoma. Pathol Int 48: 818-823.

1428. Lin CS, Wang WJ, Wong CK (1990). Acral melanoma. A clinicopathologic study of 28 patients. Int J Dermatol 29: 107-112.

1429. Lin P, Jones D, Dorfman DM, Medeiros LJ (2000). Precursor B-cell lymphoblastic lymphoma: a predominantly extranodal tumor with low propensity for leukemic involvement. Am J Surg Pathol 24: 1480-1490.

1430. Lindelof B, Sigurgeirsson B, Wallberg P, Eklund G (1991). Occurrence of other malignancies in 1973 patients with basal cell carcinoma. J Am Acad Dermatol 25: 245-248.

1431. Link MP, Roper M, Dorfman RF, Crist WM, Cooper MD, Levy R (1983). Cutaneous lymphoblastic lymphoma with pre-B markers. Blood 61: 838-841.

1432. Lipford EHJr, Margolick JB, Longo DL, Fauci AS, Jaffe ES (1988). Angiocentric immunoproliferative lesions: a clinicopathologic spectrum of post-thymic T-cell proliferations. Blood 72: 1674-1681.

1433. Lipsker DM, Hedelin G, Heid E, Grosshans EM, Cribier BJ (1999). Striking increase of thin melanomas contrasts with stable incidence of thick melanomas. Arch Dermatol 135: 1451-1456.

1434. Liu JC, Ball SF (1991). Nevus of Ota with glaucoma: report of three cases. Ann Ophthalmol 23: 286-289.

1435. Liu L, Dilworth D, Gao L, Monzon J, Summers A, Lassam N, Hogg D (1999). Mutation of the CDKN2A 5' UTR creates an aberrant initiation codon and predisposes to melanoma. Nat Genet 21: 128-132.

1436. Liu Y (1949). The histogenesis of clear-cell papillary carcinoma of the skin. Am J Pathol 25: 93-103.

1437. Lloyd AC (2000). p53: only ARF the story. Nat Cell Biol 2: E48-E50.

1438. Lloyd KM (1970). Multicentric pigmented Bowen's disease of the groin. Arch Dermatol 101: 48-51.

1439. Lloyd KM, Dennis M (196). Cowden's disease: A possible new symptom complex with multiple system involvement. Ann Intern Med 58: 136-142.

1440. Lo JS, Snow SN, Reizner GT, Mohs FE, Larson PO, Hruza GJ (1991). Metastatic basal cell carcinoma: report of twelve cases with a review of the literature. J Am Acad Dermatol 24: 715-719.

1441. Loane J, Kealy WF, Mulcahy G (1998). Perianal hidradenoma papilliferum occurring in a male: a case report. Ir J Med Sci 167: 26-27.

1442. Lober BA, Lober CW (2000). Actinic keratosis is squamous cell carcinoma. South Med J 93: 650-655.

1443. Lober BA, Lober CW, Accola J (2000). Actinic keratosis is squamous cell carcinoma. J Am Acad Dermatol 43: 881-882.

1444. Lohmann CM, Coit DG, Brady MS, Berwick M, Busam KJ (2002). Sentinel lymph node biopsy in patients with diagnostically controversial spitzoid melanocytic tumors. Am J Surg Pathol 26: 47-55.

1445. Longaker MA, Frieden IJ, LeBoit PE, Sherertz EF (1994). Congenital "self-healing" Langerhans cell histiocytosis: the need for long-term follow-up. J Am Acad Dermatol 31: 910-916.

1446. Longley BJ, Metcalfe DD (2000). A proposed classification of mastocytosis incorporating molecular genetics. Hematol Oncol Clin North Am 14: 697-701, viii.

1447. Longley BJ, Reguera MJ, Ma Y (2001). Classes of c-KIT activating mutations: proposed mechanisms of action and implications for disease classification and therapy. Leuk Res 25: 571-576.

1448. Longley BJ, Tyrrell L, Lu SZ, Ma YS, Langley K, Ding TG, Duffy T, Jacobs P, Tang LH, Modlin I (1996). Somatic c-KIT activating mutation in urticaria pigmentosa and aggressive mastocytosis: establishment of clonality in a human mast cell neoplasm. Nat Genet 12: 312-314.

1449. Longley BJJr, Metcalfe DD, Tharp M, Wang X, Tyrrell L, Lu SZ, Heitjan D, Ma Y (1999). Activating and dominant inactivating c-KIT catalytic domain mutations in distinct clinical forms of human mastocytosis. Proc Natl Acad Sci U S A 96: 1609-1614.

1450. Longley J, Duffy TP, Kohn S (1995). The mast cell and mast cell disease. J Am Acad Dermatol 32: 545-561.

1451. Longy M, Lacombe D (1996). Cowden disease. Report of a family and review. Ann Genet 39: 35-42.

1452. Lonsdale RN, Widdison A (1992). Leiomyosarcoma of the nipple. Histopathology 20: 537-539.

1453. Lopez-Guillermo A, Cid J, Salar A, Lopez A, Montalban C, Castrillo JM, Gonzalez M, Ribera JM, Brunet S, Garcia-Conde J, Fernandez dS, Bosch F, Montserrat E (1998). Peripheral T-cell lymphomas: initial features, natural history, and prognostic factors in a series of 174 patients diagnosed according to the R.E.A.L. Classification. Ann Oncol 9: 849-855.

1454. Lopriore E, Markhorst DG (1999). Diffuse neonatal haemangiomatosis: new views on diagnostic criteria and prognosis. Acta Paediatr 88: 93-97.

1455. Lowe D, Fletcher CD, Shaw MP, McKee PH (1984). Eosinophil infiltration in keratoacanthoma and squamous cell carcinoma of the skin. Histopathology 8: 619-625.

1456. Lu D, Patel KA, Duvic M, Jones D (2002). Clinical and pathological spectrum of CD8-positive cutaneous T-cell lymphomas. J Cutan Pathol 29: 465-472.

1457. Lucas P, Bogomeletz WV, Cattan A (1984). [Cutaneous localization of Hodgkin's disease. Description of 4 cases and review of the literature]. Sem Hop 60: 749-754.

1458. Lund HZ (1957). Tumors of the skin. Armed Forces Institute of Pathology: Washington.

1459. Lund HZ (1965). How often does squamous cell carcinoma of the skin metastasize? Arch Dermatol 92: 635-637.

1460. Lund KA, Parker CM, Norins AL, Tejada E (1990). Vesicular cutaneous T cell lymphoma presenting with gangrene. J Am Acad Dermatol 23: 1169-1171.

1461. Lundquist K, Kohler S, Rouse RV (1999). Intraepidermal cytokeratin 7 expression is not restricted to Paget cells but is also seen in Toker cells and Merkel cells. Am J Surg Pathol 23: 212-219.

1462. Luz FB, Gaspar TAP, Kalil-Gaspar N, Ramos-e-Silva M (2001). Multicentric reticulohistiocytosis. J Eur Acad Dermatol Venereol 15: 524-531.

1463. Lymboussaki A, Partanen TA, Olofsson B, Thomas-Crusells J, Fletcher CD, de Waal RM, Kaipainen A, Alitalo K (1998). Expression of the vascular endothelial growth factor C receptor VEGFR-3 in lymphatic endothelium of the skin and in vascular tumors. Am J Pathol 153: 395-403.

1464. Lynch ED, Ostermeyer EA, Lee MK, Arena JF, Ji H, Dann J, Swisshelm K, Suchard D, MacLeod PM, Kvinnsland S, Gjertsen BT, Heimdal K, Lubs H, Moller P, King MC (1997). Inherited mutations in PTEN that are associated with breast cancer, cowden disease, and juvenile polyposis. Am J Hum Genet 61: 1254-1260.

1465. Ma Y, Zeng S, Metcalfe DD, Akin C, Dimitrijevic S, Butterfield JH, McMahon G, Longley BJ (2002). The c-KIT mutation causing human mastocytosis is resistant to STI571 and other KIT kinase inhibitors; kinases with enzymatic site mutations show different inhibitor sensitivity profiles than wild-type kinases and those with regulatory-type mutations. Blood 99: 1741-1744.

1466. Macaulay WL (1968). Lymphomatoid papulosis. A continuing self-healing eruption, clinically benign – histologically malignant. Arch Dermatol 97: 23-30.

1467. Macgrogan G, Vergier B, Dubus P, Beylot-Barry M, Belleannee G, Delaunay MM, Eghbali H, Beylot C, Rivel J, Trojani M, Vital C, de Mascarel A, Bloch B, Merlio JP (1996). CD30-positive cutaneous large cell lymphomas. A comparative study of clinicopathologic and molecular features of 16 cases. Am J Clin Pathol 105: 440-450.

1468. Machin P, Catasus L, Pons C, Munoz J, Conde-Zurita JM, Balmana J, Barnadas M, Marti RM, Prat J, Matias-Guiu X (2002). Microsatellite instability and immunostaining for MSH-2 and MLH-1 in cutaneous and internal tumors from patients with the Muir-Torre syndrome. J Cutan Pathol 29: 415-420.

1469. Machin P, Catasus L, Pons C, Munoz J, Conde-Zurita JM, Balmana J, Barnadas M, Marti RM, Prat J, Matias-Guiu X (2002). Microsatellite instability and immunostaining for MSH-2 and MLH-1 in cutaneous and internal tumors from patients with the Muir-Torre syndrome. J Cutan Pathol 29: 415-420.

1470. Mackenzie DH (1957). A clear-cell hidradenocarcinoma with metastases. Cancer 10: 1021-1023.

1471. MacKie RM (2000). Malignant melanoma: clinical variants and prognostic indicators. Clin Exp Dermatol 25: 471-475.

1472. MacKie RM, Bray CA, Hole DJ,

Morris A, Nicolson M, Evans A, Doherty V, Vestey J (2002). Incidence of and survival from malignant melanoma in Scotland: an epidemiological study. Lancet 360: 587-591.

1473. MacKie RM, English J, Aitchison TC, Fitzsimons CP, Wilson P (1985). The number and distribution of benign pigmented moles (melanocytic naevi) in a healthy British population. Br J Dermatol 113: 167-174.

1474. MacKie RM, McHenry P, Hole D (1993). Accelerated detection with prospective surveillance for cutaneous malignant melanoma in high-risk groups. Lancet 341: 1618-1620.

1475. Macmillan A, Champion RH (1971). Progressive capillary haemangioma. Br J Dermatol 85: 492-493.

1476. MacSweeney F, Desai SA (2000). Inflammatory pseudotumour of the sub-cutis: a report on the fine needle aspiration findings in a case misdiagnosed cytologically as malignant. Cytopathology 11: 57-60.

1477. Maeda Y, Izutani T, Yonese J, Ishikawa Y, Fukui I (1998). Pyogenic granuloma of the glans penis. Br J Urol 82: 771-772.

1478. Maehama T, Dixon JE (1998). The tumor suppressor, PTEN/MMAC1, dephosphorylates the lipid second messenger, phosphatidylinositol 3,4,5-trisphosphate. J Biol Chem 273: 13375-13378.

1479. Magana M, Sangueza P, Gil-Beristain J, Sanchez-Sosa S, Salgado A, Ramon G, Sangueza OP (1998). Angiocentric cutaneous T-cell lymphoma of childhood (hydroa-like lymphoma): a distinctive type of cutaneous T-cell lymphoma. J Am Acad Dermatol 38: 574-579.

1480. Maggini M, Petrelli G (1984). Malignant melanoma mortality in Italy: 1955-1978. Eur J Cancer Clin Oncol 20: 1321-1323.

1481. Magnus K (1973). Incidence of malignant melanoma of the skin in Norway, 1955-1970. Variations in time and space and solar radiation. Cancer 32: 1275-1286.

1482. Magnus K (1981). Habits of sun exposure and risk of malignant melanoma: an analysis of incidence rates in Norway 1955-1977 by cohort, sex, age, and primary tumor site. Cancer 48: 2329-2335.

1483. Magrath IT, Bhatia K (1997). Pathogenesis of small noncleaved cell lymphomas (Burkitt's lymphoma). In: The Non-Hodgkin's Lymphomas, Magrath IT, ed., Arnold: London , pp. 385-409.

1484. Magro CM, Crowson AN, Kovatich AJ, Burns F (2001). Lupus profundus, indeterminate lymphocytic lobular panniculitis and subcutaneous T-cell lymphoma: a spectrum of subcuticular T-cell lymphoid dyscrasia. J Cutan Pathol 28: 235-247.

1485. Mahalingam M, Bhawan J, Finn R, Stefanato CM (2001). Tumor of the follicular infundibulum with sebaceous differentiation. J Cutan Pathol 28: 314-317.

1486. Mahalingam M, Goldberg LJ (2001). Atypical pilar leiomyoma: cutaneous counterpart of uterine symplastic leiomyoma? Am J Dermatopathol 23: 299-303.

1487. Mahalingam M, LoPiccolo D, Byers HR (2001). Expression of PGP 9.5 in granular cell nerve sheath tumors: an immunohistochemical study of six cases. J Cutan Pathol 28: 282-286.

1487A. Mahre E (1963). Malignant melanomas in children. Arch Pathol Microbiol Scand 59: 184-193.

1488. Maiorana A, Nigrisoli E, Papotti M (1986). Immunohistochemical markers of sweat gland tumors. J Cutan Pathol 13: 187-196.

1489. Maitra A, McKenna RW, Weinberg AG, Schneider NR, Kroft SH (2001). Precursor B-cell lymphoblastic lymphoma. A study of nine cases lacking blood and bone marrow involvement and review of the literature. Am J Clin Pathol 115: 868-875.

1490. Maize JC, Jr., McCalmont TH, Carlson JA, Busam KJ, Kutzner H, Bastian BC (2005). Genomic Analysis of Blue Nevi and Related Dermal Melanocytic Proliferations. Am J Surg Pathol 29: 1214-1220.

1491. Majewski S, Jablonska S (1995). Epidermodysplasia verruciformis as a model of human papillomavirus-induced genetic cancer of the skin. Arch Dermatol 131: 1312-1318.

1492. Majewski S, Jablonska S (2002). Do epidermodysplasia verruciformis human papillomaviruses contribute to malignant and benign epidermal proliferations? Arch Dermatol 138: 649-654.

1493. Maldonado JL, Fridlyand J, Patel H, Jain AN, Busam K, Kageshita T, Ono T, Albertson D, Pinkel D, Bastian BC (2003). Determinants of BRAF mutations in primary melanomas. J Natl Cancer Inst 95: 1878-1890.

1494. Maldonado JL, Timmerman L, Fridlyand J, Bastian BC (2004). Mechanisms of cell-cycle arrest in Spitz nevi with constitutive activation of the MAP-kinase pathway. Am J Pathol 164: 1783-1787.

1495. Maloney ME, Jones DB, Sexton FM (1992). Pigmented basal cell carcinoma: investigation of 70 cases. J Am Acad Dermatol 27: 74-78.

1496. Mambo NC (1983). Eccrine spiradenoma: clinical and pathologic study of 49 tumors. J Cutan Pathol 10: 312-320.

1496A. Mancianti ML, Clark WH, Hayes FA, Herlyn M (1990). Malignant melanoma simulants arising in congenital melanocytic nevi do not show experimental evidence for a malignant phenotype. Am J Pathol 136: 817-829.

1497. Mancini L, Gubinelli M, Fortunato C, Carella R (1992). Blue nevus of the lymph node capsule. Report of a case. Pathologica 84: 547-550.

1498. Mancini RE, Quaife JV (1962). Histogenesis of experimentally produced keloids. J Invest Dermatol 38: 143-181.

1499. Manente L, Cotellessa C, Schmitt I, Peris K, Torlone G, Muda AO, Romano MC, Chementi S (1997). Indeterminate cell histiocytosis: a rare histiocytic disorder. Am J Dermatopathol 19: 276-283.

1500. Mangini J, Li N, Bhawan J (2002). Immunohistochemical markers of melanocytic lesions: a review of their diagnostic usefulness. Am J Dermatopathol 24: 270-281.

1501. Mansson-Brahme E, Johansson H, Larsson O, Rutqvist LE, Ringborg U (2002). Trends in incidence of cutaneous malignant melanoma in a Swedish population 1976-1994. Acta Oncol 41: 138-146.

1502. Manstein CH, Gottlieb N, Manstein ME, Manstein G (2000). Giant basal cell carcinoma: a series of seven T3 tumors without metastasis. Plast Reconstr Surg 106: 653-656.

1503. Mao X, Lillington D, Child F, Russell-Jones R, Young B, Whittaker S (2002). Comparative genomic hybridization analysis of primary cutaneous B-cell lymphomas: identification of common genomic alterations in disease pathogenesis. Genes Chromosomes Cancer 35: 144-155.

1504. Mao X, Lillington D, Scarisbrick JJ,

Mitchell T, Czepulkowski B, Russell-Jones R, Young B, Whittaker SJ (2002). Molecular cytogenetic analysis of cutaneous T-cell lymphomas: identification of common genetic alterations in Sezary syndrome and mycosis fungoides. Br J Dermatol 147: 464-475.

1505. Mao X, Lillington DM, Czepulkowski B, Russell-Jones R, Young BD, Whittaker S (2003). Molecular cytogenetic characterization of Sezary syndrome. Genes Chromosomes Cancer 36: 250-260.

1506. Mao X, Orchard G, Lillington DM, Russell-Jones R, Young BD, Whittaker SJ (2003). Amplification and overexpression of JUNB is associated with primary cutaneous T-cell lymphomas. Blood 101: 1513-1519.

1507. Marcil I, Stern RS (2000). Risk of developing a subsequent nonmelanoma skin cancer in patients with a history of nonmelanoma skin cancer: a critical review of the literature and meta-analysis. Arch Dermatol 136: 1524-1530.

1508. Marghoob AA (2002). Congenital melanocytic nevi. Evaluation and management. Dermatol Clin 20: 607-16, viii.

1509. Marghoob AA, Swindle LD, Moricz CZ, Sanchez Negron FA, Slue B, Halpern AC, Kopf AW (2003). Instruments and new technologies for the in vivo diagnosis of melanoma. J Am Acad Dermatol 49: 777-797.

1510. Margo CE, Grossniklaus HE (1995). Intraepithelial sebaceous neoplasia without underlying invasive carcinoma. Surv Ophthalmol 39: 293-301.

1510A. Margo CE, Mulla ZD (1998). Malignant tumors of the eyelid: a population-based study of non-basal cell and non-squamous cell malignant neoplasms. Arch Ophthalmol 116: 195-198.

1511. Margolis RJ, Tong AK, Byers HR, Mihm MCJr (1989). Comparison of acral nevomelanocytic proliferations in Japanese and whites. J Invest Dermatol 92: 222S-226S.

1512. Mariatos G, Gorgoulis VG, Laskaris G, Kittas C (1999). Epithelioid hemangioma (angiolymphoid hyperplasia with eosinophilia) in the oral mucosa. A case report and review of the literature. Oral Oncol 35: 435-438.

1513. Mariatos G, Gorgoulis VG, Laskaris G, Kittas C (2001). Epithelioid haemangioma (angiolymphoid hyperplasia with eosinophilia) in the inner canthus. J Eur Acad Dermatol Venereol 15: 90-91.

1514. Mark GJ, Mihm MC, Liteplo MG, Reed RJ, Clark WH (1973). Congenital melanocytic nevi of the small and garment type. Clinical, histologic, and ultrastructural studies. Hum Pathol 4: 395-418.

1515. Marks R (1987). Nonmelanotic skin cancer and solar keratoses. The quiet 20th century epidemic. Int J Dermatol 26: 201-205.

1516. Marks R, Foley P, Goodman G, Hage BH, Selwood TS (1986). Spontaneous remission of solar keratoses: the case for conservative management. Br J Dermatol 115: 649-655.

1517. Marks R, Rennie G, Selwood TS (1988). Malignant transformation of solar keratoses to squamous cell carcinoma. Lancet 1: 795-797.

1518. Marsden J, Allen R (1987). Widespread angiokeratomas without evidence of metabolic disease. Arch Dermatol 123: 1125-1127.

1519. Marsh DJ, Coulon V, Lunetta KL, Rocca-Serra P, Dahia PL, Zheng Z, Liaw D,

Caron S, Duboue B, Lin AY, Richardson AL, Bonnetblanc JM, Bressieux JM, Cabarrot-Moreau A, Chompret A, Demange L, Eeles RA, Yahanda AM, Fearon ER, Fricker JP, Gorlin RJ, Hodgson SV, Huson S, Lacombe D, LePrat F, Odent S, Toulouse C, Olopade OI, Sobol H, Tishler S, Woods CG, Robinson BG, Weber HC, Parsons R, Peacocke M, Longy M, Eng C (1998). Mutation spectrum and genotype-phenotype analyses in Cowden disease and Bannayan-Zonana syndrome, two hamartoma syndromes with germline PTEN mutation. Hum Mol Genet 7: 507-515.

1520. Marsh DJ, Dahia PL, Zheng Z, Liaw D, Parsons R, Gorlin RJ, Eng C (1997). Germline mutations in PTEN are present in Bannayan-Zonana syndrome. Nat Genet 16: 333-334.

1521. Marsh DJ, Kum JB, Lunetta KL, Bennett MJ, Gorlin RJ, Ahmed SF, Bodurtha J, Crowe C, Curtis MA, Dasouki M, Dunn T, Feit H, Geraghty MT, Graham JMJr, Hodgson SV, Hunter A, Korf BR, Manchester D, Miesfeldt S, Murday VA, Nathanson KL, Parisi M, Pober B, Romano C, Tolmie JL, Trembath R, Winter RM, Zackai EH, Zori RT, Weng LP, Dahia PLM, Eng C (1999). PTEN mutation spectrum and genotype-phenotype correlations in Bannayan-Riley-Ruvalcaba syndrome suggest a single entity with Cowden syndrome. Hum Mol Genet 8: 1461-1472.

1522. Martel P, Laroche L, Courville P, Larroche C, Wechsler J, Lenormand B, Delfau MH, Bodemer C, Bagot M, Joly P (2000). Cutaneous involvement in patients with angioimmunoblastic lymphadenopathy with dysproteinemia: a clinical, immunohistological, and molecular analysis. Arch Dermatol 136: 881-886.

1523. Martin-Lopez R, Feal-Cortizas C, Fraga J (1999). Pleomorphic sclerotic fibroma. Dermatology 198: 69-72.

1524. Martin Flores-Stadler E, Gonzalez-Crussi F, Greene M, Thangavelu M, Kletzel M, Chou PM (1999). Indeterminate-cell histiocytosis: immunophenotypic and cytogenetic findings in an infant. Med Pediatr Oncol 32: 250-254.

1525. Martin RC, Edwards MJ, Cawte TG, Sewell CL, McMasters KM (2000). Basosquamous carcinoma: analysis of prognostic factors influencing recurrence. Cancer 88: 1365-1369.

1526. Martinez-Mir A, Gordon D, Horev L, Klapholz L, Ott J, Christiano AM, Zlotogorski A (2002). Multiple cutaneous and uterine leiomyomas: refinement of the genetic locus for multiple cutaneous and uterine leiomyomas on chromosome 1q42.3-43. J Invest Dermatol 118: 876-880.

1527. Marzano AV, Berti E, Paulli M, Caputo R (2000). Cytophagic histiocytic panniculitis and subcutaneous panniculitis-like T-cell lymphoma: report of 7 cases. Arch Dermatol 136: 889-896.

1528. Masback A, Olsson H, Westerdahl J, Ingvar C, Jonsson N (2001). Prognostic factors in invasive cutaneous malignant melanoma: a population-based study and review. Melanoma Res 11: 435-445.

1529. Mascaro JM (1963). Consideration sur les tumeurs fibro-epitheliales. Le syringofibroadenome. Ann Dermatol Syphilol 90: 146-153.

1530. Massa MC, Fretzin DF, Chowdhury L, Sweet DL (1984). Angiolymphoid hyperplasia demonstrating extensive skin and mucosal lesions controlled with vinblastine therapy. J Am Acad Dermatol 11: 333-339.

1531. Massi D, Carli P, Franchi A, Santucci

M (1999). Naevus-associated melanomas: cause or chance? Melanoma Res 9: 85-91.
1532. Massi G, LeBoit PE (2004). Histology of Naevi and Melanoma. Steinkopff Verlag: Darmstadt, Berlin.
1533. Massone C, Chott A, Metze D, Kerl K, Citarella L, Vale E, Kerl H, Cerroni L (2004). Subcutaneous, blastic natural killer (NK), NK/T-cell, and other cytotoxic lymphomas of the skin: a morphologic, immunophenotypic, and molecular study of 50 patients. Am J Surg Pathol 28: 719-735.
1534. Mathers ME, O'Donnell M (2000). Squamous cell carcinoma of skin with a rhabdoid phenotype: a case report. J Clin Pathol 53: 868-870.
1535. Mathews GJ, Osterholm JL (1972). Painful traumatic neuromas. Surg Clin North Am 52: 1313-1324.
1536. Mathiak M, Rutten A, Mangold E, Fischer HP, Ruzicka T, Friedl W, Propping P, Kruse R (2002). Loss of DNA mismatch repair proteins in skin tumors from patients with Muir-Torre syndrome and MSH2 or MLH1 germline mutations: establishment of immunohistochemical analysis as a screening test. Am J Surg Pathol 26: 338-343.
1537. Mathis ED, Honningford JB, Rodriguez HE, Wind KP, Connolly MM, Podbielski FJ (2001). Malignant proliferating trichilemmal tumor. Am J Clin Oncol 24: 351-353.
1538. Matt D, Xin H, Vortmeyer AO, Zhuang Z, Burg G, Boni R (2000). Sporadic trichoepithelioma demonstrates deletions at 9q22.3. Arch Dermatol 136: 657-660.
1539. Mazoujian G, Pinkus GS, Haagensen DEJr (1984). Extramammary Paget's disease – evidence for an apocrine origin. An immunoperoxidase study of gross cystic disease fluid protein-15, carcinoembryonic antigen, and keratin proteins. Am J Surg Pathol 8: 43-50.
1540. Mazur MT, Shultz JJ, Myers JL (1990). Granular cell tumor. Immunohistochemical analysis of 21 benign tumors and one malignant tumor. Arch Pathol Lab Med 114: 692-696.
1541. McAlvany JP, Jorizzo JL, Zanolli D, Auringer S, Prichard E, Krowchuk DP, Turner S (1993). Magnetic resonance imaging in the evaluation of lymphangioma circumscriptum. Arch Dermatol 129: 194-197.
1542. McBride SR, Leonard N, Reynolds NJ (2002). Loss of p21(WAF1) compartmentalisation in sebaceous carcinoma compared with sebaceous hyperplasia and sebaceous adenoma. J Clin Pathol 55: 763-766.
1543. McCalmont TH (1996). A call for logic in the classification of adnexal neoplasms. Am J Dermatopathol 18: 103-109.
1544. McCalmont TH (1998). Analysis of the anatomic distribution of adnexal neoplasms suggests a preponderance of lesions of folliculosebaceous lineage. J Cut Pathol 25: 506.
1545. McCalmont TH, Brinsko R, LeBoit PE (1991). Melanocytic acral nevi with intraepidermal ascent of cells (MANIACs): A reappraisal of melanocytic lesions from acral sites. J Cut Pathol 18: 378.
1546. McCalmont TH, Salmon PJM, Geisse JK, Grekin RG (1997). Desmoplastic squamous and adenosquamous carcinoma. 60 examples of an overlooked pattern of epithelial malignancy. J Cutan Pathol 24: 111.
1546A. McCarthy SW, Scolyer RA, Palmer AA (2004). Desmoplastic melanoma: a diagnostic trap for the unwary. Pathology 36: 445-451
1547. McClain KL, Leach CT, Jenson HB, Joshi VV, Pollock BH, Parmley RT, DiCarlo FJ, Chadwick EG, Murphy SB (1995). Association of Epstein-Barr virus with leiomyosarcomas in children with AIDS. N Engl J Med 332: 12-18.
1548. McCluggage WG, Fon LJ, O'Rourke D, Ismail M, Hill CM, Parks TG, Allen DC (1997). Malignant eccrine spiradenoma with carcinomatous and sarcomatous elements. J Clin Pathol 50: 871-873.
1549. McCluggage WG, Walsh MY, Bharucha H (1998). Anaplastic large cell malignant lymphoma with extensive eosinophilic or neutrophilic infiltration. Histopathology 32: 110-115.
1550. McCormack CJ, Kelly JW, Dorevitch AP (1997). Differences in age and body site distribution of the histological subtypes of basal cell carcinoma. A possible indicator of differing causes. Arch Dermatol 133: 593-596.
1551. McDonagh JER (1912). A contribution to our knowledge of the naevoxanthoendothelioma. Br J Dermatol 24: 85-99.
1552. McGovern TW, Litaker MS (1992). Clinical predictors of malignant pigmented lesions. A comparison of the Glasgow seven-point checklist and the American Cancer Society's ABCDs of pigmented lesions. J Dermatol Surg Oncol 18: 22-26.
1553. McGovern VJ (1983). Melanocytic lesions of glabrous skin. In: Melanoma: Histological Diagnosis and Prognosis, McGovern VJ, ed., Raven Press: New York , pp. 125-136.
1554. McGregor JM, Crook T, Fraser-Andrews EA, Rozycka M, Crossland S, Brooks L, Whittaker SJ (1999). Spectrum of p53 gene mutations suggests a possible role for ultraviolet radiation in the pathogenesis of advanced cutaneous lymphomas. J Invest Dermatol 112: 317-321.
1555. McKee PH, Fletcher CD, Stavrinos P, Pambakian H (1990). Carcinosarcoma arising in eccrine spiradenoma. A clinicopathologic and immunohistochemical study of two cases. Am J Dermatopathol 12: 335-343.
1556. McKee PH, Wilkinson JD, Black MM, Whimster IW (1981). Carcinoma (epithelioma) cuniculatum: a clinico-pathological study of nineteen cases and review of the literature. Histopathology 5: 425-436.
1557. McKinley E, Valles R, Bang R, Bocklage T (1998). Signet-ring squamous cell carcinoma: a case report. J Cutan Pathol 25: 176-181.
1558. McLelland J, Chu T (1988). Dermatofibrosarcoma protuberans arising in a BCG vaccination scar. Arch Dermatol 124: 496-497.
1559. McMenamin ME, Fletcher CD (2002). Reactive angioendotheliomatosis: a study of 15 cases demonstrating a wide clinicopathologic spectrum. Am J Surg Pathol 26: 685-697.
1560. McNiff JM, Cooper D, Howe G, Crotty PL, Tallini G, Crouch J, Eisen RN (1996). Lymphomatoid granulomatosis of the skin and lung. An angiocentric T-cell-rich B-cell lymphoproliferative disorder. Arch Dermatol 132: 1464-1470.
1561. McNiff JM, Eisen RN, Glusac EJ (1999). Immunohistochemical comparison of cutaneous lymphadenoma, trichoblastoma, and basal cell carcinoma: support for classification of lymphadenoma as a variant of trichoblastoma. J Cutan Pathol 26: 119-124.
1562. McNutt NS (1998). "Triggered trap": nevoid malignant melanoma. Semin Diagn Pathol 15: 203-209.
1563. McNutt NS, Urmacher C, Hakimian J, Hoss DM, Lugo J (1995). Nevoid malignant melanoma: morphologic patterns and immunohistochemical reactivity. J Cutan Pathol 22: 502-517.
1564. Medema RH, Kops GJ, Bos JL, Burgering BM (2000). AFX-like Forkhead transcription factors mediate cell-cycle regulation by Ras and PKB through p27kip1. Nature 404: 782-787.
1565. Meeker JH, Neubecker RD, Helwig EB (1962). Hidradenoma papilliferum. Am J Clin Pathol 37: 182-195.
1566. Megahed M, Scharffetter-Kochanek K (1993). Acantholytic acanthoma. Am J Dermatopathol 15: 283-285.
1567. Mehlman MA (1991). Dangerous and cancer-causing properties of products and chemicals in the oil refining and petrochemical industry: Part I. Carcinogenicity of motor fuels: gasoline. Toxicol Ind Health 7: 143-152.
1568. Mehregan AH (1964). Apocrine cystadenoma. A clinicopathologic study with special reference to pigmented variety. Arch Dermatol 90: 274-279.
1569. Mehregan AH (1975). Lentigo senilis and its evolutions. J Invest Dermatol 65: 429-433.
1570. Mehregan AH, Brownstein MH (1978). Pilar sheath acanthoma. Arch Dermatol 114: 1495-1497.
1571. Mehregan AH, Hashimoto K, Rahbari H (1983). Eccrine adenocarcinoma. A clinicopathologic study of 35 cases. Arch Dermatol 119: 104-114.
1572. Mehregan AH, Lee KC (1987). Malignant proliferating trichilemmal tumors – report of three cases. J Dermatol Surg Oncol 13: 1339-1342.
1573. Mehregan AH, Mehregan DA (1993). Malignant melanoma in childhood. Cancer 71: 4096-4103.
1574. Mehregan DA, Gibson LE, Mehregan AH (1992). Malignant blue nevus: a report of eight cases. J Dermatol Sci 4: 185-192.
1575. Mehregan DA, Mehregan AH (1993). Deep penetrating nevus. Arch Dermatol 129: 328-331.
1576. Mehregan DR, Hamzavi F, Brown K (2003). Large cell acanthoma. Int J Dermatol 42: 36-39.
1577. Mehregan DR, Mehregan AH, Mehregan DA (1992). Benign lymphangioendothelioma: report of 2 cases. J Cutan Pathol 19: 502-505.
1578. Mejia R, Dano JA, Roberts R, Wiley E, Cockerell CJ, Cruz PDJr (1997). Langerhans' cell histiocytosis in adults. J Am Acad Dermatol 37: 314-317.
1579. Mendonca GA (1992). [Increasing risk of skin melanoma in Brazil]. Rev Saude Publica 26: 290-294.
1580. Mene A, Buckley CH (1985). Involvement of the vulval skin appendages by intraepithelial neoplasia. Br J Obstet Gynaecol 92: 634-638.
1581. Mentzel T, Calonje E, Fletcher CD (1993). Dermatomyofibroma: additional observations on a distinctive cutaneous myofibroblastic tumour with emphasis on differential diagnosis. Br J Dermatol 129: 69-73.
1582. Mentzel T, Kutzner H (2003). Haemorragic dermatomyofibroma (plaque-like dermal fibromatosis): clinicopathological and immunohistochemical analysis of three cases resembling Kaposi's sarcoma. Histopathology .
1583. Mentzel T, Kutzner H, Rutten A, Hugel H (2001). Benign fibrous histiocytoma (dermatofibroma) of the face: clinicopathologic and immunohistochemical study of 34 cases associated with an aggressive clinical course. Am J Dermatopathol 23: 419-426.
1584. Mentzel T, Partanen TA, Kutzner H (1999). Hobnail hemangioma ("targetoid hemosiderotic hemangioma"): clinicopathologic and immunohistochemical analysis of 62 cases. J Cutan Pathol 26: 279-286.
1585. Mentzel T, Requena L, Kaddu S, Soares de Aleida LM, Sangueza OP, Kutzner H (2003). Cutaneous myoepithelial neoplasms: clinicopathologic and immunohistochemical study of 20 cases suggesting a continuous spectrum ranging from benign mixed tumor of the skin to cutaneous myoepithelioma and myoepithelial carcinoma. J Cutan Pathol 30: 294-302.
1586. Mentzel T, Wadden C, Fletcher CD (1994). Granular cell change in smooth muscle tumours of skin and soft tissue. Histopathology 24: 223-231.
1587. Menzies SW, Westerhoff K, Rabinovitz H, Kopf AW, McCarthy WH, Katz B (2000). Surface microscopy of pigmented basal cell carcinoma. Arch Dermatol 136: 1012-1016.
1588. Merkow LP, Burt RC, Hayeslip DW, Newton FJ, Slifkin M, Pardo M (1969). A cellular and malignant blue nevus: a light and electron microscopic study. Cancer 24: 888-896.
1589. Mesnard JM, Devaux C (1999). Multiple control levels of cell proliferation by human T-cell leukemia virus type 1 Tax protein. Virology 257: 277-284.
1590. Metcalf JS, Maize JC, LeBoit PE (1991). Circumscribed storiform collagenoma (sclerosing fibroma). Am J Dermatopathol 13: 122-129.
1591. Metry DW, Dowd CF, Barkovich AJ, Frieden IJ (2001). The many faces of PHACE syndrome. J Pediatr 139: 117-123.
1592. Metzger S, Ellwanger U, Stroebel W, Schiebel U, Rassner G, Fierlbeck G (1998). Extent and consequences of physician delay in the diagnosis of acral melanoma. Melanoma Res 8: 181-186.
1593. Metzler G, Schaumburg-Lever G, Hornstein O, Rassner G (1996). Malignant chondroid syringoma: immunohistopathology. Am J Dermatopathol 18: 83-89.
1594. Meyer TK, Rhee JS, Smith MM, Cruz MJ, Osipov VO, Wackym PA (2003). External auditory canal eccrine spiradenocarcinoma: A case report and review of literature. Head Neck 25: 505-510.
1595. Meyerson LB (1971). A peculiar papulosquamous eruption involving pigmented nevi. Arch Dermatol 103: 510-512.
1596. Micali G, Innocenzi D, Nasca MR (1997). Cellular blue nevus of the scalp infiltrating the underlying bone: case report and review. Pediatr Dermatol 14: 199-203.
1597. Michal M (1998). Cellular blue naevi with microalveolar pattern – a type of naevus frequently confused with melanoma. Pathol Res Pract 194: 83-86.
1598. Michal M, Baumruk L, Skalova A (1992). Myxoid change within cellular blue naevi: a diagnostic pitfall. Histopathology 20: 527-530.
1599. Michal M, Kerekes Z, Kinkor Z, Ondrias F, Pizinger K (1995). Desmoplastic cellular blue nevi. Am J Dermatopathol 17: 230-235.
1600. Michal M, Lamovec J, Mukensnabl P, Pizinger K (1999). Spiradenocylindromas of the skin: tumors with morphological fea-

tures of spiradenoma and cylindroma in the same lesion: report of 12 cases. Pathol Int 49: 419-425.
1601. Michel S, Hohenleutner U, Stolz W, Landthaler M (1999). Acquired tufted angioma in association with a complex cutaneous vascular malformation. Br J Dermatol 141: 1142-1144.
1602. Michelson HE (1933). Nodular subepidermal fibrosis. Arch Dermatol Syphilol 27: 812-820.
1603. Middel P, Hemmerlein B, Fayyazi A, Kaboth U, Radzun HJ (1999). Sinus histiocytosis with massive lymphadenopathy: evidence for its relationship to macrophages and for a cytokine-related disorder. Histopathology 35: 525-533.
1604. Miettinen M (1995). Keratin 20: immunohistochemical marker for gastrointestinal, urothelial, and Merkel cell carcinomas. Mod Pathol 8: 384-388.
1605. Miettinen M (2003). Malignant and potentially malignant fibroblastic and myofibroblastic tumors. In: Diagnostic Soft Tissue Pathology, Miettinen M, ed., Churchill Livingston: New York , pp. 189-204.
1606. Miettinen M, Holthofer H, Lehto VP, Miettinen A, Virtanen I (1983). Ulex europaeus I lectin as a marker for tumors derived from endothelial cells. Am J Clin Pathol 79: 32-36.
1607. Mihm MC, Clark WH, Reed RJ, Caruso MG (1973). Mast cell infiltrates of the skin and the mastocytosis syndrome. Hum Pathol 4: 231-239.
1608. Mihm MC, Googe PB (1990). Vulvar nevus with atypism. In: Problematic Pigmented Lesions: A Case Method Approach, Mihm MCJr, Googe PB, Tong AK, eds., Lea & Febiger: Philadelphia , pp. 221-239.
1609. Mihm MC, Jr., Clemente CG, Cascinelli N (1996). Tumor infiltrating lymphocytes in lymph node melanoma metastases: a histopathologic prognostic indicator and an expression of local immune response. Lab Invest 74: 43-47.
1610. Mihm MC, Jr., Googe PB (1990). Problematic pigmented lesions. Lea & Febiger: Philadelphia.
1611. Milburn PB, Brandsma JL, Goldsman CI, Teplitz ED, Heilman EI (1988). Disseminated warts and evolving squamous cell carcinoma in a patient with acquired immunodeficiency syndrome. J Am Acad Dermatol 19: 401-405.
1612. Milburn PB, Sian CS, Silvers DN (1982). The color of the skin of the palms and soles as a possible clue to the pathogenesis of acral-lentiginous melanoma. Am J Dermatopathol 4: 429-433.
1613. Milde P, Brunner M, Borchard F, Sudhoff T, Burk M, Zumdick M, Goerz G, Ruzicka T (1995). Cutaneous bacillary angiomatosis in a patient with chronic lymphocytic leukemia. Arch Dermatol 131: 933-936.
1614. Miliauskas JR (1994). Myxoid cutaneous pleomorphic fibroma. Histopathology 24: 179-181.
1615. Miller AM, Sahl WJ, Brown SA, Young SK, Quinlan CM, Patel PR, Benbrook DM, Naylor MF (1997). The role of human papillomavirus in the development of pyogenic granulomas. Int J Dermatol 36: 673-676.
1616. Miller RW, Rabkin CS (1999). Merkel cell carcinoma and melanoma: etiological similarities and differences. Cancer Epidemiol Biomarkers Prev 8: 153-158.
1617. Miller SJ (2000). The National Comprehensive Cancer Network (NCCN) guidelines of care for nonmelanoma skin cancers. Dermatol Surg 26: 289-292.
1618. Mills AE (1989). Rhabdomyomatous mesenchymal hamartoma of skin. Am J Dermatopathol 11: 58-63.
1619. Mills SE, Cooper PH, Fechner RE (1980). Lobular capillary hemangioma: the underlying lesion of pyogenic granuloma. A study of 73 cases from the oral and nasal mucous membranes. Am J Surg Pathol 4: 470-479.
1619A. Milton GW, Shaw HM, Thompson JF, McCarthy WH (1997). Cutaneous melanoma in childhood: incidence and prognosis. Australas J Dermatol 38 Suppl 1: S44-S48.
1620. Miracco C, Pacenti L, Santopietro R, Laurini L, Biagioli M, Luzi P (2000). Evaluation of telomerase activity in cutaneous melanocytic proliferations. Hum Pathol 31: 1018-1021.
1621. Miracco C, Raffaelli M, de Santi MM, Fimiani M, Tosi P (1988). Solitary cutaneous reticulum cell tumor. Enzyme-immunohistochemical and electron-microscopic analogies with IDRC sarcoma. Am J Dermatopathol 10: 47-53.
1622. Mirza I, Macpherson N, Paproski S, Gascoyne RD, Yang B, Finn WG, Hsi ED (2002). Primary cutaneous follicular lymphoma: an assessment of clinical, histopathologic, immunophenotypic, and molecular features. J Clin Oncol 20: 647-655.
1623. Misago N, Ackerman AB (1999). Trichoblastic (basal-cell) carcinoma with trichilemmal (at the bulb) differentiation. Dermatopathology, practical & conceptual 5: 200-204.
1624. Misago N, Narisawa Y (2000). Sebaceous neoplasms in Muir-Torre syndrome. Am J Dermatopathol 22: 155-161.
1625. Mishima Y (1970). Cellular blue nevus. Melanogenic activity and malignant transformation. Arch Dermatol 101: 104-110.
1626. Mishima Y, Mevorah B (1961). Nevus Ota and nevus Ito in American Negroes. J Invest Dermatol 36: 133-154.
1627. Mittelbronn MA, Mullins DL, Ramos-Caro FA, Flowers FP (1998). Frequency of pre-existing actinic keratosis in cutaneous squamous cell carcinoma. Int J Dermatol 37: 677-681.
1628. Miyamoto Y, Ueda K, Sato M, Yasuno H (1979). Disseminated epidermolytic acanthoma. J Cutan Pathol 6: 272-279.
1629. Modly C, Wood C, Horn T (1989). Metastatic malignant melanoma arising from a common blue nevus in a patient with subacute cutaneous lupus erythematosus. Dermatologica 178: 171-175.
1630. Moller R, Reymann F, Hou-Jensen K (1979). Metastases in dermatological patients with squamous cell carcinoma. Arch Dermatol 115: 703-705.
1631. Mones JM, Ackerman AB (1984). Proliferating trichilemmal cyst is a squamous-cell carcinoma. Dermatopathology, practical & conceptual 4: 295-310.
1632. Mones JM, Ackerman AB (2003). Melanomas in prepubescent children: review comprehensively, critique historically, criteria diagnostically, and course biologically. Am J Dermatopathol 25: 223-238.
1633. Montagna W (1962). The Structure and Function of Skin. 2nd ed. Academic Press: New York.
1634. Montagna W, Hu F, Carlisle K (1980). A reinvestigation of solar lentigines. Arch Dermatol 116: 1151-1154.
1635. Montonen O, Ezer S, Laurikkala J, Karjalainen-Lindsberg ML, Thesleff I, Kere J, Saarialho-Kere U (1998). Expression of the anhidrotic ectodermal dysplasia gene is reduced in skin cancer coinciding with reduced E-cadherin. Exp Dermatol 7: 168-174.
1636. Mooi WJ (2001). Histopathology of Spitz naevi and "Spitzoid" melanomas. Curr Top Pathol 94: 65-77.
1637. Mooi WJ (2001). The expanding spectrum of cutaneous blue nevi. Curr Diagn Pathol 7: 56-58.
1638. Mooi WJ (2002). Spitz nevus and its histologic simulators. Adv Anat Pathol 9: 209-221.
1639. Moon TE, Levine N, Cartmel B, Bangert JL, Rodney S, Dong Q, Peng YM, Alberts DS (1997). Effect of retinol in preventing squamous cell skin cancer in moderate-risk subjects: a randomized, double-blind, controlled trial. Southwest Skin Cancer Prevention Study Group. Cancer Epidemiol Biomarkers Prev 6: 949-956.
1640. Mooney MA, Barr RJ, Buxton MG (1995). Halo nevus or halo phenomenon? A study of 142 cases. J Cutan Pathol 22: 342-348.
1641. Moore AY (2001). Cutaneous warts. In: Human Papillomaviruses: Clinical and Scientific Advances, Sterling JC, Tyring SK, eds., Arnold: London .
1642. Moraillon I, Rybojad M, Chemaly P, Bourrillon A, Morel P (1993). [Congenital multiple cutaneous Abrikossof tumors]. Ann Dermatol Venereol 120: 816-818.
1643. Mordehai J, Kurzbart E, Shinhar D, Sagi A, Finaly R, Mares AJ (1998). Lymphangioma circumscriptum. Pediatr Surg Int 13: 208-210.
1644. Moreno A, Lamarca J, Martinez R, Guix M (1986). Osteoid and bone formation in desmoplastic malignant melanoma. J Cutan Pathol 13: 128-134.
1645. Moreno C, Jacyk WK, Judd MJ, Requena L (2001). Highly aggressive extraocular sebaceous carcinoma. Am J Dermatopathol 23: 450-455.
1646. Moreno C, Requena L, Kutzner H, de la Cruz A, Jaqueti G, Yus ES (2000). Epithelioid blue nevus: a rare variant of blue nevus not always associated with the Carney complex. J Cutan Pathol 27: 218-223.
1647. Morgan JM, Carmichael AJ, Ritchie C (1996). Extramammary Paget's disease of the axilla with an underlying apocrine carcinoma. Acta Derm Venereol 76: 173-174.
1648. Mori M, Manuelli C, Pimpinelli N, Mavilia C, Maggi E, Santucci M, Bianchi B, Cappugi P, Giannotti B, Kadin ME (1999). CD30-CD30 ligand interaction in primary cutaneous CD30(+) T-cell lymphomas: A clue to the pathophysiology of clinical regression. Blood 94: 3077-3083.
1649. Mori O, Hachisuka H, Sasai Y (1990). Proliferating trichilemmal cyst with spindle cell carcinoma. Am J Dermatopathol 12: 479-484.
1650. Morier P, Merot Y, Paccaud D, Beck D, Frenk E (1990). Juvenile chronic granulocytic leukemia, juvenile xanthogranulomas, and neurofibromatosis. Case report and review of the literature. J Am Acad Dermatol 22: 962-965.
1651. Morman MR, Petrozzi JW (1980). Cutaneous Hodgkin's disease. Cutis 26: 483-4, 491.
1652. Morrell DS, Esterly NB (2001). Solitary, lobulated, firm nodule. Pediatr Dermatol 18: 356-358.
1653. Mortier L, Marchetti P, Delaporte E, Martin de Lassalle E, Thomas P, Piette F, Formstecher P, Polakowska R, Danze PM (2002). Progression of actinic keratosis to squamous cell carcinoma of the skin correlates with deletion of the 9p21 region encoding the p16(INK4a) tumor suppressor. Cancer Lett 176: 205-214.
1654. Mortimore RJ, Whitehead KJ (2001). Dermatomyofibroma: a report of two cases, one occurring in a child. Australas J Dermatol 42: 22-25.
1655. Morton DL, Wen DR, Wong JH, Economou JS, Cagle LA, Storm FK, Foshag LJ, Cochran AJ (1992). Technical details of intraoperative lymphatic mapping for early stage melanoma. Arch Surg 127: 392-399.
1655A. Morton DL, Thompson JF, Cochran AJ et al. (2005) Interim results of the multicenter selective lymphadenectomy trial (MSLT-I) in clinical stage melanoma. J Clin Oncol 23: 7500
1656. Motley R, Kersey P, Lawrence C (2002). Multiprofessional guidelines for the management of the patient with primary cutaneous squamous cell carcinoma. Br J Dermatol 146: 18-25.
1657. Moy RL, Moy LS, Matsuoka LY, Bennett RG, Uitto J (1988). Selectively enhanced procollagen gene expression in sclerosing (morphea-like) basal cell carcinoma as reflected by elevated pro alpha 1(I) and pro alpha 1(III) procollagen messenger RNA steady-state levels. J Invest Dermatol 90: 634-638.
1658. Moyes CD, Alexander FW (1977). Mucosal neuroma syndrome presenting in a neonate. Dev Med Child Neurol 19: 518-534.
1659. Mrak RE, Baker GF (1987). Granular cell basal cell carcinoma. J Cutan Pathol 14: 37-42.
1660. Mraz-Gernhard S, Natkunam Y, Hoppe RT, LeBoit P, Kohler S, Kim YH (2001). Natural killer/natural killer-like T-cell lymphoma, CD56+, presenting in the skin: an increasingly recognized entity with an aggressive course. J Clin Oncol 19: 2179-2188.
1661. Muche JM, Lukowsky A, Asadullah K, Gellrich S, Sterry W (1997). Demonstration of frequent occurrence of clonal T cells in the peripheral blood of patients with primary cutaneous T-cell lymphoma. Blood 90: 1636-1642.
1662. Muller-Hermelink HK, Catovsky D, Montserrat E, Harris NL (2001). Chronic lymphocytic leukaemia/small lymphocytic lymphoma. In: World Health Organization Classification of Tumours. Pathology and Genetics of Tumours of Haematopoietic and Lymphoid Tissues, Jaffe ES, Harris NL, Stein H, Vardiman J, eds., IARC Press: Lyon , pp. 127-130.
1663. Mulliken JB, Fishman SJ, Burrows PE (2000). Vascular anomalies. Curr Probl Surg 37: 517-584.
1664. Mulvany NJ, Sykes P (1997). Desmoplastic melanoma of the vulva. Pathology 29: 241-245.
1665. Munn SE, McGregor JM, Jones A, Amlot P, Rustin MH, Russell JR, Whittaker S (1996). Clinical and pathological heterogeneity in cutaneous gamma-delta T-cell lymphoma: a report of three cases and a review of the literature. Br J Dermatol 135: 976-981.
1666. Murakami I, Gogusev J, Fournet JC, Glorion C, Jaubert F (2002). Detection of molecular cytogenetic aberrations in langerhans cell histiocytosis of bone. Hum Pathol 33: 555-560.

Naevus angiokeratoticus 242
Naevus flammeus 240
Naevus fuscoceruleus ophthalmomaxillaris 96
Naevus incipiens 104
Naevus keratoangiomatosus 242
Naevus lipomatosus 253
Naevus of Ito 79, **96**
Naevus of Ota 79, 82, **96**
Naevus of spindled and/or epithelioid cells 114
Naevus of Sun 96
Naevus sebaceous 125, 141
Naevus sebaceous of Jadassohn 144
Naevus spilus (congenital speckled lentiginous naevus) 104
Naevus vascularis unius lateralis 242
Naevus with architectural disorder 105
Naevus with focal dermal epithelioid component 100
Nail dystrophy 175
NAME syndrome 103, 291
Naturopathic medicines 32
Necrosis en masse 123
NER See Nucleotide excision repair
Nerve sheath myxoma/neurothekeoma **270**
Nerve sheath tumours 231
Neurilemmomatosis 223
Neurocutaneous melanocytosis 79
Neuroendocrine carcinoma of the skin 272
Neurofibroma 231, 258, 260
Neurofibromatosis 78, 222, 223, 265
Neurofibromatosis type 1 (NF1) 78, 81, 223, 275, 278
Neurofibromatosis type 1 b (NF1b) 223, 278
Neurofibromatosis type 2 (NF2) 223
Neurofibromatosis type 2 b (NF2b) 278
Neurofilament 269
Neurofollicular hamartoma 158
Neuroma **265**, 266
Neuromuscular hamartoma 253
Neurotization 98
Neurotropism **76**, 77, 78
Neutropaenia 193
Nevoxanthoendothelioma 222
NF1 See neurofibromatosis type 1 (NF1)
NF2 See Neurofibromatosis type 2 (NF2)
NGFR 275
Nickel 213
NK/T-cell lymphoma 191
NKI/C-3 69, 78, 81, 269, 270
Nodular amelanotic melanoma 43
Nodular angioblastic hyperplasia with eosinophilia and lymphofolliculosis 237
Nodular basal cell carcinoma **16,** 19
Nodular hidradenocarcinoma 131

Nodular hidradenoma 143
Nodular lymphocyte predominant Hodgkin lymphoma (NLPHL) 207
Nodular melanoma 55, 56, **68**, 73, 74, 119, 262
Non-cutaneous melanoma 63
Non-diabetic cutaneous xanthomatosis 224
Non-encapsulated neuroma 265
Non-Hodgkin lymphoma 204, 205
Non-inflammatory halo naevi 119
Non-Langerhans-cell (LC) histiocytosis 222
Non-melanoma skin cancer (NMSC) 11, 12
Non-neuroendocrine small cell carcinoma 268
Non-regressing lipodystrophy centrifugalis abdominalis 240
Normocholesterolemic xanthomatosis 224
Npm-alk protein (p80) 181
Nuclear pseudoinclusions 69
Nucleolar organizing regions (AgNORs) 87
Nucleotide excision repair (NER) 282-284

O

Ocular melanocytosis 79, 82
Oculodermal melanocytosis 79, 96
Odontogenic keratocysts 287
OKM1 220
OKT6 223
Oral contraceptives 80
Oral florid papillomatosis 22
Orange skin 227
Orbital melanoma 79
Organ transplantation 20, 34, 202
Ossification 128, 149, 253
Ossifying dermatofibroma with osteoclast-like giant cells 262
Osteoarthrosis 257
Osteolytic skull lesions 218
Osteoporosis 227
Otitis media 218
Ovarian fibroma 285, 286, 287
Ozone layer 55

P

p14ARF 278, 280, 281
p15 197, 246
p16 32, 63, 108, 197, 219, 278, 279
P16/INK4 278
p16INK4A 280, 281
p19(ARF) 279

p21 69, 219
p21 WAF1 69
p62 172
P75 260
P75 (low-affinity nerve growth factor receptor) 260
Paget disease 28, 72, 129, 135, 136, 138
Paget disease of breast **136**
Paget disease (extramammary, EPD) **136,** 161
Pagetoid dyskeratosis 138
Pagetoid melanocytosis 85
Pagetoid melanoma 66
Pagetoid reticulosis **173**
Pagetoid reticulosis of the Ketron-Goodman type 185
Pagetoid Spitz naevus 138
Pagetoid upward migration 86, 89
Pagetoid variant of Bowen disease 28
Pale cell acanthoma 43
Pale scar-like lesions 13
Palisaded, encapsulated neuroma (PEN) **265**
Palisading pattern 265
Palmar pits 155
Palmar-plantar-subungal-mucosal melanoma (P-S-M melanoma) 73
Palmo-plantar keratoderma 142, 175
Palpable migratory arciform erythema 212
Pan T-cell markers 192
Pancreatic cancer 279
Pan-cytokeratin 273
Pancytopenias 182, 218
Pan-muscle actin (HHF-35) 252
Panniculitis 182, 183, 184, 185, 200
Papillary apocrine gland cyst 139
Papillary thyroid carcinoma 80
Papillary tubular adenoma 145, 146
Papillomatosis 22, 23, 31, 33, 37, 38, 40, 42, 44, 242
Papillomatosis cutis carcinoides 22, 23
Parakeratosis 27, 30, 31, 36, 41, 44, 47, 59, 112, 155, 171, 215, 216
Parakeratosis variegata 171, 216
Parapsoriasis 171, **215**, 216
Parapsoriasis - Large patch type, with or without poikiloderma **215**
Parapsoriasis en grandes plaques poikilodermiques 171, 216
Parapsoriasis en plaques (Brocq disease) 215, 216, 171
Parapsoriasis lichenoides 171, 216
Parasitosis 228
PATCHED1 14, 287
Pautrier microabscesses 170, 190
PCFCL 196, 197
PCNA 21, 46, 69, 81, 87, 172
Peanut agglutinin (PNA) 223